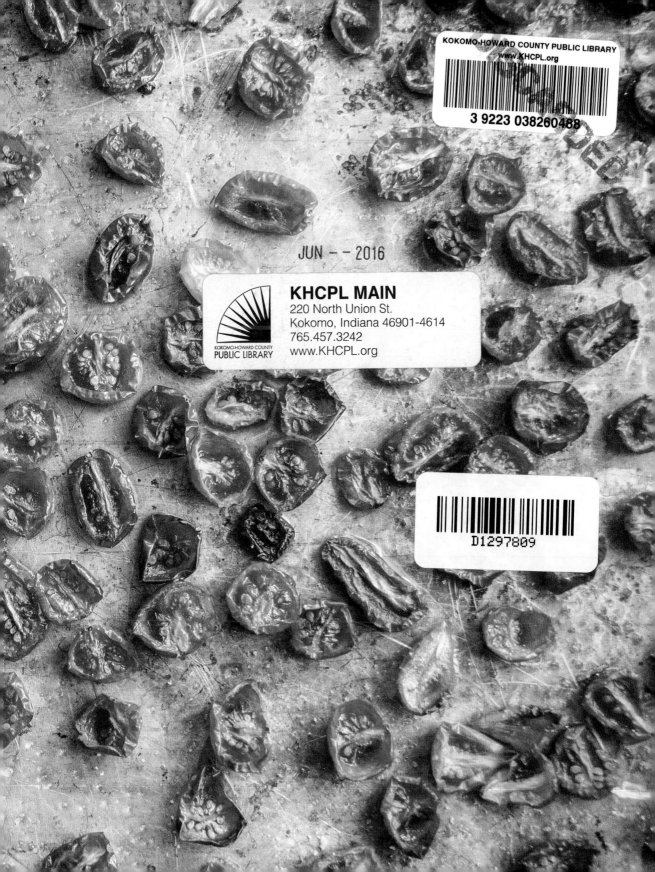

pure delicious

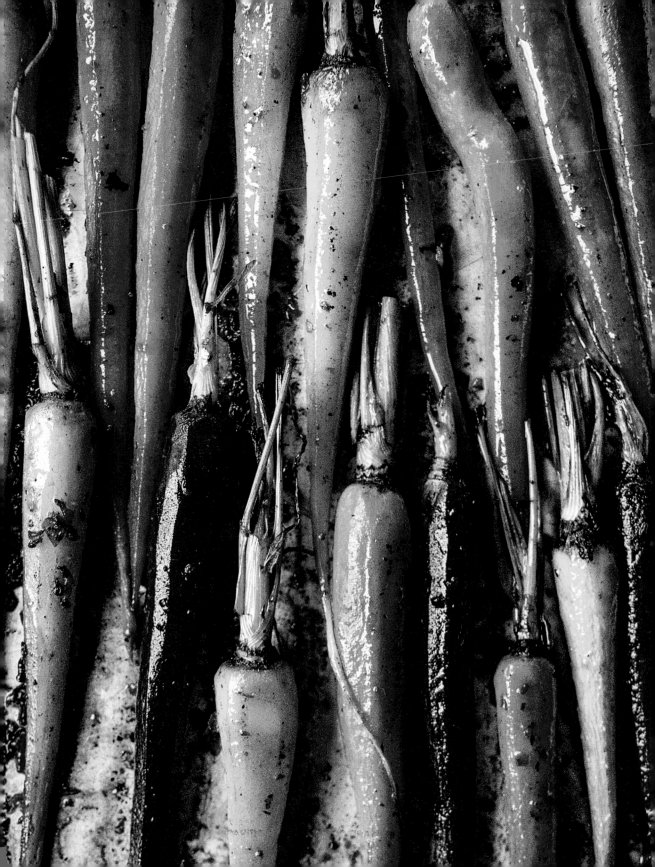

pure delicious

HEATHER CHRISTO

More than **150** Delectable Allergen-Free Recipes
without gluten, dairy, eggs, soy, peanuts, tree nuts,
shellfish, or cane sugar

PAM KRAUSS BOOKS · AVERY
an imprint of Penguin Random House
New York

PAM KRAUSS BOOKS • AVERY
an imprint of Penguin Random House LLC
375 Hudson Street
New York, New York 10014

Most Avery books are available at special quantity discounts for bulk purchase
for sales promotions, premiums, fund-raising, and educational needs.
Special books or book excerpts also can be created to fit specific needs.
For details, write SpecialMarkets@penguinrandomhouse.com.

Library of Congress Cataloging-in-Publication Data

Christo, Heather, author.
Pure delicious / Heather Christo. —First edition.
p.   cm
Includes index.
1. Food allergy—Diet therapy. I. Title.
RC588.D53C45   2016   2015035231
641.5'6318—dc23

ISBN 978-0-553-45925-8

Printed in the United States of America
1 3 5 7 9 10 8 6 4 2

Book and jacket design: La Tricia Watford

Photographs on pages 8, 20, 33, and 44 © Katie M. Simmons

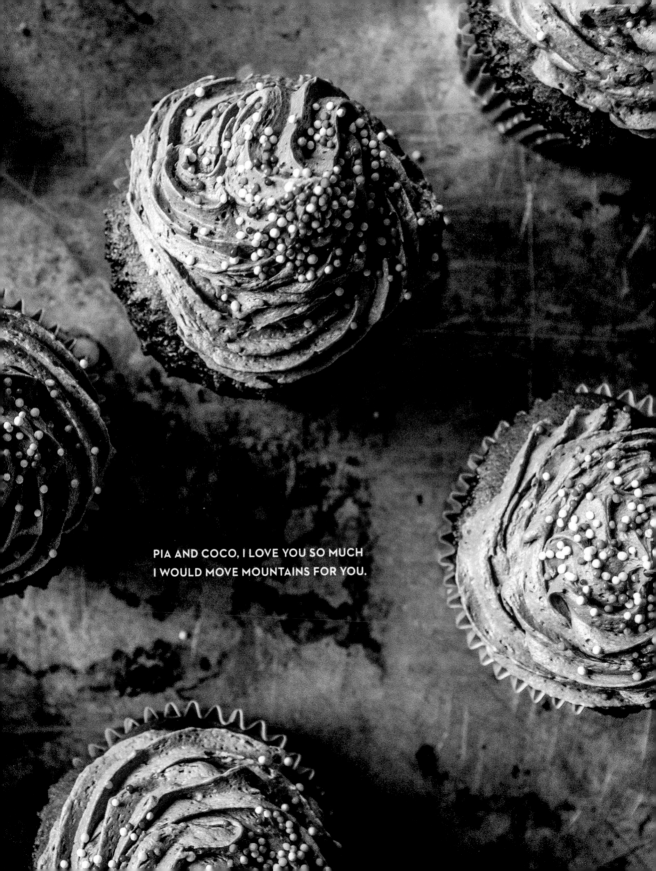

PIA AND COCO, I LOVE YOU SO MUCH
I WOULD MOVE MOUNTAINS FOR YOU.

contents

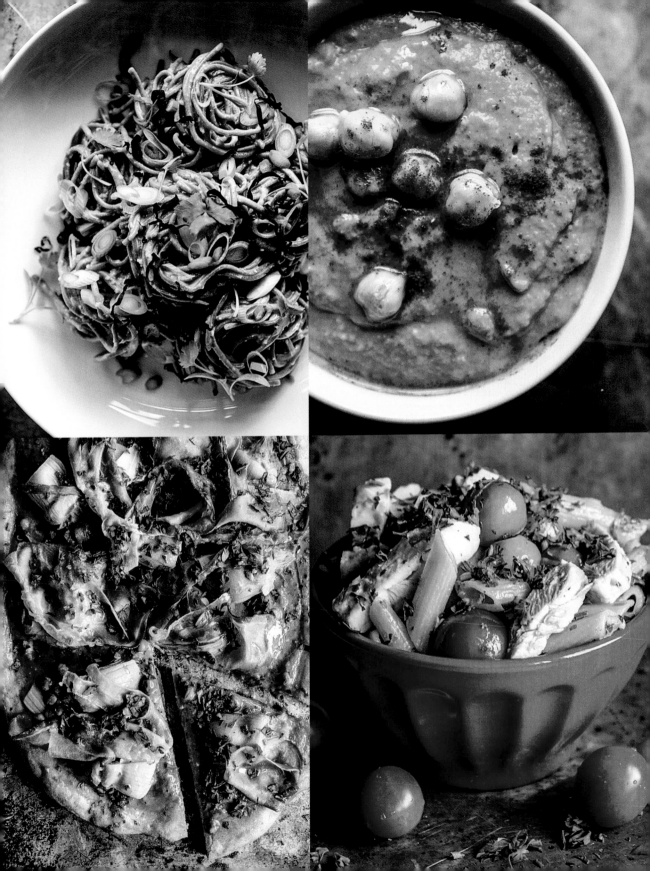

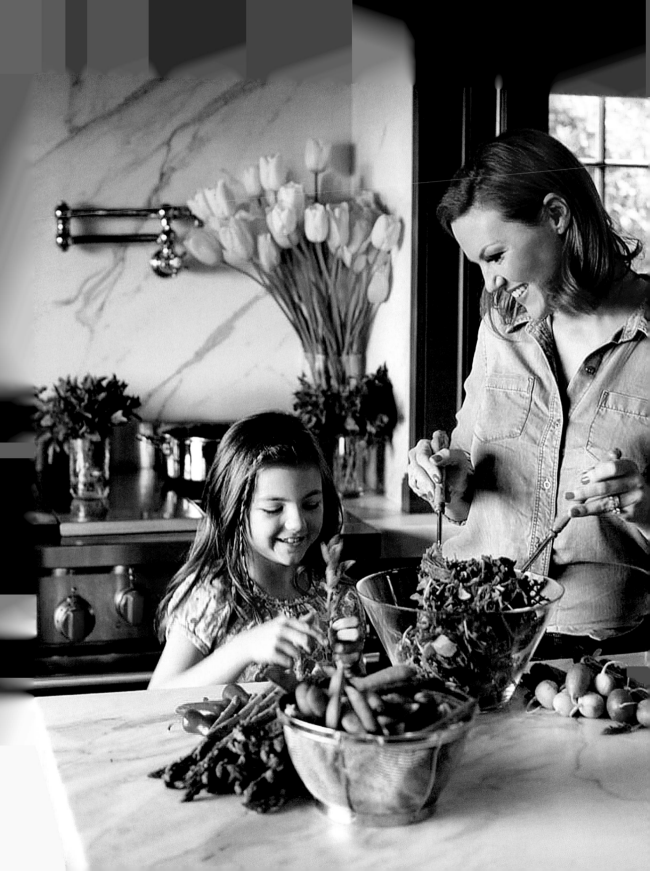

introduction

I wrote this book for you. Those of you who have food allergies or sensitivities, or have family members or friends with allergies; those of you who suspect that eating a cleaner, healthier diet may alleviate some of your pesky (or dramatic) health issues; and any of you on prescribed anti-inflammatory diets who are tired of subsisting on chicken breasts and steamed vegetables. I get it. I am you, my children are you, my mother is you, and I couldn't care about you and this issue more.

My own journey began when my daughter Pia was five and had a health crisis that resulted in a trip to the emergency room, which snapped me out of a cynical fog. I realized that food sensitivities and allergies were not just some "fad" to roll my eyes at, but indeed played a much larger role in our personal lives and health. I was forced to admit something I really did not want to be true: what we eat matters and food allergies cannot be medicated away.

I had no idea then that this realization would transform my life, my career, and the health and well-being of me and my entire family in such a positive way. I could see only the challenges, the deprivations, the disappointments my family and I would face. But I knew something had to change—and you probably do, too.

Until I decided to take control of my family's health by completely revising the way we all eat, I had been completely in the dark about the food-allergy epidemic we are in the middle of; that *inflammation* is the culprit and that food can trigger it; and taking control of our lives and health, by eliminating the constant doctor visits and low-level (at best) ill health and discomfort, is downright *empowering*. I want to help you see this new way of eating as the path to health and food—in your own kitchen, under your own control, according to your own needs—as the most important line of defense against illness. I wrote this book to share the lessons I (and my girls) learned the hard way, and to share the shortcuts I found and recipes I developed that have made the transition to clean eating not only manageable, but enjoyable.

I am not a doctor, nutritionist, or health expert. I wrote this as a mother and a chef. I will introduce you to an eight-week elimination program designed to clear your body of the most common allergens and inflammation-causing food sources.

Perhaps you've been prescribed such a diet before by a doctor or nutritionist but failed to stick to it because the food was, frankly, bland and boring, and just made you long for the foods you could no longer eat. That's where this one differs. You'll be cooking and eating amazingly delicious food that makes you look forward to mealtimes, and that, I believe, you'll want to continue eating for life.

Why eight weeks? Your body needs this time to completely eliminate these allergens from your body—even as little as 10 mg of some of them. And though there are tests for many allergens, as I will explain, there are mixed opinions as to the reliability of their results, and those expensive tests are not always covered by insurance. So even if you use testing as a starting point for your journey, doing an elimination diet is still the best gauge of which foods irritate your body. I will guide you through eight weeks of eating meals completely free of the most common allergens, and then show you how to reintroduce these foods and figure out which ones do and don't work well for your body, and which ones have even been wreaking havoc on your system.

In our case, we found that the symptoms Pia had suffered from since infancy—colic and stomachaches, ear infections, chronic constipation, eczema, rashes, hives, migraines, sinus infections, mystery ailments—were entirely gone within eight weeks, along with a host of other complaints for the whole family!

I also address the three biggest challenges for families dealing with food sensitivities:

- getting used to new ingredients and more home-cooking than you might be accustomed to

- helping kids (and yourself!) through the changes

- adjusting to social situations

Throughout this book you'll find helpful information about the most common food allergens and where they are hiding, quick-reference icons to help you make menu decisions at a glance, and weekly planners.

Best of all, my eight-week plan will give you (and your family) a structure that allows you to focus, plan, assess, and incorporate all the steps necessary to make the transition relatively smooth. By the end of the eight weeks, my family and I found that we had created a "new normal" for ourselves. And that normal looks a whole lot better than the "old normal," in which we attributed all manner of health issues to stress, hormones, germs, or genetics. Now we feel energetic and healthy and our immune systems seem to be better than ever, with ailments like headaches, GI trouble, and even head colds rare occurrences. You can achieve the same for yourself and your family, and enjoy every bite of the process.

Changing the way we eat is a difficult, emotional transition. I know you still love beautiful, delicious food and I know you're busy. I've created the recipes and tips in the pages that follow with that in mind. It's my hope that this book will become the dog-eared bible for anyone faced with the need to make a lasting transition to a new way of eating—and a whole new life.

....

NOTE: I use the term "food allergies" throughout the book, but there are important distinctions to be made between allergies, intolerances or sensitivities, and disease, which I discuss in more depth on pages 16–17.

....

chapter 1
our story of transformation

I don't want to have any cliff-hangers here. In fact, I'll put my conclusions right up front:

- People struggling with their health *can* become whole and happy.

- What you put in your body is the key.

- The process takes time and dedication.

- It's totally worth it!

Here's the story of how I got there.

THE WAKEUP CALL

Seeing my daughter Pia writhing and screaming on the floor of the emergency room forced me to reconsider a thought I had been stubbornly refusing to confront for years: *This could be food allergies.*

As a busy mother, chef and blogger, wife to a good-bread-and-cheese-loving Greek husband, and fun-loving friend whose career and social life revolved around food, I found the idea of food as a health hazard threatening, both personally and professionally. But standing in one of the most respected children's hospitals in the world, seeing our little girl in so much pain, and everyone around her so apparently helpless to bring her relief, snapped me into another reality.

The attack, which consisted of severe abdominal pain and dry heaving, started at my parents' house. I was freaking out, but I knew I could rely on my parents to tell me objectively if I was overreacting—after all, they had raised four children, had five grandchildren, and are totally no-nonsense. When I saw that they were panicked, too, I raced Pia to the ER.

After several hours of testing, Pia's pains subsided, but the test results came up completely inconclusive. In the end, the ER doc literally shrugged and said, "Maybe she needs to poop more?"

Seriously?! At that moment I just set my jaw and "channeled my instincts," wracking my brain for anything that had ever caused me terrible stomachaches as a child. And suddenly it came to me: dairy.

Pia was five then. She had been sick *a lot* since she was born, almost always had an earache or a sinus infection, and had suffered through multiple trips to the ER and urgent care center. We were serious regulars at the pediatrician's office, and she was prescribed antibiotics six to eight times a year.

None of her doctors could agree on what was wrong with her. I was told she had eczema—for which she was given steroid creams. Her stomachaches and constipation "had to be" because she was not consuming enough fiber—so we should give her fiber supplements. Or maybe her stomach was hurting because she was "stressed out" (cue the gross mom-guilt). Her sinus infections and earaches were due to "seasonal allergies" and it was recommended that she take Claritin—every day for the rest of her life. And when that didn't work and the symptoms overwhelmed her, they would just prescribe antibiotics, again. She eventually became allergic to half of them from overuse, so the doctors would just try another. Each symptom was treated individually, but we were never given an overall diagnosis for why this little girl simply never felt entirely well.

There in the ER room, I began to put the pieces together. I had been diagnosed "lactose intolerant" by my own pediatrician when I was about Pia's age. In the early eighties, though, this "trouble" with milk was seen as just an annoyance, a trivial detail to accommodate when possible. It mainly meant my poor mom might have to cook a different meal for me than what she was cooking for my three siblings (which *wasn't* going to happen), or that occasionally she would drop a container of very expensive Mocha Mix (fake milk) into the shopping cart. Mostly people just told me to "toughen up." There was an industry-fueled pressure in the air, too. Remember the slogan: *Milk. It does a body good*? If I didn't drink cow's milk, I would never "grow tall and strong," so more often than not I would find myself drinking the glass of milk set before me despite my body's protests.

And so I spent a lot of time as a child crying with stomachaches after dinner. In my late teens and early twenties I was plagued with a fresh influx

of terrible stomach pain and constant heartburn. I was put on the B.R.A.T. diet (bananas, rice, applesauce, and toast) and then had multiple endoscopies to identify the source of my pain and the inflammation they found in my stomach and esophagus. After five years without a definitive diagnosis, discomfort became my new normal. Not one doctor ever suggested it could be due to what I was eating. But now, all these years later, watching Pia go through something similar, a lightbulb turned on.

Back home, I started writing down everything she ate and her reactions, and it didn't take long for my suspicions to be borne out: dairy did indeed give her stomachaches, but when combined with gluten (think macaroni and cheese, grilled-cheese sandwiches, quesadillas, pizza) it was even more intense. I had my marching orders.

In September Pia started kindergarten and ventured into a whole new way of life. I was so motivated to help her feel good at this critical stage and fix what was going on with her that I completely cut out dairy in her meals and started experimenting with cutting gluten here and there, too.

For a while it seemed to help, but then a few weeks into the school year I had to pick Pia up early after she had been sent to the school office—with neck pain. *Neck pain*? After she got home and had a nap, she felt better, so I didn't read too much into it.

But that night we went to one of our favorite restaurants, which happens to serve the best pita bread on the planet. Even though I'd been limiting her gluten to some extent, after the bad day she'd had I decided to make an exception for that amazing bread. Ten minutes after she dove into the pita basket she was writhing in pain, screaming about her painful neck and fuzzy eyes!

I finally recognized that she was describing the beginnings of a migraine headache (for a five-year-old, the base of her skull was her neck; "fuzzy eyes" was her way of describing the auras associated with vision-altering migraines). At that moment it could not have been more obvious to me that she was allergic to wheat or gluten.

GETTING TESTED

Having heard others' stories about skeptical doctors, I went to Pia's pediatrician well armed with evidence and examples of her reactions to suspected allergens. To his credit he was surprisingly open to the idea of testing and ordered a preliminary (though not very detailed) food-specific allergy blood test that measured her IgG levels (IgG, short for Immunoglobulin G, is a type of antibody) when exposed to the thirteen most common foods in the American diet. When the results came back a few weeks later, reality started to sink in. She was allergic to twelve of the thirteen tested foods.

But they had no idea how to help us further and couldn't give a diagnosis or a plan of action because the test is not approved by the FDA. Due to the lack of information they had at their disposal and their inexperience on the topic, they were uncomfortable giving me advice on how to proceed. I think the pediatrician's exact words were, "I'm sorry, I don't know what to say."

So I cut dairy and gluten and a few other common allergens that had popped up on the IGg test

from her diet, hoping the answer was just that simple. Sadly, things in Allergy World are rarely that straightforward. Her symptoms persisted, particularly a chronic congestion and postnasal drip that caused her to clear her throat again and again. In fact, the constant throat clearing had become so reflexive that it was distracting and disruptive at home and at school. When we took her to the doctor to see what was going on, we were told it looked like Tourette's syndrome and that Pia needed to work with a behavioral therapist! That was the true turning point. I started researching MDs, specialists, naturopaths—anyone with an opinion about food allergies—who might be able to help us. Eventually we found our way to Dr. Kelly Baker, ND, at the IBS Treatment Center in Seattle, where they treat irritable bowel syndrome and do food-allergy testing. Filling out intake forms as we waited to see the doctor, I had a real wakeup call as I scanned the list of dairy-allergy symptoms:

- abdominal pain
- gas
- acne
- headaches
- ADD/ADHD
- heartburn
- anxiety
- indigestion
- arthritis
- anemia
- canker sores
- irritability
- constipation
- irritable bowel
- diarrhea
- joint pain
- ear infections
- osteoporosis
- fatigue
- poor immunity
- fibromyalgia

Check, check, check. And I'm not talking about Pia—*that list was me*. I had almost every single symptom.

Meanwhile, our younger daughter, Coco, had also begun to suffer from terrible stomachaches and facial rashes. At four years old she was the most constipated child I had ever seen, and it had also been suggested that she was developing asthma. Since I now knew that most children's allergies are inherited from one or both parents, I realized that Coco and I would need to be tested, too. This is where you probably ask, "What about your husband? Didn't Pete want to be tested too?" Well, no, he didn't. He still waffles with whether or not he wants to do it, depending on if his heartburn is flaring up or not. I share this with you because it is real life. Not everyone is going to want to get on board. He is really respectful of our diet in the home and is a team player with the kids and our health, but each person has to decide to do this for themselves. He admittedly feels great when he eats in conjunction with us, and terrible when he does not, but he has not made the permanent leap yet.

So right before Christmas 2013, the three of us went through the extensive and specific blood-3

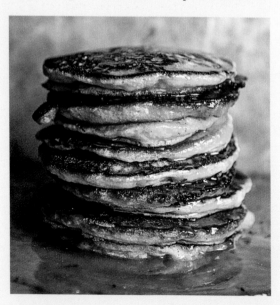

antibody ELISA testing (see page 15) that assessed our reactions to 160 foods, spices, and herbs. And then, doing what any normal person facing the knowledge that she might never be able to eat certain foods again would do, we gorged over the holidays.

January found us all sick and exhausted, not just from our holiday binge but from the shocking test results. Among my allergens:

- cow and goat dairy
- eggs
- pineapple, bananas, passion fruit, kiwi (highly, triggering, bordering on anaphylaxis)
- coffee beans, vanilla beans (there go the lattes)
- whole wheat, gluten, flaxseed
- black pepper, bean sprouts, lima beans, navy beans
- clams, scallops

PIA TESTED POSITIVE FOR THESE:

- cane sugar, eggs, cow and goat dairy, ginger, curry, and garlic
- oranges, grapefruit, pineapple, cranberries
- gluten, whole wheat, rye, flax, spelt, barley, Kamut (a variety of wheat)
- psyllium (think of all those fiber supplements)
- hazelnuts, peanuts
- string beans, lima beans, navy beans, coffee beans, soy

AND COCO HAD HER OWN LIST:

- gluten, whole wheat, spelt, Kamut
- eggs, cow and goat dairy
- oranges and cranberries

With so many foods to avoid, how was I possibly going to feed my family? Even garlic was on the verboten list, along with virtually all of my Greek husband's traditional family foods! And what about my blog readers? Some of my most popular posts that year were recipes for Cheese-and-Cream Baked Potatoes, Skillet-Baked Stuffed Rigatoni, cheese-dripping Caprese Soup, and Slutty Halloween Brownies.

As upsetting as the prospect of living without all those foods was, I knew I had to find out what would happen if we did. Having been openly skeptical about the very existence of food allergies—I had been known to smirk at those who went on about what I privately dubbed their "New Age" allergies—I knew I may have to eat crow. I had to put our health before my ego. Drawing on my skills as a chef as well as the true grit and determination of a mother who loves her children, I vowed to dismantle our routines, habits, and social lives, and then rebuild them on a new, sturdier, healthier foundation, piece by piece.

That January, we went cold turkey on all of the items on our ELISA test. The whole family went gluten, dairy, egg, soy, and cane sugar free, and then we had various other ingredients that we individually avoided based on our results.

A WORD ABOUT TESTING

Let me save you a lot of time. If you start researching, you'll find opinions on all sides about ELISA (enzyme-linked immunosorbent assay), a blood-draw test for inflammation and response from three different antibodies IgG, IgE and IgA for up to 160 foods and herbs and spices); finger-prick enzyme tests; and smaller panels of antibody tests (like the one Pia originally received)—all approaches with both detractors and champions—and other even more controversial forms of testing such as muscle testing and hair analysis and on into multiple woo-woo theories and products.

Differences between and definitions of allergies, sensitivities, intolerances, and inflammation are in flux and sometimes hotly debated. The Food Allergy Research and Education (FARE) website is a good place to get an overview, but much is still unknown. The one thing that everyone seems to agree on at this point is this: If you have a life-threatening allergy to, say, peanuts or shellfish or strawberries, you already know to avoid those foods at all cost. For those with more subtle or more chronic reactions, the avoid-and-reintroduce approach is inexpensive and pretty reliable: take suspect foods out of your diet for a while, and then add them back in one at time and see what happens. For me, the ELISA was helpful because it motivated me to get serious about eliminating suspect foods and gave me a starting point. (And I should note that the test was expensive, and insurance paid only for my girls' testing, not mine.) My real conviction came from the drastic improvements I saw as the result of my own experimentation and tracking.

AMAZING RESULTS WITHIN EIGHT WEEKS

Within three days, Pia's stomachaches stopped. Within a week, her skin rashes had cleared up and she had no more headaches. Within two weeks, her eyes were no longer puffy and their dark circles had faded, normal healthy bathroom habits resumed, and her nasal congestion and constant throat clearing began to wane.

I also noticed that her wild emotional swings, which I had chalked up to "being a little girl," seemed to even out. While she would normally cry every afternoon and be drooping with exhaustion after school, she started coming home in a great mood and full of energy. She was a different girl!

Sound hard to believe? All I can say is, I began this journey as a nonbeliever who considered food-allergy nuts fussy, demanding, and self-absorbed, whereas *I* was all about cooking with abandon and eating with passion and loving life through all the senses! Little did I know I was dulling our senses by chronically stressing our systems.

WHAT WE LEARNED

For simplicity and ease, I use the term "allergies" when I talk about reactions to foods. It's good shorthand that everyone seems to understand. That said, there are distinctions that can be made between different kinds of food reactions.

I learned that my girls and I had typical *allergic* reactions to many foods. A true "food allergy" causes an immune system or histamine reaction within two hours of eating the offending food.

When the food enters the body, the immune system identifies the food as a harmful substance. It then produces antibodies to fight off the substance. This process begins in a chemical reaction that leads to common food-allergy symptoms as the result of increased histamine levels in the body. Histamine reactions cause inflammation in tissue where food-allergy symptoms typically appear, such as the sinuses, stomach, and lungs. Reactions encompass such symptoms as a tingling or itching mouth; swelling of the lips, tongue, throat, or face; and hives, wheezing, or difficulty breathing. Anaphylaxis, or a severe inability to breathe, is the most extreme of these reactions, and it can result in death.

We learned that, in addition to hereditary factors, food *allergies*—which cause immune-system histamine responses and inflammatory responses—can be triggered by chronic overexposure, and that with so many common allergens like wheat, soy, and cane sugar being used as fillers in processed foods, even people who avoid fast food and "junk" can be getting ongoing overexposure to them.

A food *intolerance* or *sensitivity*, which is thought *not* to involve an immune response, will not have an immediate or histamine reaction but will have a delayed reaction after ingesting them that will come on anywhere from a few hours to a couple of days later and is not immediately life threatening. The symptoms can vary widely, and typically include inflammatory responses, joint pain, nausea or vomiting, gas, bloating, diarrhea, constipation, gut tenderness, heartburn, headaches, mood swings, or skin issues. While those are the "typical" reactions, the secondary effects of food intolerances appear to be even more far-reaching. For example, my dentist noticed a remarkable difference in the health of my teeth and gums within eight weeks of my new eating style, and the symptoms of my diagnosed ADD—restlessness, terrible difficulty with focusing, and anxiety—are pretty much gone. I have a genetic predisposition to rheumatoid arthritis on both my maternal and paternal sides (my mom suffers from it) and I started to develop symptoms in my twenties. Today, unless I have a gluten slip, these symptoms seem to be at bay.

Celiac disease is something different still, a hereditary autoimmune disorder so severe that even the consumption of microscopic amounts of gluten can cause damage to the small intestines. Contrary to popular belief, though, celiac symptoms are not necessarily more pronounced than those associated with gluten intolerance. In fact 50 percent of people with celiac have no digestive symptoms at all. Most people simply don't associate their nondigestive symptoms with the celiac diagnosis until those symptoms go away after eliminating gluten. It is estimated that one in one hundred people suffer from celiac (although I know ten personally, so I suspect that estimate is low), with only about one-third of them being diagnosed. It is also important to note that celiac disease runs in families, with first- and second-degree relatives being at an increased risk for the disease.

THIS IS VERY IMPORTANT! If you suspect that you may have celiac disease or if you have any relatives with celiac disease, get tested BEFORE you start this plan. If you have been off gluten for even a few weeks, you *cannot* get an accurate celiac reading. Learn from our mistakes—we went about this in the wrong order, and now,

unless we eat gluten for eight to twelve weeks straight and then get tested, we will never know definitively if we are celiac.

THE SOBERING TRENDS

My family is hardly unique. Consider the following statistics:

- Nearly one in five households has at least one member who suffers from a food allergy or intolerance, and those with known food allergies are mostly people under thirty-five.

- Nearly 40 percent of children with food allergies have a history of severe reactions, and over 30 percent have multiple food allergies.

- Potentially deadly food allergies affect one in thirteen children, and the incidence of such allergies is rising quickly.

- The *New York Times* reported in 2014 that 28 percent of Americans say they are reducing or eliminating gluten from their diets. That is 91 million people, and gluten is actually the third most prevalent allergy or intolerance after cow dairy and eggs.

- Food allergies are the most common cause of anaphylaxis (a degree of sensitivity that can send you into shock within seconds or minutes and is potentially fatal), and numbers are trending upward.

Yet many physicians remain in the dark. Even though it's been a decade since the FDA passed a consumer protection act identifying "The Big 8" food allergens—gluten, dairy, eggs, soy, tree nuts, peanuts, shellfish, and fish—doctors often seem baffled or indifferent if you mention food allergies. I'm not trying to vilify the medical community. I honestly believe that current medical school curriculums simply don't prepare doctors to diagnose or treat food allergies and sensitivities, and that my doctors (and my daughters) genuinely didn't know that the symptoms for which we had been (over)treated for years might disappear with a change of diet.

For most people, eight weeks seems to be about how long it takes for symptoms to clear out completely and the body to begin to stabilize. In our case, we started seeing results almost immediately.

TAKING THE LEAP

Once you have mentally committed to embarking on this journey and feel that you understand what it will entail, you need to make sure that you prepare. It is essential to have an open dialogue with your primary care physician before you begin this or any other dietary modification. They will be as interested in the outcome as you are. But if this journey has taught me anything, it's that being open-minded to a holistic, well-rounded approach to self-care is crucial for long-term health, which may mean you also need to seek out an alternative practitioner whose practice can provide you with the additional support that you need.

After eight weeks of completely avoiding potential trigger foods, you will typically find that your body's natural sensitivity will be restored. Instead of minor reactions to foods that you have spent a lifetime building up immunity to, you will have a true reaction, and you may find that if

you deviate even slightly on a problem food, your system will clearly let you know what it does not like. Before the diet change, eating eggs would give me a stomachache; after the diet change and reintroduction of eggs, even a microscopic amount would almost immediately result in vomiting. I strictly avoid eggs now. Gluten and vanilla bean give me a sore throat, crazy runny nose, and sinus congestion, while a smidge of dairy activates a round of bloating and an acne breakout that I want no part of ever again. Clams cause such bloating and pain that my stomach looks like I am five months pregnant—not cute. You get the picture.

Perhaps you're thinking that making your body that sensitive to trigger foods is a mistake, and that it is easier to regularly indulge in those foods and irritate the body to keep a low level of resistance and avoid a more dramatic reaction. But I argue that this is just plain wrong. If your body has a severe reaction to a food just because you haven't eaten it for a while, *it is trying to tell you something*. I have chosen to listen to that kind of message from my body, because, frankly, I am hoping to avoid chronic inflammation, illness, and the diseases that inflammation has the potential to cause, such as cancer, heart disease, stroke, diabetes, kidney disease, immune repression, and more. This is bigger than just avoiding a stomachache.

No one fully understands yet just how far reaching inflammation is, how exactly food triggers work, what testing is reliable, or how long it can take for a person's immune system to recover from a lifetime of daily assaults. We are just beginning to realize how devastating chronic inflammation can be on our health and bodies. A new generation of food scientists, medical researchers, and home cooks are spearheading a promising new wave of research into ongoing questions about inflammation. New understandings are unfolding every month. Still, you don't have to wait years for the science to come together, or to find out which theories were on target and which were full of holes. Millions of people are discovering that *choices we can make in our own kitchens* can have a hugely beneficial impact on our physical and mental health.

You have to be accountable for your own diet and well-being. No one is going to stop you from eating your trigger foods—there are no food police looking over your shoulder, and you don't need a license to buy even the things that elicit the most severe reactions. It's all up to you. But here is how I think of food: It's either medicine that fuels a healthy, happy life, or poison that will drag you down and deplete you, preventing you from living a happy, healthy life. It's your job to figure out which foods go into which category for your body's and your family's optimal health. When you think about all the things that our bodies do for us, daily and throughout our lives, it doesn't seem like such a sacrifice to eat this way—you are simply taking care of yourself at the highest level. You will very quickly come to realize that the rewards drastically outweigh the sacrifices. And when you can enjoy the alternative versions I've created of our favorite "normal" treats—healthier versions of cookies, cakes, and pasta dishes—the sacrifices truly are few and far between.

EVERYONE IS DIFFERENT

While the recipes in this book are made without the main culprits of common allergies and inflammation, it would not be possible to create food that is 100 percent allergen-free for everyone. Every person is different. My husband realized that he has a really hard time digesting garlic, as do my mom and several of my girlfriends. Foods that "don't agree with" a person are likely not something he or she should be eating. Maybe you know someone who gets sick or hungover from a glass or two of wine or a bite of guacamole—that's a reaction, too. When you come right down to it, we all have a personal list of foods we know make us feel off the next day in one way or another, but because we enjoy them (or the context they are served in), we are willing to "pay the price" for eating them. But I think we have to ask ourselves what that price really is. Is it a problem for just a day, or is it much more far reaching over time and in its long-term effects? I think of what our family's problem foods were doing to our moods, energy, time, and resources, and the answer seems clear to me.

As for the rest of us, the benefits of avoiding the foods on our "reaction lists" were astounding:

My eczema and rosacea cleared up, and my twenty-year affliction with cystic acne cleared up.

My monthly migraines, which I had suffered since the age of twelve, went away.

The swelling, soreness, and restriction in my hands that had been diagnosed as pre-arthritis subsided.

I started sleeping eight to nine hours at night (in a row!), which had not happened since I was a kid.

My ADD symptoms retreated to the point that I am no longer taking medication for it.

My heartburn is gone and my digestion is better than I imagined was possible!

I had gotten so used to discomfort that it seemed normal.

Coco felt relief from stomachaches and chronic constipation within a few days on the new regimen. Three weeks in, the mysterious bumps and rashes on her face and neck were gone. Her "asthma" symptoms come on only if she accidentally stumbles into some dairy.

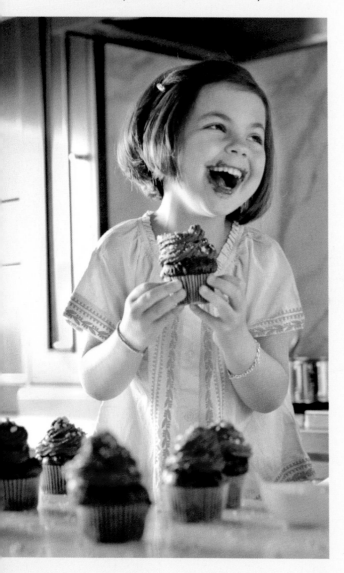

Pete, just along for the ride, lost 25 pounds in three months, even though he was actually eating more food than he had been before. (Leave it to men!) He also stopped snoring—thank God!—and no longer suffers from heartburn and indigestion when he eats on the program.

In our family, everything improved: our moods, the quality of our sleep, our energy levels, mobility, focus—the changes were dramatic and undeniable. We laugh more, have more energy, and spend *much* less time (and money) at the doctor. Being sick is now the exception rather than the rule.

As for me—a woman whom anyone would have considered healthy and normal two years ago—I feel like a 2.0 version of my old self. In shedding so many old health nuisances I have accessed a new wellspring of energy that lets me live life more fully. I have more physical energy to exercise and keep up with my young children, and more mental energy to devote to my passions. And I am finally living happily in my body without the ever-present dread of wanting to "lose a few pounds." For the first time in my life I eat as much as I want (within the confines of my allergies/intolerances) and am maintaining a body size I feel great about.

Sound good? Are you ready to say good-bye to many pesky health irritations? Sleep better, look better, feel better? Tackle this program, eat bountifully, and watch the weeks (and weight!) fall away. I humbly hope this story helps you make the adjustment, and encourages you to get out there and live your best life.

chapter 2
the food elimination diet

The Food Elimination Diet is the heart of the process of figuring out what your body thrives on and what is dragging it down. If you are one of the lucky people who already knows exactly what makes you sick, then you can skip this part and head straight to the recipes! But for everyone still struggling to figure out which food culprit is to blame for your aches and pains, or someone who has only just come to realize it's possible food could be the missing link between themselves and their best health, this elimination diet is your path to that discovery.

WHAT, *EXACTLY*, IS AN ELIMINATION DIET?

A food elimination diet is basically a controlled trial-and-error experiment. You stop eating suspect foods, give your system time to settle and heal, and then bring the eliminated foods back on board, one food at a time, to see how you handle it. It should really be called an elimination-and-reintroduction plan, because that is what you are doing: taking a food completely out of your diet, and then reintroducing it to your now rested system. A rested system is one that has stopped fighting food irritants on a day-to-day basis and begun to rebuild and restore its natural immunity. When you reintroduce a food to this clean slate, your reaction will be more pronounced, making the connection between cause and effect crystal clear.

An elimination diet is less expensive and more accurate than any other type of testing you can go through. It is your best chance to let your body speak to you. And while this diet cuts out eight highly allergic foods in an attempt to help 90 percent of you easily find your culprit, many of you will find that the healed body may have more to say to you than you think. After two months of cutting out dairy and gluten in sympathy with my daughter, and long before I was tested and did my own elimination diet, that slight break in digestive stress was enough for my body to give me my first major briefing. I discovered I am violently allergic to kiwifruit. I had not eaten it in ages, for no particular reason, when I had some fresh-pressed kiwi juice at a hotel buffet. I took a teaspoon-sized sip and dropped to the ground. It felt as though I had been pepper sprayed and my throat immediately began to swell shut as I gasped to take a breath through my uncontrollable coughing. By a quirk of fate I happened to have some liquid Benadryl in my purse and, with a double dose, was able to control the swelling until I could get some help. To say it was out of left field is an understatement. With the introduction of the elimination diet, vanilla bean seeds, passion fruit, flaxseed, pineapple, and banana all revealed themselves to cause pretty severe throat and skin reactions, even though they were not the focus of or even remotely part of the elimination diet I was following. My body was reset enough to start kicking up a fuss when anything it wasn't interested in tolerating came knocking.

When you finish your elimination diet, the best-case scenario is that you might discover you have only one problem food, and that by making the decision to live without it, you can begin to get your life back. It's also possible you will discover that your body needs a rest from certain foods and that, once allowed to recover and rebuild, your body will be able to tolerate those foods again, in moderation and with eyes wide open about the trade-offs.

The worst that can happen is you identify a real allergy or stubborn sensitivity to several foods, and in that case, you have the two hundred recipes in this book to help you hop right over the obstacles and get back to near normalcy in a couple of months, instead of struggling with poor health for the rest of your life.

During the process of the elimination diet, it is important to remember that you are completely in control, and to be successful in the diet, you must be diligent. While "a little cheating here and there" may not seem like a big deal, in fact it is tantamount to throwing all your hard work out the window. I'm not saying this to be harsh or judgmental, it just is what it is.

It takes a while to wrap your mind around this reality, and until you do, connecting cause and effect will be impossible. That said, it's probable that you will go off the rails along the way, and it really helps to cultivate a little self-acceptance. *I learn a tremendous amount each time I slip up (usually by accident). There is nothing more frustrating than feeling awful after eating something that you could have avoided, but such incidents serve as great reminders why I don't want to live my life feeling that way and what a stark contrast it is to the state of feeling healthy and allergen-free.* Remind your kids and yourself often: "We're doing a really good job, and it's going to pay off!" or "A little setback is not going to stop us!" Be your own best cheerleader and then climb back on the wagon.

WHY THESE EIGHT FOOD GROUPS IN PARTICULAR?

Ninety percent of all food allergies in the United States are caused by the "Big 8": dairy, eggs, gluten, soy, tree nuts, peanuts, shellfish, and fish (see chart, pages 24–25). You will notice that the only one of the "Big 8" used in my recipes is fish. Fish is a healthy and prominent part of our diet, and I prefer to eat it more often than other forms of animal protein. Fish allergies tend to be lifelong, with 60 percent of sufferers discovering their allergies as children and 40 percent as adults, so many of you would already know if you had them. However, if you believe you may have a fish allergy, or have a close relative with a fish allergy, then you may not want to include fish and fish products in your diet. (It is important to note that there is no relationship between allergies to shellfish and allergies to fish—you can be allergic to one or the other, or both.) Corn is another food some people have sensitivity to, although I do use it in a few of my recipes as well. If either of these foods is of concern for you, don't worry; the overwhelming majority of the recipes in this book will be just fine for you. Just read the ingredient lists carefully before you choose your menus.

One ingredient that is not widely recognized as an allergen but that I no longer use in my home cooking is cane sugar. Cane sugar is one of the most prevalent ingredients in the American diet, and you will find it in just about every single packaged food in your market. The massive overconsumption of cane sugar is its own epidemic, and more and more people are finding that its negative effects run deeper than a sugar crash. Whether sensitivities and allergies to cane sugar are resulting from overexposure or genetic predispositions, they are happening all the same. Many naturopathic doctors who dispense the ELISA tests will tell you that it is consistently in the top six most common antibody reactions. I can attest to this—it happens to be an allergy trigger for Pia and an inflammatory trigger for many, and let me tell you, it is very real. I wanted to include it in this program so those who know they have a problem with cane sugar will have recipe solutions and, for those of you who are open to the idea, a chance to explore other ways of sweetening your food. (But please don't misinterpret this as encouragement to indulge in artificial sweeteners like aspartame, saccharine, and sucralose—I do not use them or endorse the use of them in any way.)

WHY EIGHT WEEKS?

Eight weeks is what my doctor and many doctors who have experimented with longer and shorter time periods have found serves their patients best. Eight weeks is enough time to let the body really clear out, rest, and reset, and for people to get a real feel for a different way of eating. Truth be told, gluten can stick in the body for several months longer than this, but eight weeks will certainly be enough time to get an accurate reaction from your body on its tolerance level. Less than that is a lot of work without the real benefits. We are dealing with a lifetime of habits, and the fact that it takes *only* eight weeks is a testament to how amazing our bodies are, once they have the right healing environment.

HOW TO REINTRODUCE FOODS AND WHAT TO WATCH FOR

You probably don't have to do this diet forever (but you could still eat amazing food at every meal if you do!). The reintroduction period is about adding eliminated foods back in to your cleansed healthy body to see which ones can stay and which ones have to go, potentially forever.

This part is really important to understand: if you reintroduce more than one food at a time, you will never really know what causes what! You have to be very disciplined in that regard: only introduce one food, and record your sleep quality, moods, digestion, skin, energy level, mental focus, aches and pains, etc., for at least three to four days.

FREE FOR ALL—EVERY RECIPE IN *PURE DELICIOUS* IS FREE OF THE FOLLOWING KNOWN ALLERGENS

DAIRY

This is the most common allergen in infants and young children, and some would argue in adults as well. The most prevalent and precarious dairy allergies are typically an immune reaction to the caseins and whey proteins found in dairy. Much less prevalent is (the usually genetically predetermined) lactose intolerance. This is characterized by an inability of the body to process the milk sugar lactose. The lactose intolerance type of dairy allergy is three times more likely in those of South Asian descent. Dairy can be anaphylactic, but more common allergic reactions to dairy can include symptoms in the GI tract, skin, or airways, typically within an hour of ingestion or less. Lactose-intolerant reactions are more typically based in the stomach and intestines.

GLUTEN

Reactions to gluten are diverse. They can be as severe as anaphylaxis; a range of skin symptoms like hives and rashes; and/or stomach and GI effects like nausea, vomiting, bloating, cramping, and diarrhea. Sinus and lung issues are also common, since the nasal and lung tissues can become inflamed, leading to a stuffy or runny nose, sneezing, and postnasal drip as well as wheezing and asthmatic coughing. Headaches and joint swelling are also common complaints. Many reactions occur instantly, though others might not be noticed until the morning after. A gluten allergy or sensitivity can also be triggered environmentally by cosmetics or beauty products, depending on how sensitive you are.

SHELLFISH

"Shellfish" encompasses two families: crustaceans and mollusks. Crustacean shellfish allergies (to lobster, crab, crawfish, prawns, and shrimp) tend to be more severe as well as more common, with lobster, crab, and shrimp causing the majority of reactions. Mollusks is a much larger group that includes scallops, clams, mussels, oysters, marine snails, and abalone as well as octopus and squid. Those allergic to mollusks may find that they also have reactions to nondietary invertebrates like cockroaches and dust mites. If you are allergic to one group, you may be able to eat from the other without being affected. You may also find that only one or two species affect you from one of the groups, but depending on the severity of your reaction, you should be careful to make sure it is not the whole group. Shellfish are interesting in that 60 percent of people with a shellfish allergy do not discover it until adulthood. Once you have it, it is a lifelong allergy. Shellfish reactions are varied and range from anaphylaxis to severe reactions such as shortness of breath or a hoarse throat, repetitive coughing, trouble swallowing, face swelling, pale-blue coloring, and dizziness or confusion. Less severe reactions can include heartburn, vomiting, stomach cramps, bloating, and diarrhea.

CANE SUGAR

The most common symptoms of a cane sugar allergy are nasal and respiratory issues. The histamine reaction causes the sinus tissue to become inflamed and swollen, which then causes excessive mucus. The mucus can compound, causing sinus headaches, as well as stuffy and runny noses, postnasal drip, and puffy swollen eyes. The throat can also become inflamed causing a hoarse throat, chronic coughing, and even affecting breathing and causing asthmatic symptoms like wheezing. If the exposure is ongoing, the compounded mucus can eventually turn into an infection of the sinuses. Cane sugar reactions can also come in the form of skin reactions like hives and rashes.

PEANUTS

Peanuts, a member of the legume family, have a high trigger rate of anaphylaxis. Between 25 and 40 percent of individuals with a peanut allergy are also reactive to at least one tree nut, though not always to other legumes such as soy. Up to 20 percent of peanut-allergic people find they grow out of the allergy or that the allergy becomes far less severe. For people who are most sensitive to peanuts, even trace amounts or, in rare cases, peanut particles in the air can cause severe reactions. Anaphylactic symptoms are almost instantaneous, as are less severe histamine reactions like itchy skin, throat, and mouth or welts. Peanuts can also cause nausea or a stuffy or runny nose.

SOY

Soybeans are part of the legume family, although having an allergy to soy does not mean you have a greater chance of being allergic to other members of the legume family such as peanuts or beans. Rarely, anaphylaxis can occur as a reaction to soy, but other more common reactions range from hives and an "itchy mouth" to nausea, vomiting, and diarrhea. A stuffy nose, wheezing, and asthmatic coughing are also often associated with this allergy.

EGGS

Eggs are the second most prevalent food allergy. It is more common to be allergic to proteins in the egg white than the egg yolk. Eggs can cause anaphylaxis. While skin and airway reactions can occur as soon as the egg is ingested, most egg reactions tend to reveal themselves in the stomach and intestines, and the severity and time frame can vary from almost immediate to up to forty-eight hours after ingestion.

TREE NUTS

Along with peanuts and shellfish, this is one of the food categories most likely to cause anaphylaxis. Tree nuts include walnuts, almonds, hazelnuts, cashews, pistachios, pecans, pine nuts, and Brazil nuts. Tree nuts do *not* include peanuts or sesame seeds, although those too can be allergens. Most people with tree nut allergies discover the allergy in childhood, and roughly 90 percent experience a lifelong allergy. It is important to note that siblings and children of tree nut–allergic people are at an increased risk for tree nut allergies. These allergies can range in severity from anaphylaxis to other histamine reactions like shortness of breath; itching; or swelling of the throat, face, eyes, or mouth. They can also trigger abdominal pain, vomiting, and diarrhea. For extra-sensitive people, nut particles in the air and tree nut oils may be just as likely to cause a reaction as ingestion. Tree nut oils can be found in beauty products, lotions, and soaps, so always check labels.

Eating a piece of cheesy pizza (no matter how badly you want it) will infuse your body with gluten and dairy (and possibly eggs, cane sugar, and soy) all at once, making it impossible to tell which ingredient is the culprit when you feel sick afterward.

You need to continue to eat pure foods and wait the three to four days after reintroducing a food, really paying attention to what your body does and how you feel. Once you've given that food a thumbs-up or thumbs-down, move on to the next one. The idea is that your body will be your ultimate guide to what it does or does not want.

One day, try eating eggs for breakfast, and if you feel okay, then have eggs the next day, too, to make sure you don't get a reaction. A few days later, have some gluten-free soy sauce and edamame with your sushi to test your reaction to soy. A few days after that, you can eat a piece of cheese or drink some milk and see what happens. Just don't do it all at once!

Any histamine reactions that occur quickly will be obvious, but others will require more observation and a day or two. For example, when I did my elimination diet I included a few things not on this list of eight (due to my ELISA testing), including coffee. The first time I added coffee back in, nothing happened, and I thought I was in the clear—but after the second day in a row, I was horribly nauseated, and that was followed up with a crippling headache and nasty mood swings! After that clear illustration of its effects on me, no way did I want to go back to my four-cup-a-day habit.

When it comes to your children, look for less obvious reactions such as changes to their skin (bumpy arms, rashes, hives), energy (lethargy, hyperactivity), mood swings (tantrums or crying jags), sleeping habits, and bathroom habits. Since we can't experience it for them, try to pay careful attention and ask a lot of questions about how they are feeling. If they do have a reaction, it will be a major aha moment for them, too. I will never forget the first time Coco ate a piece of bread after completing her elimination diet and developed a raised, itchy, peeling red rash around her throat that looked like a collar. She "got it" even before the stomachaches started, and now she simply doesn't ask for bread anymore.

GOOD JOURNALING

I can't stress how helpful journaling can be at this point in your process. It is pretty difficult to keep track of all this in your head, especially if you are tracking for more than one person. I also find that if your memory or resolve gets a little weak with time, you can refer to your reaction notes and remember exactly what happens to you after you indulge in say, that cup of coffee. . . .

You want to write down exactly what you ate and then jot down any and all physical reactions or changes, as well as changes in sleep or mood, that stand out to you over the next few days. There may be nothing bad, but if there is, trust me, you will notice.

DIVING DEEPER

If you're one of the 10 percent who don't find their answers within these eight foods or find only some of them, then two things may have happened: one, you discovered other sensitivities or allergies along the way (like myself with all those tropical fruits), or two, you have decided to use this elimination diet as the foundation for diving deeper into other possible allergies.

Of course, the experiment could go on longer than expected if your problem food isn't one of the eight tested at first. You might be one of those who can't eat garlic, or strawberries, or paprika, or celery. But by the time you have tested the eight most common problem foods, you will have trained yourself to pay attention, and will find it easier to start making connections between what you ate yesterday and how you feel today. You may have to dig deeper to test other foods, or go for the next level of blood tests. It is sleuth work. But what isn't? We are constantly paying attention and making connections in order to improve our lives. Food testing just happens to require a bit of structure. Keep your eyes on the prize, and your efforts will pay off.

UNCOMMON ALLERGIES

I thought it worth sharing with you some foods and spices that, while less common allergens, are prevalent enough that they come up again and again in ELISA testing and may help find that needle in a haystack if you are struggling.

- Vanilla bean, coffee beans (not caffeine), cacao beans (pure chocolate), honey

- Sesame seeds, fruit seeds, chestnuts

- Beef, lamb, poultry, pork

- Baker's yeast, brewer's yeast, wine

- Ancient grains like Kamut, millet, and quinoa

- Kiwi, pineapple, bananas (It is worth noting that kiwi, pineapple, and bananas are a trifecta of allergies. Passion fruit is also related. If you find that two of them bother you, it is almost certain that the third will. And if you have all three, then you are almost surely sensitive or allergic to latex as well.)

- Strawberries, citrus fruits, cranberries, avocados, apples (and even apple skins), melons, papaya

- Celery, carrots, potatoes, yams, bell peppers, tomatoes

- Beans, all types, from lima and broad beans to green beans

- Coriander, celery, caraway, fennel, nutmeg (which is a seed, not a nut), and mace (made from the outer layer of the nutmeg seed), cinnamon, saffron, mustard, paprika, red pepper, poppy seeds, black pepper, pink peppercorns (the latter is linked to people with cashew allergies)

- Ginger, curry, onions, garlic

- Psyllium, black or green tea, licorice, spirulina, ginseng

- Pits and seeds of citrus fruits

- Buckwheat (actually a grass, not a grain)

WHERE ALLERGENS HIDE

Many of the foods we eat every day have all types of hidden allergens in them, and even a very small amount can completely derail your health. Ten milligrams of a food allergen—about the size of a bread crumb—is enough to inflame your system for as long as six to eight weeks. Shocking, isn't it!?

And yet these potential allergens lurk everywhere. Did you know, for example, that the wax used to coat non-organic apples and cucumbers is full of dairy proteins? A few bites of an apple may not cause a sudden reaction, but it can prolong the aggravation to your system. Did you know that many chewing gums have gluten in them? Or that anywhere you see "modified food starch" in an ingredient list, you should assume it is wheat or barley? Soy can hide in tea bags and lactose in melatonin supplements. Ten percent of wines are filtered with eggs and dairy. All this makes it easy for allergens to go undetected. Check condiment labels closely; Dijon mustard and Worcestershire sauce, for instance, may contain sugars. Many Asian condiments like garlic chili sauce, sambal oelek, and sriracha contain sugar. Unless you know the source of the sweetener (agave, pure maple syrup, honey, beet sugar, corn or rice syrup, date sugar, palm sugar, stevia, or molasses) you can guess it's cane sugar.

COMMON SOURCES OF HIDDEN GLUTEN

I find gluten to be one of the easier things to avoid. It's by far the most well-known allergen, and things are more and more often labeled when they are gluten-free. When you are at a restaurant and can't read the labels, just be diligent about making sure there isn't any gluten lurking in soups or sauces, as flour can be used as a thickener. You also have to watch out for soy sauce, which is predominantly wheat. Soy sauce is added to lots of sauces and even salad dressings, so make sure you read the labels or ask.

Malt vinegar

Brewer's yeast

Baking spray

Processed lunch meats and meatballs/meat loaf

Imitation crabmeat (such as that used in California rolls)

Tobiko (flying fish roe used in sushi)

Some vegetarian meat substitutes (like veggie burgers)

Frozen french fries

Soy sauce, hoisin sauce, oyster sauce (they also contain soy)

Licorice and red licorice

Gummy candy

Play-Doh (be sure your children wash their hands after using it if they have a sensitivity to gluten)

Some vitamins and medications (be sure to ask your pharmacist)

Many packaged sauces, soups, and salad dressings, including xanthan gum (see page 34)

COMMON SOURCES OF HIDDEN DAIRY

I have found dairy the most difficult allergen to avoid when eating out. I have had waitstaff and chefs ask me if "no dairy" includes butter, and have been "dairy-bombed" many times by a nonvigilant kitchens. Butter, along with salt, is used lavishly and universally in restaurant kitchens to create those rich, lush flavors we all look for when we are paying good money for a special meal; asking a restaurant to cook without either is like asking a drummer to play with one drumstick. So unless you are crystal clear that you are including butter among the things you must not eat, you may get a "dairy-free" meal full of butter. In defense of the restaurants, which certainly have no wish to make their patrons sick, it's not surprising that they get confused, because some people avoid dairy because of an allergy to milk proteins and others because of sensitivity to milk sugars, and those in the latter camp can eat butter, which is low in sugars, or lactose. The bottom line is that most any restaurant meal will include butter somewhere along the line unless you insist otherwise, so it's important to be specific with your waitstaff: "No milk products or butter, please."

Salad dressings

"Health bars," protein powders, and anything that contains whey protein or powdered milk

Some medications and supplements like melatonin

Any product whose label includes butter, milk or milk solids, ghee, curds

Casein and caseinates

Hydrolysates

Lactalbumin

Lactate solids

Lactic yeast

Lactitol monohydrate

COMMON SOURCES OF HIDDEN EGG

I have found that the most commonly used egg product is mayonnaise. Many people add mayonnaise (or aioli, a flavored mayonnaise) to sauces, salad dressings, and dips. Egg is also a common binder, so it's almost a given that it's in every type of meatball, meat loaf, pressed meat, and things like fritters and veggie cakes. And unless you know a gluten-free baked good definitely doesn't have eggs, you should assume it does. Some other places egg might be hidden include:

Candied nuts

Marshmallows

Processed meats and meatballs/meat loaf

"Velveted" Chinese meat or seafood dishes ("velveting" is a cooking technique in which ingredients are cooked in a sauce of egg whites and cornstarch)

Salad dressings

Flu shots and vaccines (you can request an egg-free shot, although they are usually reserved for those who have a histamine reaction to eggs, like facial or throat swelling)

Any product whose label includes albumin, globulin, lecithin, livetin, lysozyme, vitellin, or ovoglobulin

COMMON SOURCES OF HIDDEN SOY

Soy seems to be the sneakiest of the allergens. The obvious versions like soy sauce and soy products, such as tofu and edamame, are easy enough to find, but soy can be hidden in preservatives and obscure places like "artificial flavorings," which are in nearly every packaged food. The great news is that all products covered by FDA labeling laws must be labeled if they contain soy. An interesting note: Vegetable oil derived from soy is safe for all but the most extremely soy-allergic individuals.

Tempeh

Tamari

Miso

Soy lecithin

Edamame

Tobiko (flying fish roe used in sushi)

Artificial flavorings

Vegetable broth

Vegetable gum (a thickener)

Vegetable starch

Tea bags (check labels)

Some vitamins and supplements (ask your pharmacist or read labels)

chapter 3
a kitchen that supports you

Since getting our allergy diagnoses, I have completely changed the way I shop, cook, and feed my family. It wasn't always easy, but I can honestly say I have never felt as much in control of my own health and the future health of my children as I do now. I've been able to create a new food lifestyle for us without sacrificing taste, satisfaction, or the pleasure of eating well. I won't pretend we don't occasionally miss the joys—short-lived though they may be—of eating badly. But hey, doesn't everyone?

Nor will I pretend that any of us embraced the challenge of completely upending the way we ate enthusiastically or even willingly. Pia was sullen and quietly sad, while Coco had outright temper tantrums over the foods she could no longer have. As a mother it was heartrending to see them deprived not just of treats, but of basic foods other children were eating.

So being a chef and a recipe developer, I did the only thing that made sense—I got to work in the kitchen. It took time, patience, a lot of experimentation, and a true desire to understand the new set of ingredients I had at my disposal. I had to reinvent the wheel with virtually every aspect of cooking. I couldn't accept that my children would never again be able to have a cupcake or slice of pizza, so my goal was to re-create the foods they craved in a way that was safe for them to eat. All children want to fit in

with their peers; to be labeled as different can be embarrassing or painful. Watching your entire class pigging out on birthday cake while you sit there with an apple is no fun, and I wanted to spare my girls from those feelings. (Um, am I projecting?)

Pizza was the first makeover I tackled, and I tried out close to twenty variations before hitting on the one I considered truly delicious. Now when Pia's class has Pizza Party Tuesdays, she can bring her own pizza and not feel left out.

Doughnuts were next on the wish list. After a lot of trial and error, I found that using fruit and vegetable purées helped me make moist and tender baked doughnuts that were delicious and completely satisfied the cravings of my little ones. I got to send Coco to preschool with them so she felt included on "doughnut day."

Bread, muffins, and waffles followed, as well as homemade breakfast cereals so that we could occasionally indulge in a warm and comforting weekend breakfast.

Nailing the perfect cupcakes was an exciting hurtle. When I finally got a gluten-free vegan chocolate cupcake recipe that worked, Pia was over the moon. It made me teary to see how excited she was to have a beautiful chocolate cupcake to take to a friend's birthday party so she wouldn't miss out.

We found joy in savory treats, too, and being able to include chicken nuggets and french fries on the menu now and then made the kids feel much more comfortable with the "new normal." Coco's favorite food on earth, potstickers, led me on a quest to make wonton wrappers with rice flour when I couldn't find a gluten-free commercial substitute. And I'm proud to say that in every instance I consider my "newfangled" version of these beloved dishes every bit as delectable as the original.

MAKING THE CHANGE

The most important part of the whole transition is setting up your family to succeed. You've got to start by cleaning out all the unsafe foods and strive to restock the kitchen not only with safe foods but also less-processed foods. There is undoubtedly a long period of discovery—a lot of ingredients you may never have tried, much less cooked and baked with. But in the spirit of starting anew, try to embrace the excitement of shaking things up with a whole new arsenal of healthy ingredients.

Without a doubt, there has been a direct connection between cleaning up our kitchen and successfully cleaning up our diet! Once you start taking the steps toward positive changes, it is surprising how quickly and easily the rest of the dominoes fall. Truth is, I had been trying to get more organized and efficient in my kitchen for, well, forever. Making the transition to an allergen-free kitchen provided the push I needed to make life-changing and lasting adjustments that have only made my life easier and healthier.

EASIER, NOT HARDER

Though it may sound counterintuitive, when you transition to a way of cooking that relies primarily on whole foods and straightforward preparation techniques, not only will your cooking become more streamlined, but you'll be simplifying your kitchen and gaining counter space! I found I was actually using fewer appliances and gadgets than before and enjoying the time and taste benefits of less-complicated ingredients. My microwave has been moved to the basement for occasional use, and I retired my bread maker, panini press, and pasta roller (you wouldn't believe how much real estate I have opened up in my kitchen cabinets!), and many of the cooking techniques feel more pure and straightforward.

One of the solutions for keeping things easy is to embrace the idea of *prepare-ahead food*. Once you get in a rhythm of making foods to eat at a later date, you'll see that it's a huge time-saver and relief to have a multitude of ready-to-eat foods in the pantry, fridge, and freezer at all times. In the pantry for example, this meant having the base of many of my family's favorite baked goods already prepared, cake-mix style. If you make banana bread, for instance, scoop and dump the dry ingredients for an extra recipe into an airtight container for next time. In the refrigerator, this means having dips and fresh vegetables ready for snacking, or containers of grain salads and soups that could be easily served or heated for a fast and convenient meal.

Meal plans, recipes, and grocery lists also help to keep you organized and make the whole process of cooking much more straightforward. You don't want to get home from a long day at work or of shuttling your kids around with no food and no game plan. Those are the situations that lead to meltdowns and delivery pizza. Try to start every week with a meal plan, even if it covers only a few days. Shop for those meals and think ahead about lunches and snacks at the same time.

This idea of trading a few extra minutes to preserve your energy and perhaps your sanity is especially important in the early stages of this process. It's easy to flounder around, uncertain about what to make, and it is important that you have the right ingredients on hand so you don't feel helpless. Planning out your meals ahead of time will eliminate grocery store panic, aimless wandering, and wasteful overbuying, and hopefully encourage more streamlined shopping.

A TRIGGER-FREE ENVIRONMENT

Clearing triggers out of your kitchen has to be the first step. It's nearly impossible to succeed in a house full of temptation and cross-contamination. My food mantra is: If it's not in the house, it can't be there to tempt you. If you have a hard time letting go of something (as I

did with my fancy chocolate bars), imagine it as something that threatens you, like a mosquito or a hairy spider in your space: just claim your rightful territory and get it out the door.

The first step in changing our diet was to go to the source of the allergies: the fridge and pantry. For us, tossing the eggs, butter, and cheese from the refrigerator, while unpleasant, was pretty straightforward. You can give these things to a friend or neighbor, but just tossing them can be kind of a house-cleansing ritual—cathartic and symbolic.

The pantry is another matter. Once you pile up the pasta, cereal, breads, crackers, cookies, pancake mix, cake mix, chocolate bars, and a multitude of other packaged goods, you may realize that you have been consuming more processed foods than you thought—probably a *lot* more. It can be eye-opening to discover how much wheat, gluten, soy, cane sugar, eggs, and dairy were hidden in the small print of the foods you have been eating every week. And I'm not judging. For goodness' sake, if you saw what came out of my "pastry chef's" pantry, you would know I'm in no position to be pointing fingers.

Consider donating any unopened packages to your local food bank and toss the rest. Now we can go about rebuilding your pantry.

Where you once kept pounds and pounds of dried semolina (wheat) pasta, you now have room for all kinds of gluten-free grains and dried goods: oats, polenta, millet, rice, quinoa, and rice-, corn- and quinoa-based pasta, as well as buckwheat noodles (buckwheat is actually a seed that is unrelated to wheat). Stock up on corn tortillas and tapioca- and rice-based fresh-roll wrappers. Dried beans and rice can become new staples.

Fill plastic containers or mason jars with your own homemade muffin, waffle, pizza crust, pancake, doughnut, and cupcake mixes.

If you're a baker (like me), you're going to be giving your pastry-making pantry quite a face-lift and investing in some new types of flours. Millet, sorghum, oat, coconut, brown and white rice flours, and tapioca and potato starch will take the place of your old all-purpose, pastry, and bread flours. These tend to be sold in small bags that can leak, so if you bake often, transfer them from their original packaging to canisters or jars that you can stack to save space and avoid mess. (If you don't bake much, leave them in the original packaging or be sure to add an expiration date to your container, as some of these grains can become rancid over time.) Other baking necessities are unsweetened chocolate, stevia-sweetened vegan chocolate bars, and allergen-free chocolate chips. I recommend coconut by the boatload: cans of coconut milk and cream and coconut oil, as well as shredded unsweetened coconut. Beet, palm, and coconut sugar; maple syrup; honey; and agave are great sweeteners, and sunflower butter and various seeds are great to have on hand.

Are you thinking, "That's a lot of stuff—how do you expect me to buy all of that at once!?" You're right—it is a lot of new stuff, and it would be expensive to buy all these replacement ingredients in a single shopping trip. Don't panic. Take a deep breath and remember that you only need to buy what you will eat. If you've been making meal plans as I suggest, you'll know when you need to add to your pantry, and you can build it as you go. After a while, these ingredients will become as familiar to you as the things you used to buy, and you will find it is a pretty even swap. Just go slowly and with intention; there is no need to buy a new ingredient just on the off chance you may want to use it someday.

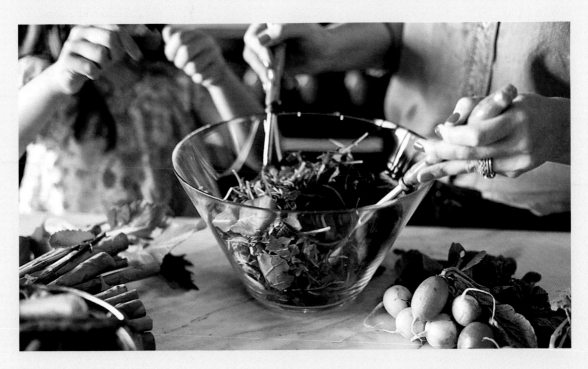

COCONUT OIL. I go through this stuff at what some people might consider an alarming rate—ninety-seven jars alone in the making of this cookbook. I use it for everything from sweets to savory dishes, and it is my cooking and baking oil of choice. I also prefer coconut oil spray for preparing baking dishes because of its slightly sweet flavor (but you can certainly use vegetable oil spray in its place, if you prefer).

I use coconut oil because my body likes it and because it's versatile and delicious, but it also offers many health benefits. For one thing, it is nature's richest natural source of lauric acid, which has powerful antimicrobial properties. To put things in perspective, coconut oil contains 50 percent lauric acid, and the next highest source of lauric acid is breast milk, at 10 percent. There is also much recent interest in the possible connections between coconut oil and healthy brains. So much interest and anecdotal evidence, in fact, that the National Institute on Aging started a double-blind clinical trial (the results of which will be published in 2016) to study coconut oil for the treatment of mild and moderate Alzheimer's disease! That's something that runs in my family, so I'll be keeping an eye on the results of that study.

OLIVE OIL. My second oil of choice is extra-virgin olive oil. Long touted for its healthy fat and health benefits that range from cardiovascular health and prevention of cancer to anti-inflammatory properties and immune system strength. I also love the taste. Vegetable oil is best for baking because it doesn't interfere with the flavor of your pastry, and grape-seed is wonderful in dressing and sauces when you don't want that strong olive oil flavor.

COCONUT MILK AND CREAM. I use these versatile dairy replacers in many sweet and savory preparations and always keep a variety of forms on hand: refrigerated unsweetened coconut milk in a carton, canned coconut milk and canned coconut cream in the pantry. I don't personally use reduced-fat, or "lite," coconut milk in my recipes, as they seem watered down to me, but you can certainly make that substitution if you prefer. Coconut cream may be a bit trickier to come by than the other two, but if you live near a Trader Joe's, you're in luck; their canned coconut cream has a really thick texture and very rich flavor, and I use it as the base for ice cream, chocolate ganache, whipped cream, and many other things. If you don't live near one, coconut cream is also sold on Amazon.

BOB'S RED MILL GLUTEN-FREE ALL-PURPOSE FLOUR. This is my favorite all-purpose gluten-free baking blend, a great shortcut for some recipes that don't require a custom blend of ingredients.

GARBANZO BEAN FLOUR is a great binder and thickener. The flour adds moisture and is packed with fiber, protein, and iron.

BOB'S RED MILL ASSORTED FLOURS. For the aforementioned custom flour blends, Bob's Red Mill is also my go-to source. They make everything from rice, oat, millet, and sorghum flours to binders like xanthan gum, and they are widely available in supermarkets as well as natural foods stores.

XANTHAN GUM. I use this food stabilizer and thickener in very small amounts to give baked goods the elasticity or stickiness they need to mimic the texture of gluten-based foods. Basically the xanthan gum helps to make gluten-free baked goods chewy instead of crumbly. Note, however, some people with sensitivities to wheat, corn, dairy, or soy may have a reaction to xanthan gum, as all of those may be used to cultivate the bacterium from which it is derived.

GLUTEN-FREE ROLLED OATS. These are used as a binder and base for granola, cookies, and bars. Plus, I just love oatmeal.

PUMPKIN AND SWEET POTATO PURÉES. Unsweetened canned pumpkin and sweet potato purées find their way into many of my baked goods. Both are a great binder, add moisture, and are full of fiber and vitamins. It's pretty easy to make your own purée when pumpkins are in season. If you are going to make your own sweet potato purée, I prefer the orange-fleshed variety and will roast mine in the oven at 400°F for 45 minutes. Alternatively, you could microwave one for 5 to 8 minutes, rotating them halfway through.

BEET SUGAR. Because one of my daughters is severely allergic to cane sugar, I almost always use beet sugar in recipes that call for cane sugar. It can be substituted 1:1, and it has given us a ton of freedom to experiment with baked goods while avoiding cane sugar. We order NOW Foods' organic non-GMO beet sugar online, but you can also buy American Crystal Sugar brand or White Satin white sugar, brown sugar, and confectioners' sugar, all of which are made with beet sugar. They are sold at many grocery stores and bulk and restaurant supply stores. I have also made my own confectioners' sugar by "puréeing" 1 cup of granulated beet sugar and 1 tablespoon of cornstarch together in a blender on high until fluffy (note that you will have to sift several times to get a fine result). Similarly, you can make a substitute for brown sugar by beating 1 cup of granulated beet sugar with 1 tablespoon of molasses with an electric mixer until uniform. You can also substitute palm and coconut sugars, but they are not as sweet as cane or beet sugar.

AGAVE, HONEY, AND MAPLE SYRUP. I use these to sweeten foods anytime they don't compromise the structure of a dish with too much liquid. For that reason, I use them rarely in baking, but often in cooking. They produce a more natural sweet flavor and they don't make your blood sugar spike in the same way that refined white sugar can. If you are vegan, feel free to substitute agave for the honey in otherwise vegan recipes.

PUMPKIN AND SUNFLOWER SEEDS. Use these in place of nuts in pesto, cereal, cookies, and snack bars. They are crunchy and delicious and full of protein and fiber.

SUNFLOWER BUTTER. Ground sunflower seeds make a good replacement for peanut butter in sauces and baked goods.

CHOCOLATE AND CHOCOLATE CHIPS. For cooking chocolate and chips I like Enjoy Life brand chocolate, which is free of everything on our "no" list except cane sugar. If you need to strictly avoid cane sugar (like Pia and I do), Amore Di Mona brand chocolate is sweetened with agave and available on their website or on Amazon. I buy it in bar form and chop the bars into chunks to use instead of chocolate chips. There are a few other chocolate chip brands that are gluten-free and vegan and sweetened with stevia, but always make sure you check the label for soy. Vegan chocolate bars are widely available, although they are not always marketed as vegan (look for cocoa percentages in the 80 percent or higher range). Unsweetend chocolate has no dairy in it.

COCONUT AMINO ACIDS. This is a soy-free, gluten-free substitute for soy sauce or tamari.

APPLE CIDER VINEGAR. I use this in combination with unsweetened coconut milk to create a faux buttermilk that adds great flavor, moisture, and tenderness to baked goods. Apple cider vinegar also boasts incredible health benefits ranging from antibiotic effects to topical and internal anti-inflammatory benefits.

CHIA SEEDS. Chia seeds are an incredible superfood that is very high in fiber and nutrients for a relatively small amount of calories. When they are mixed with hot water, chia seeds form a gel that is an excellent binder and substitute for eggs. One tablespoon of chia seeds mixed with three tablespoons hot water is a direct substitution for one large egg.

CANNED GARBANZO BEAN LIQUID (ALSO KNOWN AS AQUAFABA). This may sound weird, but the liquid that comes from canned garbanzo beans is an amazing egg replacer that also adds moisture. I use this in the pizza crust recipe on page 190 as well as in breadsticks and Hamburger Buns (page 178) and even chewy molasses cookies (page 284). Three tablespoons of aquafaba is a direct substitution for one large egg.

DEHYDRATED POTATO FLAKES. Sometimes known as dried mashed potatoes or potato buds, which are 100 percent real potatoes. These are amazing for binding (like in meatballs) and for tenderness (like in pizza crust).

These are easy to find at the grocery store just make sure you get plain, not flavored.

VEGAN BUTTER. Soy-free vegan butter creates a creamy flavor and texture that is superior to coconut oil or any other fat in many baking recipes. Most stores carry several varieties—read the label to be sure it is soy-free.

GLUTEN-FREE BEER. You'll find a bit of beer in many of my baking recipes because the carbonation gives a fantastic lift and yeasty flavor that I can't achieve any other way. It gives waffles (page 322) just the right fluffiness. Plus, I keep it in the fridge because sometimes I just want a beer (see the sidebar on page 54).

PACKAGED BROTHS. Whenever my recipes call for broth, you may use vegetable or chicken broth interchangeably. I just use whatever I have in my pantry. When buying packaged stocks and broths, do take time to read labels! Many broths and stocks have added ingredients you will want to avoid like cane sugar or soy.

KOSHER SALT AND (LACK OF) BLACK PEPPER. I use Diamond kosher salt for everything—cooking, baking, you name it. Be aware, though, that kosher salt does not measure out the same as table salt, and that other brands, like Morton's, can be significantly "saltier," so always add salt to your own taste. You may also notice that I do not call for black pepper in any of these recipes. I have never subscribed to the idea that everything seasoned with salt must also be seasoned with pepper, and not just because it turns out I am allergic to black pepper, a more common problem than you would imagine. If you don't have a problem with pepper and really miss it, you may certainly add pepper to taste, but try eating without it for a while. You may not notice its absence as much as you'd think.

FRESH CHILE PEPPERS. I use a lot of fresh chiles in my cooking. Besides being delicious, they are incredibly good for you, offering immense amounts of nutrients in a small package. I previously thought that I could not tolerate spicy food, but it turns out the dairy, eggs, and wheat were ulcerating my esophagus and GI track, not the chiles. Something to think about for those of you who have uttered the well-known "I love spicy food, it just doesn't like me." Also, see Aloe Vera, at right, for naturally healing your whole GI tract.

TAHINI. I use sesame paste and sesame seeds in some of my recipes, something I note because many people who have serious nut allergies also have sesame allergies.

GARLIC. Personally, I am obsessed, but my daughter and husband can't eat garlic. If you find that you have crazy heartburn after eating it, you probably shouldn't, either. When I need to leave it out of a recipe, I add extra onions or something else like a pinch of red pepper flakes or a little lemon juice to supply that kick garlic provides.

CORN. Many Americans have trouble with corn and it is most definitely used as filler in a wide range of processed foods. For that reason, even though corn is not one of the "Big 8," only a handful of these recipes contain corn and all note clearly when it is included.

VEGAN AND SOY-FREE PROTEIN POWDER. I add this to most of my smoothies in the morning because as an adult I need protein with my carbs. It gives me staying power and energy to get through exercise and my daily routine. You may have to experiment with finding one that works for your diet and your taste buds, but it can be a great addition to your diet when you do. Be aware that this is not a closely monitored industry, so going online where you can carefully read labels and reviews is helpful.

ALOE VERA. You know how aloe vera soothes your skin? Drinking aloe vera juice helps heal the tissues on the inside of the body, too. We are addicted in my family, and I add an ounce or two to any of the smoothies in the drink section or just take a shot of it in the morning. My favorite brand is AloeCure, which is organic (I like Regular, and my kids like the Grape flavor, which is sweetened with stevia).

APPLIANCES AND TOOLS

Good tools that work well and are versatile help save time and give your kitchen that humming-along-smoothly feeling. While my stand mixer was once my most used kitchen appliance, I now find that I am reaching for my blender and food processor far more often. Here are the ones I consider essential:

BLENDER. Hands-down the appliance I rely on the most—this puppy is used ten times a day to make smoothies, salad dressings, dips, soups, and cake batters.

FOOD PROCESSOR. Another item you will use often. Minced foods, dips, dough, and marinades are really easy to make with a food processor.

HANDHELD ELECTRIC BEATERS. If you don't have a stand mixer, don't worry. Handheld beaters work perfectly well for whipping up frothy coconut cream or smooth and shiny chocolate ganache.

VEGETABLE SPIRALIZER. This inexpensive contraption uses a mandoline plate and a variety of perforated plates to turn your veggies into paper-thin rounds or spaghetti-like strings that sauces cling to well. It makes veggies a lot more exciting to eat.

SHARP KNIVES. A chef's knife, a paring knife, and a serrated knife can make all the difference in the world when it comes to efficient (and safe) preparation of your ingredients.

ZESTER. Fresh citrus zest is a fantastic addition to lots of recipes, and a zester makes collecting it without scraping off the bitter pith fast and easy. (Try to buy organic citrus if you're going to eat the zest!)

RASP. Great for citrus, and even better for grating garlic, ginger, jalapeño, and onion super-fine for sauces.

MEASURING CUPS AND SPOONS. There is no such thing as "a pinch of this or that" in gluten-free baking. You must be precise— really precise! Make sure you have a sturdy set of measuring cups and spoons.

CANDY THERMOMETER. Frying at the correct temperature ensures a crispy result that doesn't absorb much oil.

PLASTIC PINT AND QUART TAKEOUT CONTAINERS. My favorite easy-to-get containers for keeping an organized and efficient pantry. I also use them for pantry items, and also to keep portions of fast and easy ready-to-eat dishes in the fridge so we're not tempted to reach for less healthy choices. Last night's leftovers all go into the containers labeled with a Sharpie and are put on the center shelf so I can easily see what is available.

RESEALABLE PLASTIC BAGS. These are very helpful for all kinds of things. I fill bags with freshly cut vegetables for snacking and quick access when I'm making meals. In my freezer you'll find bags filled with cookies, chicken fingers, potstickers, and frozen chopped fruit ready for smoothies. They

are perfect for piping doughnut batter in pans, too.

PINT PAPER FREEZER CONTAINERS. These are the small paper containers with lids that you would find at the soup bar at your local grocery store or when you buy ice cream by the pint. I fill these with homemade sorbets and ice creams but they are also microwave friendly and convenient for food storage in lunch boxes when the kids need to be able to just compost or trash the container. I order these online or pick them up at my local restaurant supply store.

THE FREEZER. Your freezer is a great tool that can help you be more organized and efficient. When I go to the trouble of making something like cookies or dumplings, I want a lot of return on my effort. Freezing helps me achieve that. To double the quantity only takes a little extra time in the moment, but will save me tremendously in the future. My freezer is full of things like homemade waffles, soups, homemade chicken nuggets, potstickers, brownies, and cookies.

(You can even pack frozen cookies in lunches, as they will have thawed by lunchtime.) You will find that the freezer is one of the best ways to take advantage of your time and efforts in this process.

chapter 4
helping kids transition

When you have a child with food allergies or eating restrictions, it is important to put things in perspective. The mental, physical, and emotional health of your child are at stake. If it had been just me who was diagnosed, I might have pushed it under the rug and gone on about my business in mediocre health rather than disrupt my whole family's way of life.

But now, armed with the knowledge that making such significant changes would actually help us to grow together as a healthy and cohesive unit, I would never make that choice. And whether it is all of you who choose to eat this way, or just you catering to your children who have allergies, set the example. Not only is it healthier physically, it's easier emotionally when the family works and eats together as a team. Can you imagine how it would feel for your kids to watch their parents eating foods that not only make them sick, but that are so hard for them to give up? Trust me, it will mean *everything* to them to know they have partners in learning how to eat safely and, just as important, learning to advocate for themselves.

For the first few months after my diagnosis, I hid behind my children's needs, embarrassed to speak up on my own behalf or deal with the judgment of others, especially since I'd been a naysayer for all those years. But four months into the transition, I got incredibly sick after failing to divulge my allergies at a work function. I dragged my swollen, ravaged body back home expecting to fall into bed. Instead, I had an epiphany. Just as important as teaching my children the right foods to eat is showing them that they can and should be honest and open about what they need. Hiding something you can't help or acting embarrassed about it is not the behavior I want to model for them. Taking control of their own health and figuring out how to make the best of a difficult situation is what I want them to take away from this.

MAINTAINING NORMALCY

If *you* seem at peace with your new normal, your kids and your community are more likely to take it in stride without judgment. You should be able to travel, have life experiences, and live in joy, unhindered or dictated by what you *can't* eat. Try to keep the focus on what you *can* eat.

When it comes to your children, I think it is okay to go out of your way to help them maintain normalcy with their peers. You can send them to birthday parties with their own cupcakes. Ask their teachers to e-mail you when there will be treats in class and have batches of cookies and brownies stored in the freezer for your child to bring to school. (Those make-ahead freezer tricks really come in handy when you need a cookie fast!) And I cannot stress preparation and thinking ahead enough. For example, I know it is Pizza Day at school the first Tuesday of every month for my children, so that means it is Pizza Night at home the first Monday of every month, with extra slices for the lunch box the next morning. Not a big sacrifice when we all love pizza anyway.

I think that through this process, you will find that your kids will grow in flexibility and acceptance as well as compassion. They will understand what it means to take care of their bodies and their health. They will learn to advocate for themselves and others. They may learn to "look out for" siblings and friends, and to lend to support when needed. They will learn to adapt to circumstances that are beyond their control, and most important, they will learn empathy. These are all qualities I have seen being awakened in my own children, and I believe you will see them in yours, too.

REWARD AND TRACKING SYSTEMS

Children love to keep track of their progress and earn rewards for their hard work. I don't see it as bribery, but as motivation. As adults we monitor our progress and goals in life and reward ourselves. I like to do the same for my children.

Whether you employ charts with stickers, or a point system, or a jar with marbles, choose a technique that is exciting to your children and realistic for you. Decide on the types of occasions that will warrant "points" and how many points you need to earn to receive larger "prizes." The specifics are totally up to your family.

Especially in the beginning, you will just want to get through certain situations that are new for them without a total meltdown. Let's take birthday parties at school, for example, or the fact that your child can't order her favorite buttered noodles at your regular haunt. There will probably be tears and maybe some begging. Those situations suck. First-world problems, I know, but they become parenting issues just the same. The bottom line is that some kind of reward system can be enormously helpful in getting through those first eight weeks. You don't need to promise ponies or shopping sprees, but small rewards (stickers, temporary tattoos, extra screen time, a sparkly pencil) for getting through small hurdles and larger ones (family movie night, a gift card, or a new app) for getting through large blocks of time without fighting the new program. And every step of the way, reassure them that you are doing this for them and their health. The truth is, it won't be that hard. Whether they are young or teenagers, they will be able to tell the difference almost immediately in how much better they feel. And trust me, the first time they fall off the wagon and get sick, the point will be driven home more clearly than you could ever make it: they will be horrified. These are teachable moments, so be on the lookout.

BUILDING COMMUNITY

When your kids are at home, everyone will be invested in making this transition as easy and successful as possible. Out in the real world, though, it's a different matter. Building a supportive community is imperative, especially when dealing with children. Talk to your extended family and caregivers immediately and in depth about what you are doing and why. Having grandparents, aunts and uncles, cousins, and close family friends on board is nonnegotiable. Many gatherings of family or friends revolve around food, so address the changes immediately and firmly with whoever is hosting. Be clear that there is no room for "creative interpretation" of the situation. By stressing that this is about the health of the children, you can keep cynics focused on what is important: the kids.

Babysitters, nannies, and day-care employees may also need educating. Don't be embarrassed to leave them very clear instructions. I also recommend talking to your children's teachers and the appropriate office staff at school. And don't forget to update your child's health records and list in detail their food allergies and symptoms for the nurse's office.

If you think that this might be a pain for your children's teachers, you may be surprised by how receptive and helpful they can be. During our "research phase," Pia's kindergarten teacher went as far as to write down what Pia was eating and not eating and how she felt afterward, and then closely monitor that Pia was staying on-program even after the research phase had ended. It was obvious to her that Pia was more focused and had good, steady energy throughout the day instead of the daily roller coaster of emotions and health ailments she exhibited previously. And if you ask your teachers to drop you an e-mail in the event that there is going to be a special occasion (a lunch or a birthday treat) at school the next day, most will be happy to oblige. Stress to the teacher that this is about helping to create a healthy child who will ultimately be a better, more attentive student and member of the class.

When your children have playdates, make sure that the parents know about the allergies. If you feel that the special request might be an imposition or that your requests aren't being taken as seriously as you'd hope, just send a snack with them.

For every adult who undermines your child's health by trying to sneak them candy because they "don't believe in food allergies" (and I've definitely found myself in this situation), there are a ton of people who just want to help these kids to get healthy and stay that way. And the great news is that with every passing month, your kids will be more self-assured and comfortable with saying what they can and can't eat.

The truth is that food allergies are no rarity anymore. Each year my own children have several more kids in their classes who are diagnosed with allergies and even celiac disease. It is nice to be able to trade recipes and tactics with the other parents—I guarantee they are out there and will appreciate the camaraderie as well.

SCHOOL LUNCH PREP

If you have a child of school age, you probably dread packing lunches. My mother always found it a chore, and I am pretty sure it is a universal pain in the ass. But there are ways to make it easier on yourself because, truth be told, you can't just toss a few processed-food snack-packs in the lunch boxes or give your kids money to buy hot lunch. Those are simply no longer options most of the time. Instead, try to make meals and snacks do double-duty. Your child's lunches may be a little less traditional than your standard sandwich, apple, and cookie—but that's just fine. And if you do decide to make homemade sandwich bread, they can have sandwiches for a few days in a row.

When you cook, always consider how leftovers and extras could be repurposed later in the week or frozen for later use in the lunch box. When you make muffins or banana bread, immediately wrap some for a few lunches later in the week. Roast chicken and turkey leftovers can be lunch box regulars, and whenever you serve the kids pasta for dinner, fill their lunchbox containers for the next day at the same time. I also am fond of doubling up on the after-school smoothies and pouring the extra into metal water bottles that I stash in the freezer. In the morning you can put that frozen smoothie in a lunch box, and by lunchtime it will have thawed to a perfect slushy consistency. You can also pack things like veggies and hummus, and if you have adventurous eaters, any of the grain salads in this book make a healthy and filling lunch. Buy a good-quality thermos for soup that won't leak and really keeps the contents hot—you will use it often.

COOKING DINNER *WITH* YOUR KIDS

There are so many ways kids benefit when their parents cook at home. Not only does it establish routine (which is comforting), but it allows the kids to be involved in caring for their own health and learning skills that will stand them in good stead forever. Look for opportunities for them to help out, to learn valuable life lessons (even if only by osmosis), and to practice counting and dexterity. Kids get a much better understanding of where their food comes from and how life is feeding life when they see the "before" (piles of fresh veggies, herbs, and greens, or bowls of flour and stir-ins) become the "after" (steaming soups and flaky baked treats). Consider, too, that every aroma wafting from the kitchen is a life memory in the making. Just try to tell me that the smell of apples and cinnamon cooking or tomato sauce simmering doesn't immediately press your nostalgia button.

Also, a great tip: Not long after the girls were diagnosed, we realized how difficult it was for them to remember everything (it takes a while for young children to get the hang of things). One very helpful solution was that we purchased them old-fashioned medical ID bracelets. On one side we wrote, "I have severe food allergies!" On the other side (albeit in very small print), we listed the foods that they are not to eat. This accomplished two things: If they were with an adult who was unsure about what to feed them, they could simply read the bracelet, and it also seemed to make some of the more dubious adults take things more seriously.

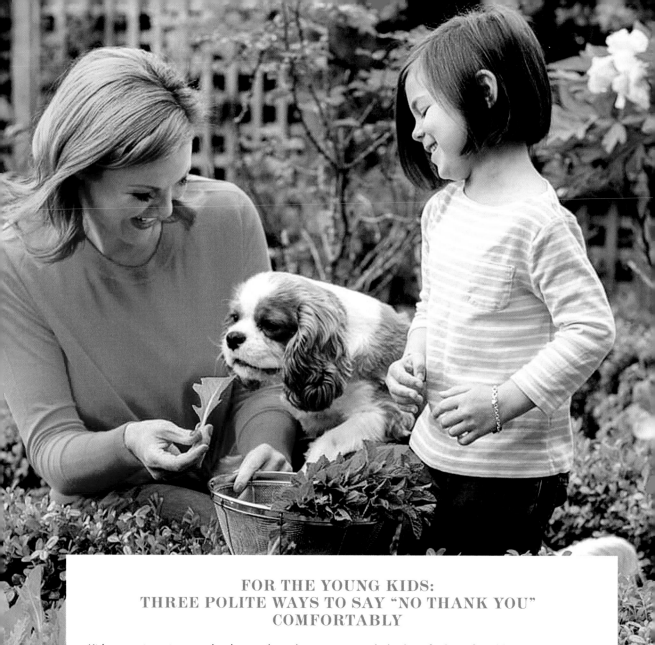

FOR THE YOUNG KIDS:
THREE POLITE WAYS TO SAY "NO THANK YOU" COMFORTABLY

Kids sometimes just need to be taught a phrase or two to help them feel comfortable saying no. (And it's very hard for skeptics to undermine polite children who know what they can and can't eat!) Brainstorming with your kids about actual situations can really help them feel empowered and self-accepting. These are some of the lines my little girls use on a regular basis:

"No thank you, I am allergic to that, but thank you for asking."

"It looks delicious, but I am afraid I'm allergic to that food."

"I hope you don't mind, I brought my own snacks! I just want to make it easier for everyone!"

chapter 5
eating out

Restaurants have become a huge part of many people's lives. For happy hours, Friday and Saturday nights, brunch, work lunches, and family celebrations, restaurants are just about impossible to avoid, and honestly, why would you want to? You can absolutely eat on-program and still go out and enjoy yourself. You just need to have a few tricks up your sleeve!

AVOIDING THE PITFALLS

These days it is not uncommon for a server in a restaurant to inquire if any of your party has food allergies, which is a *huge* step in the right direction. But just because the kitchen is aware that allergies exist doesn't mean they are familiar with your *particular* allergies, or that even a well-meaning server can remember a long list that you rattle off verbally. If you have food allergies that cause anaphylaxis, you need to let the kitchen know in advance of arriving if possible, to make sure it is safe for you to eat there. (For example, someone with a severe nut allergy may not be able to tolerate particles in the air and the kitchen will tell you if they are comfortable serving you.) If you are allergic to anything unusual or to a great many ingredients, I suggest you have a card listing them printed up. We made laminated fluorescent-green double-sided cards (about the size of a business card) with Coco's allergies on one side and Pia's on the other. They save the poor waitstaff from having to come back and double-check on ingredients every few minutes. (We also pass them out to all caretakers, teachers, and relatives who may take them out to eat or for handy reference.) I also cannot stress this enough: Do not assume anything about what is in a dish based on a menu description. In fact, assume it *is* cooked in butter and laced with gluten and everything else you aren't having. Even being a professional chef who prides myself on being able to "assume" what is in dishes based on the menu, this is typically how I have gotten myself in trouble.

When you head out for the first time, review what you will be doing with your kids, and clarify how they can show good manners and empowerment in the experience (pack along some stickers or whatever your positive reinforcements are).

I have worked as a waitress and in restaurant kitchens, so I am very thoughtful when it comes to communicating with the waitstaff and kitchen staff. My emphatic advice is: BE POLITE! It's really true that you catch more flies with honey, you know? It is important to be clear about your needs, but also to be patient with the staff and realize that while you are the customer, in a busy establishment taking the time to make adjustments for your needs is an accommodation that deserves acknowledgment and thanks.

WHAT TO ORDER?

As long as you are up front about your allergies and use common sense when ordering, you can typically find a way. At this point I feel I can find something to eat at pretty much any restaurant I visit. That said, some cuisines present bigger challenges than others. Here are some tips for ordering at different types of restaurants:

Classic American: Steer toward grilled fish, steaks, pork, chicken, and big salads, hold the cheese.

Steak Houses: Any grilled meat or fish, plain baked potatoes, french fries, salads, sides of vegetables (just make sure you say no butter, and check the sauces!).

Thai Food: Curries are typically safe, as is pad thai with no egg or peanuts. Order chicken, pork, or beef instead of tofu. The summer or fresh rolls with tapioca skin and rice noodles are good, too, but forgo the dipping sauce. Beware of things like "garlic sauce" or "chili sauce"—anything with a brown tinge probably has soy sauce in it.

Japanese: Sushi is great. Bring your own bottle of coconut amino acids to use in place of soy sauce.

Be sure to be aware of any of the salads or sauces, which almost always have soy sauce or ponzu sauce in them.

Mexican: This is one of the easiest cuisines to indulge in. While *mostly* naturally gluten-free, make sure that you tell your server about your allergies, and be on the lookout for cheese or crema. Choose corn tortillas over flour tortillas and make sure that there is no hidden dairy in the guacamole or flour or nuts in the mole sauce. Ask to have your margarita sweetened with agave instead of sugar.

Mediterranean: Go for the grilled meats, fish, or kebabs or souvlaki. Beware of pressed meatball kebabs, which may be thickened with bread or egg. Dips like baba ghanoush and hummus should be safe as well as some varieties of dolmas (seasoned rice wrapped in grape leaves) and Greek salad without the feta. Luckily, most dishes are cooked with olive oil, but be on the lookout for yogurt and eggs, which are used in many Greek soups and sauces such as avgolemono and tzatziki.

Italian: Stick to antipasto (minus the cheese) and simple salads, vegetables, and grilled meats. Many restaurants now serve gluten-free pastas, so if the sauce is fair game, you can indulge to your heart's content. You most likely need to avoid risotto and gnocchi, which, while gluten-free most likely have dairy (risotto) and egg (gnocchi).

Once you have found a few places that work for you, it pays to become a regular. The staff will get to know you, and having your needs attended to will be no big deal at all. It never hurts to be known as a generous tipper when you need to be generously accommodated, too!

chapter 6
eight weeks to a new normal

Are you ready to get together your game plan for the next eight weeks? I've explained why you need to start your "new normal" with an elimination diet and exactly what you will be eliminating, but now we can add some additional structure and detail to the process. Eliminating allergens from your life is about more than just cooking great, purely delicious food; it's a full-on lifestyle commitment, and one that may present some choppy water and rocks that must be navigated around. This chapter will give you a step-by-step road map to transitioning your pantry, your home, and your social life to a cleaner, more supportive, and healthier lifestyle.

Each of the eight weeks you'll be following the elimination diet, you'll progress one step closer to a happy, healthy, allergen-free lifestyle, with significant milestones along the way. I have included every tip and helpful shortcut I have come across in my own process to make things easier.

As I mentioned earlier, you'll be doing a fair amount of cooking—no doubt more than you might be accustomed to.

One last word of advice: The day before you start, I recommend a "Last Supper" of sorts.

Have your fried eggs, your double-cheese pizza, and whatever else you feel you must get out of your system before saying good-bye to the foods you know are making you unwell. It is really important to get into the right headspace before embarking on this journey, and if scarfing down a bag of doughnut holes or a pan of gooey nachos is what it takes, then so be it. Enjoy yourself, and then get ready to turn your back on instant gratification for the next eight weeks. Because I'm betting that by the end of that time, you probably won't even want to let those foods back into your pristine temple of a body.

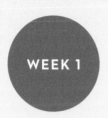

WEEK 1

clean and restock
your kitchen

This first week is the big push, your chance to start fresh. Out with the old, in with the new. The place to start is making over your pantry to reflect your new lifestyle. Keeping a healthy kitchen is an ongoing process that will reflect your health, your progress, and your changing tastes, and there's more involved here than just chucking out a few open packages of cereal and pasta.

If you have chosen a start day of Monday, you will want to get organized on Sunday so you are prepared for the week. Start your morning by getting online and ordering things that might be hard to get locally. Get comfy, gather your list, find your credit card, and bookmark each ordering page as you come to it so it will be easy to reorder. Support niche businesses when you can, but also know that you can find a lot of things on Amazon, including Trader Joe's brand even if you don't have Trader Joe's locally.

If you need new containers (see my tips, page 37) or want to put down new contact paper while you're at it, get them early so you have everything you need for this first week, and you can just make way for the new. You might want to coordinate with a friend who can take some of the good stuff you're getting rid of, or make time for a trip to a local charity with anything that is still sealed or usable.

Set aside a whole afternoon for emptying out and refilling your shelves, refrigerator, and freezer; don't try to do this in a couple of hours. Read the label on every single item that goes back on the shelves, and if you're not sure about an ingredient, err on the side of caution.

SUPPLIES

▸ Jars, bins, and resealable plastic bags

▸ Labels, stickers, and marking pens for noting contents on jars or canisters, and transferring the expiration dates from the original package to the container

▸ Scissors, straightedge, and contact paper (if you're going to re-line shelves), and cleaning supplies

▸ Corkboard, chalkboard, or notebook, for recording what you are eating/tracking your progress or for setting up a "reward chart" for your kids

▸ Bins, baskets, or boxes, for organizing new ingredients

STEP 1: Move everything from your pantry, cupboards, fridge, and freezer to boxes or to a surface—a table or counter (or yard!)—where you can sort the items into three categories:

▸ Discard

▸ Give away

▸ Return to the shelf

STEP 2: Deep clean, then stand back, look, and get together your game plan.

• You need hot, soapy water. Get into that refrigerator and freezer and deep clean! (Not many of us do this regularly enough anyway.) You want a fresh, clean surface to start with. And when you clear off those shelves in the pantry, take the time to really wipe them down. If you're planning to reuse that flour canister, you'll need to decontaminate it with a good, long dishwashing cycle. If you don't clean really, really well, the gluten and wheat and fine clouds of confectioners' sugar dust that tend to coat everything in the pantry will stick around. And it takes just a tiny bit of any of them to inflame your system again once it has calmed down.

- Clean other appliances. Your toaster needs to be cleaned out. Your stand mixer or beaters need to be cleaned off, as well as any other appliances that could have residual baking "goop" stuck to them. Sometimes crumbs find their way into other kitchen drawers—now is the time to clear those out.

Now that everything is clean, ask yourself . . .

- Is your pantry in the best possible spot? If your pantry or food storage cupboards are directly next to an appliance that gives off heat (oven, stove, or refrigerator), consider rearranging. The heat that these appliances give off can totally compromise the integrity of spices, oils, vinegar, and some grains.

- What will you reach for most often?

- Do you intend to do quite a bit of baking, or are you looking to keep just pantry basics? That will help you to figure out how much space and how many new products you need.

- What kind of organization will help keep you inspired and efficient? Do you like nice neat rows and see-through jars, or deep bins that

you can toss things into and riffle through? A pantry calls for orderliness, but order can look a lot of different ways.

STEP 3: Put it all back together.

If you have family members who will continue to eat foods not on the program, you will need to make sure those foods are stored in airtight containers separate from the new foods. If they need to be in the same pantry, put those foods at the bottom of the pantry, so that gravity doesn't inadvertently help sprinkle them into other foods.

Once you have replaced the items that you currently have, you will really be able to see what you need.

STEP 4: Hit the grocery store.

- Based on what you just cleared out, make a grocery list. DO NOT feel like you need to go to the store and max out your credit card buying every last "gluten-free" food product or New Age flour you see. DO buy a few intentional products that will get you through the next few days, and plenty of whole fresh foods.

- Ideally, make a meal plan, even if it is only through the next day or two. Gather the recipes (there are lots of them here) that you want to make and write a shopping list based on the ingredients you need to make those recipes. There should really only be a few new or different swap-out products, like buying coconut milk instead of regular milk. Again, buy only what your meal plan tells you you will need to get you through the next few days; you don't need to be prepared for every contingency right this minute.

- If you are ambitious and want to get baking right away, by all means get supplies for one or two specific recipes, but remember that rebuilding a baking pantry is a process.

- Give yourself enough time to do the shopping. If you rush through, you may forget items or feel panicked, leading to meltdowns and feelings of "This is too much to handle." Really, it's not! It's just different.

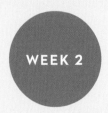

WEEK 2

set up your tracking system

Set up a good system for keep track of what is happening with your body. During this eight-week period, recording what you and/or your children eat will help you connect the dots, stay motivated, and monitor the great progress you're making.

Your first job is to write everything down. Don't go at this like you do when you track calories, selectively omitting a few things here and there to make it look good at the end of the day (um, haven't we all done this?!). With allergies, it's all about making a connection between what you put in your mouth and how it makes you feel. Reactions can be delayed, so you need to be thorough or you'll never put two and two together. Note the date and time of every single thing you eat, and notice everything you can: Skin, tummy, energy levels.

Aches, swelling, stiffness. Acne, headaches, irritability. Drowsiness, energy slumps, energy bursts. Breath (smell your own), poop (color and consistency), skin itchiness. Watch for mood shifts, bloating, gas, quality of sleep, clear or foggy thinking.

Get your children their own little notebooks, even the really young kids. Even before Pia could actually write down the words of the foods she was eating, she could draw pictures that helped jog her memory of what she had eaten during the day. Plus, during this time you should be packing their lunches so you will have a pretty solid idea of what they had during the day anyway. This is definitely an area where you could draft caretakers and teachers to help the children. You could even have them draw faces (happy, sad, sleepy, etc.) to indicate how they felt after eating.

You'll need:

A journal. This may be one notebook you carry everywhere, an endless stash of sticky notes, a giant calendar, an app on your phone, or a combination of these. You want your system to be flexible enough to access readily, because you *won't* remember what you put in your mouth and when by the end of the day. You can analyze or transfer what's on it later, but for starters, just make sure to record *everything*.

Pick a regular time to review. If you get in the habit now, you'll begin to see patterns emerge. Go over your journal notes and look for connections between when you ate things and how you felt later. This is especially fruitful when you slip or after the eight weeks of elimination when you try adding foods back in.

Be aware that everyone reacts differently. You may lose a dramatic amount of weight and have glowing skin within two weeks—or you might break out and go through withdrawals in the first few weeks. It has to do with your diet leading up to this point, your personal levels of allergy or intolerance to foods, and your personal chemistry. Have patience, know that this too shall pass, and record it all.

A rewards chart, if you're doing this with kids. Stickers, check marks, smiley faces, or a points system will help them connect the dots, too. Make separate boxes for specific goals like trying new foods, not complaining, helping in the kitchen, supporting a sibling's food choices, communicating well with a waitperson or other adult about their allergies—anything that helps them navigate the new changes and makes them feel proud of their efforts.

Reward adults, too! Whether you're giving yourself a treat or time off for you (see Celebrate Your Progress, page 54) or extending a token of thanks to a supportive teacher, grocer, waiter, or spouse, acknowledge your own progress and express gratitude to those who help you achieve your goals. It makes the whole process nicer, as well as educational.

Pick a regular time to plan. I like to choose recipes at the beginning of the week so that I can have a game plan for my grocery shopping. This helps me avoid overbuying and being wasteful. If you don't bake, then you hardly need to stock up on twelve bags of assorted flours. But if you do see yourself whipping up muffins and making Friday-night pizza, then you can check recipes and be strategic about what ingredients you need. If you must order certain foods online, you might

want to think ahead (remember shipping) and make sure you are well stocked. And remember, foods that aren't full of preservatives will spoil faster, so you want to buy in smaller amounts and use up the oldest stock first. It takes a while to get in the groove, but soon this weekly planning time will feel short and sweet.

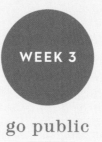

WEEK 3

go public

It's important to start letting others know about your lifestyle changes. Some need to know sooner and some whenever convenient or relevant. Take this third week to make a list of those in your world you should reach out to, and spend some time crafting appropriate messages to each of them.

Notify school authorities. If you haven't already, explain that you are following an eight-week elimination diet to test your child for food allergies and let them know what kind of accommodation you will need during this period. Besides your child's teacher, the main office and school nurse will definitely need to be notified, and I recommend having a personal conversation with them.

Tell your relatives. Those you share meals with frequently may be the hardest to tell. You can mention it oh-by-the-way in a phone call or text, or explain it after you have just fed them an allergen-free feast, or drop them a note in advance if you are being invited over to say you're doing an eight-week experiment during which you'll bring your own foods to make it easy on everyone. Your only aim is to do what is necessary to keep your family on the program, not justify everything to everyone all at once. People can (and will) get emotional about food and all the traditions tied in with it. Try not to engage at this point; wait until you have all the facts.

Draft a brief letter to your family doctors for your medical file. Hang on to this either until you see them next and can give it to them in person, or until the end of the eight weeks, when you can tweak it and then mail with a report of your results. I made a list of each food that I found I was allergic to or sensitive to, and what my reaction was in each scenario. It was shocking to see the results and the correlation to past health issues written down in black and white.

Check in with your favorite restaurants. Find out what their allergen policies are and what they need from you to make things go smoothly when you eat there.

Now brace yourself. You will get some eye rolls, some skeptical comments, and some judgment from people who may be downright pissed off at you for making these changes. Some will be acquaintances and some will be people close to you.

But guess what? It says more about them than it does about you. I don't say that because I am insensitive—I am actually the opposite. I'm so sensitive and was so gripped with fear at others' reactions that it took me almost five months to tell anyone outside of my very closest family and friends that our family had modified our diets—even though the changes were literally life altering.

But when I did, I tried really hard to focus on the outpouring of support and ignore whatever and whoever didn't support me and my family living our healthiest life. Negative reactions are usually just fear speaking—fear of losing the fun times they associate with you or of considering similar changes for their own health.

Then again, the first time you make them spaghetti and meatballs and finish it off with a glistening chocolate cake, they will let go of the notion that you've consigned yourself to a diet of gluten-free rabbit food. Just stay positive and, as I would tell my five-year-old (and occasionally remind myself), "Use your patience." The Negative Nellies are out there, but trust me: there are far greater numbers of people who are curious or excited about your trial and, eventually, the results. People love to hear success stories.

WEEK 4

stock your freezer

The real joy of the freezer (other than looking at the lined-up-Tupperware as proof of how very organized you are!) is efficiency and limiting waste. When you are juggling life, career, and family, cooking a meal from the ground up every single night is just not always a possibility. Having a well-stocked freezer offers you a shortcut. I can't recommend this enough. If you have not already implemented this technique, try one of these options this weekend:

- Make double batches of meatballs and tomato sauce and freeze them, then the next time you want it, you just have to reheat the sauce and boil the pasta.

- Freeze curries or any slow-braised meats that could stand up to being reheated. Transfer them from freezer to fridge the night before or morning of, and by dinnertime, in the time it takes to steam rice you will have hot and ready-to-serve dishes that would otherwise have taken hours to prepare.

- Make double or triple batches of pizza dough and freeze them. Pull them out the morning of to thaw by late afternoon. Let the dough come to room temperature before using. The Pizza Crust (page 190) can also be parbaked and frozen. You can just throw the frozen crust in the oven for 15 minutes to heat up, which makes it as easy as ordering delivery pizza any night.

- Make several batches of waffles at once. Cook them slightly underdone and freeze the waffles in resealable plastic bags. Pop them in the toaster in the morning.

- Freezing cookies to toss in your kids' lunches should be standard practice, whether they are "healthy cookies" or dessert.

- Make double batches of the pork potstickers (page 129), which freeze well and are super convenient. They can also be tossed into boiling soup or broth as dumplings.

- If you are just feeding one or two of you, then freezing leftover portions of soups makes dinner on a worknight really easy. They are also great for taking to work to microwave.

The freezer also lets you extend the life of any of your baked goods, and instead of dumping that last 2 cups of soup you know you won't get to for the next few days, you can pour it into a container and freeze it. And then the next time you are hanging on the refrigerator door thinking how

ABOUT FREEZING

- Be sure to cool all your food completely before placing it in the freezer. The more quickly the food freezes, the better the integrity of the food remains. Slow freezing can change the texture of the food.

- Remove as much air as possible from resealable bags when freezing

the contents, and leave space for expansion at the top of plastic or glass containers.

- Most foods can last two to three months in the freezer. Make sure you label and date all your foods, and please throw out the mystery meat from last year.

AVERAGE FREEZING TIMES:

Soup: 2 to 3 months

Pizza dough: 1 to 2 months

Baked goods: 2 to 3 months

Cooked poultry: 4 months

Raw poultry: 9 months

Cooked meat: 3 months

Raw meat or pork: 4 months

Bacon: 1 month

Cooked fish: 4 to 6 months

Raw fish: 2 to 3 months

you don't want to make lunch, you can just pull it out and heat it up. That also applies to fresh fruit that is going soft but could easily be chopped and put in the freezer for smoothies.

There is an art, though, to maintaining a freezer. Get easy-to-use and easy-to-replace (that is, recyclable) containers, and take the time to label and date everything. Some things last longer in the freezer than others, so you might want to write a "use-by" date rather than the date you froze it—it requires less thinking when you're in grab-it-quick mode.

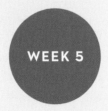

WEEK 5

invite others
into your world

Have a dinner party! Or host a brunch, or even just invite your best friends over for a super-casual BBQ—whatever you are comfortable with. Invite friends or family to your home and cook them a delicious meal, one that is in line with your new eating plan. For a long time post–allergy test, I worried that not only would no one ever have us over to dinner again, but, even worse, no one would want to come to our home for fear of going hungry or having to eat something that tasted terrible. That concern was part of what drove me to develop the recipes on my blog and in this book. I never get tired of my guests' reactions when, at the end of an indulgent and filling meal, I announce that the entire meal—from the appetizers and cocktails to the

five-course dinner, plus the dessert—was free of gluten, dairy, egg, soy, nuts, peanuts, shellfish, and cane sugar. Their shock and confusion is priceless. I always get calls or e-mails the next day from guests saying how amazing the food was—and that they didn't feel bloated or overly full afterward, even though they had overindulged. Pretty awesome.

And yes, we actually do still get invited places. I have friends who have graciously and joyfully risen to the challenge of cooking within these guidelines, sometimes even for a crowd, and found that *everyone* loved it! So you may find that you inspire others to think (and cook) outside of the box.

If a full-scale dinner party isn't your style, just keep it simple. Invite your family or friends to brunch. Make a pitcher of smoothies, muffins, or a coffee cake, and maybe some homemade granola to serve with fresh fruit and cold coconut milk. (If you want to offer Bloody Marys or mimosas, too, that's just fine!) If you're not a morning person, host a casual dinner for friends, serving roasted green salsa and chips (page 131) to start, followed by Steak Lettuce Tacos with Mango Cilantro Ginger Sauce (page 132) and Fresh Corn and Mango Salad (page 119), and maybe Chocolate Fudge Brownies (page 285) for dessert. Who wouldn't want to be invited for a meal like that?

Don't warn your guests that dinner is going to be "a little different" or make apologies for what you're not serving. (After all, if you served chicken for dinner, you wouldn't say you were sorry for not serving beef, right?) Trust me, they will probably be surprised to learn what they *haven't* just eaten and likely won't have noticed anything except how sensational the meal was until you told them.

At the end of the day, most people will take their cues from you. If you sit around telling them about how much it sucks that you can no longer eat certain foods, they are likely to perceive your new diet as one of deprivation and sacrifice. If, on the other hand, you come across as relaxed and at peace with how you are eating and living, your friends and family will quickly get on board. Positivity attracts positivity, and that is an important tool to arm yourself with as you move into a whole new phase of your life.

WEEK 6

hone and tweak

This Sunday is a time to catch your breath and reflect on the progress you've made—and how far you still need to evolve. At this point you should be feeling pretty good. Most of your old diet should have worked its way out of your system by now, and you should be seeing some of the results of your hard (and hopefully delicious!) work. Start by taking stock. Do you need to take in your clothes? If so, it might be time for a little retail therapy, or alterations to your favorite pieces. Or just try things on to see how they fit now—you might be pleasantly surprised. Write down what's going well and what's not, and have any conversations you need to have to make adjustments.

If you've had any slip-ups, acknowledge them and get back on the wagon.

Praise or love up your kids (or your supportive spouse) for their part. Have a family meeting to find out what they think about this experiment so far.

Take another look at your pantry, fridge, and freezer to see how it's working for you, or spend a little time figuring out which recipes you would still like to try, or restock your fridge or freezer with new favorites.

Perfecting this lifestyle is a process, and it takes a long time; don't expect to get everything down overnight. And have faith that it actually gets easier. Much easier. It just becomes a way of life. I don't even flinch anymore when I see a grilled cheese sandwich. The old temptation of, say, a doughnut or a cookie is so much less since I know I can just make an alternative that is equally delicious. And the truth is, the first time you go off the rails (because trust me, you will) and eat something that your *body* no longer wants any part of, you will know that *you* don't want any part of it either. I would equate it to that first time I (maybe you, too?) drank too much tequila and realized that I would deal with the repercussions for days afterward. I am a slow learner when it come to these things, but even I eventually realized that paying the price for an exception is usually just not worth it.

The longer I am at it, the better I am at avoiding pitfalls and temptations. The more carefully I read labels and understand the information they convey, the better prepared I am for living my life without road bumps. Because after six weeks or eight weeks or a year or two into this if you choose, you will have created new habits and new "normals" that vastly supersede a cheeseburger.

WEEK 7

celebrate your progress!

It's important to acknowledge the positive changes you're making—especially in the beginning when they can feel hard won. Take the focus off the food by getting a massage, buying some new songs on iTunes, or even just giving yourself permission to take a nap or go for a walk, whatever feels like an indulgence to you. New jeans in a smaller size are certainly something to celebrate. Maybe wear them on a hot date with your spouse or go out with friends for one of those gluten-free martinis! Go have fun in that new healthy body of yours.

Whatever floats your boat. Just make sure to give yourself a pat on the back for all of your hard work and dedication to achieving better health.

Of course you just might find that the greatest reward of all, the greatest celebration of your hard work, is how much better you feel. That you are living in a body that isn't as tired, or

I NEED A DRINK . . . WHAT CAN I HAVE?

There seems to be a tremendous amount of confusion over which alcoholic drinks are gluten-free. Marketing trends have only served to confuse people further, so here is the real skinny on what you can drink and what you should avoid.

BEER. Avoid beer completely unless you are drinking certified gluten-free beer (check the label!). There are many wonderful artisanal breweries making these beverages—just read your labels and do your research. There are a lot of "low-gluten" beers available that are marketed in a confusing or misleading way. You could also try hard cider, which is made from apples and is almost always gluten-free.

WINE. Wine is totally gluten-free. Well, almost. Very rarely in U.S.-made wines, they will seal the aging barrels with a wheat paste, which would give the wine a very minimal amount of gluten—probably not detectable by people with sensitivities, but definitely by those with celiac. If you are worried, or enjoy a few specific labels regularly, just call the manufacturer and ask.

HARD LIQUOR. While there are some differing opinions on whether or not all hard liquor is gluten-free, even grain-based liquors like whiskey, bourbon, and some vodkas, the distilling process should purify the liquor of all gluten. Some would argue that you can't always trust the distiller, so I would recommend going for large, well-known brands that are definitely complying with reputable distilling practices. If you swear you can tell the difference (I can't), then choose hard liquors that you know are safe, such as rum, tequila, and potato- and grape-based vodkas.

achy, or rashy. Maybe you just enjoy getting up each morning because you slept well, or are feeling trim and comfortable instead of bloated and gassy. Or you are noticing you haven't had a headache in a few weeks. Those are the true celebrations—although I also like shopping for smaller jeans.

WEEK 8

you did it! now what?

This is the last week of your eight-week program, and you should be feeling pretty dang good by now. You have cleared your body of most possible allergens and calmed inflammation, and you will probably have noticed some significant differences. Refer to your tracker and check out your specific progress. Symptoms may have diminished or disappeared entirely, and you may see differences in your joints, stomach and digestive comfort, weight, skin, sleep quality, and energy level—even your mental and emotional well-being. A visit to the doctor may show that your cholesterol numbers have improved or your blood pressure is lower.

If you did not already know exactly what your allergies or sensitivities were, now is the time to figure it out. My guess is that you have accidentally slipped up at least a tiny bit during this process and may have already discovered foods that you think are the main culprits. But no matter what, the sure way to find out how they affect your body is to eat them! That is where the reintroduction part comes into play (see page 23).

This program will give you a very good baseline for an allergen-free diet, with room for you to tweak to accommodate your own personal issues and needs. Don't forget that everyone will have a different reaction, perhaps even within your own family. For instance, Pia is far more restricted than the rest of us, so while we are respectful of her diet, we still eat nuts and peanuts and soy and occasionally cane sugar. The kids and Pete still eat clams and scallops, while I have to abstain, and they can enjoy occasional goat or sheep's-milk cheese, while I most definitely cannot. It is just part of the process of figuring out your body's chemistry.

I also have to point out that even if you are a lucky family that has little or no sensitivities to any foods but just strive to be healthier and eat cleaner, you can eat this way all the time just because it is delicious and nutritious.

So please, get into your kitchen, start cooking, and try to enjoy the process of transforming your body!

the recipes

This collection of recipes comes with absolute love and the best of intentions from my kitchen to yours. Each recipe is meant to find a place at your table and in your life in order to make things easier, healthier, and more delicious for you and your family.

My professional background includes both restaurant cooking and catering, and cooking is a true passion for me. It is not good enough simply to create a dish that is acceptable and free of irritants and allergens; it has to be great on its own merits, so that anyone who tastes it simply says, "That is delicious." No caveats, no qualifications, no making allowances for the difficulty of cooking without this or that. Just straight-up good-tasting food that is packed with naturally wholesome ingredients and nutrients. No big deal, right?

When developing these recipes, I took great pains to make sure there is a sense of balance in the flavors, pairing sweet and savory and rich, unctuous mouthfuls with just the right amount of acidic zing. And of course there is the very important visual component. Eating with your eyes is the first step to enjoying a meal, and I try not to neglect that part. By adding different colors and textures, you create such a beautiful palette, and also an exciting experience of each mouthful having a distinctive crunch or silkiness.

When working with a more restricted arsenal of ingredients, you should be bold with flavors, experimental with new ingredients, and above all open-minded. Fresh ingredients and seasonal or high-quality produce really get to be the stars when there is no rich butter sauce to drown out their flavors or steal their thunder. Fresh herbs and spices and the use of bold ethnic ingredients like harissa and curry add excitement to dishes when you are omitting other elements.

I also love that in preparing your meals at home, from scratch, you really know exactly what you are putting into your body. Reading labels is so important, but for the most part, when you are enjoying fresh foods and simple preparations, you don't *need* to read labels because you are not cooking from packages—you are using real, whole foods.

I hope you will find a set of favorite recipes that work really well for your lifestyle and others that push you to experiment and try new things! It was my goal to create recipes that will delight everyone, whether you are cooking just for yourself or for a whole group who may or may not all have food allergies. Happy cooking!

quick-reference icons

 • VEGAN

• UNDER 30 MINUTES

• KID FRIENDLY

• PALEO FRIENDLY

 • NO ADDED SUGAR

 • MAKE AHEAD

• GREAT FOR FREEZER

• HIGH FIBER

• GREAT FOR ENTERTAINING

 • GREAT FOR POTLUCKS

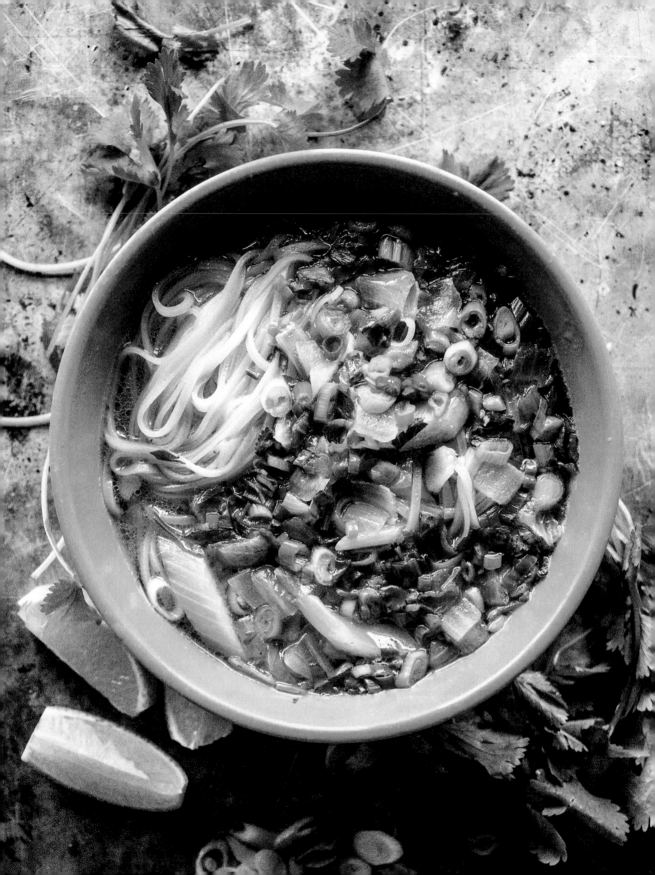

soups and chilis

There is nothing more homey than a pot of soup or chili simmering away on the stove. These recipes are my soul food and they run the gamut from fresh and light to hearty and comforting.

I love that these recipes are all pretty easy to throw together and can feed you for a few days. I tend to make double batches of the varieties that my kids like so I can really milk that pot for several meals. I also enjoy the leftovers for my own lunches or to send to school in a thermos with the girls. When my husband is out of town, I can eat from a big pot of soup for close to a week—happily, I might add! The best part about the soups is how little effort they require for such a big payoff. Oh, and it's also awesome that these tend to be low in calories and high in protein or fiber (and sometimes both). They are also filling and a great way to get vegetables into veggie-resistant family members like my husband. (Like somehow because it's cooked into a delicious soup they don't realize it's a vegetable?) And then there are the chilis and stews, which are one-pot meals. I don't feel bad if I don't make anything else when I serve these because the protein and veggies are all in there. Done and done.

◄ Asian Vegetable Noodle Soup (page 80)

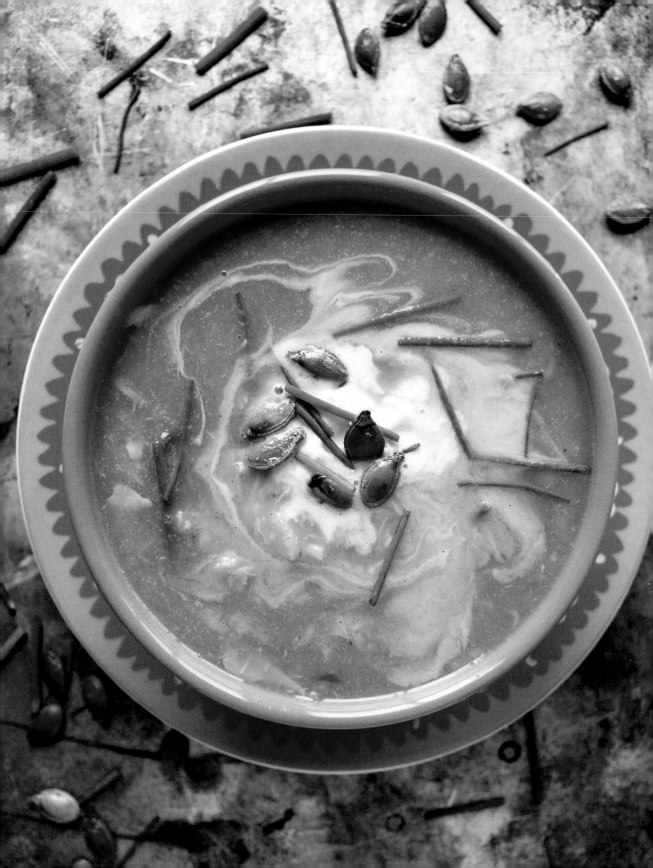

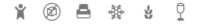

CURRIED PUMPKIN, CHICKEN, AND RICE SOUP

PREPARATION 15 MINUTES   **COOK TIME** 1 HOUR 10 MINUTES   **SERVINGS** 8

If you can get a fresh pumpkin, this is just about the best soup ever. It has all the makings of cold-weather comfort food, with pumpkin, rice, and chicken set off by the wonderful flavors of curry.

1 (3½- to 4-pound) sugar pumpkin

6 tablespoons olive oil

Kosher salt

1 yellow onion, coarsely chopped

½ cup dry sherry

4 cups chicken broth

3 tablespoons curry powder

2 cups cooked long-grain white rice (I use jasmine rice)

2 cups shredded cooked chicken

Unsweetened coconut cream and chopped fresh chives, for garnish (optional)

1 Preheat the oven to 400°F.

2 Cut the pumpkin in half through the stem and remove the seeds, setting them aside. Scrape out and discard the stringy fibers.

3 Rub the inside of the pumpkin halves with 2 tablespoons of the olive oil and sprinkle with kosher salt. Place them cut-side down on a rimmed baking sheet. Roast for 45 minutes, or until the pumpkin is tender and golden. When the pumpkin is just cool enough to handle scoop the flesh into a bowl using a large spoon. Discard the skin and set the pumpkin flesh aside.

4 While the pumpkin roasts, rinse, drain, and dry the pumpkin seeds. Place them on a rimmed baking sheet. Toss with 2 tablespoons of the olive oil and sprinkle with salt. Roast on another rack in the oven for 20 minutes, until golden brown.

5 In a heavy pot, heat the remaining 2 tablespoons olive oil over medium heat. Add the onion and cook, stirring occasionally, until the onion is soft and translucent, 5 to 7 minutes. Add the sherry and scrape up any browned bits from the bottom of the pot.

6 Add the pumpkin flesh, chicken broth, curry powder, and 2 cups water. Stir well to combine and bring to a boil over medium-high heat. Cover the pot, reduce the heat to low, and simmer for 20 minutes.

7 Working in batches, transfer the soup to a blender and carefully purée until smooth. Return the soup to the pot and reheat over medium heat.

8 Stir in the rice and shredded chicken, season with salt, and serve hot, garnished with a little coconut cream and fresh chives, if desired.

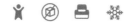

GREEK LEMON, CHICKEN, AND RICE SOUP

PREPARATION 15 MINUTES   **COOK TIME** 45 MINUTES   **SERVINGS** 4 TO 6

Avgolemono, a lemony Greek chicken soup, is one of my husband's childhood favorites. Sadly, in its original iteration, it is full of eggs. The same flavors are echoed in this play on a classic chicken and rice soup, beautifully perfumed with lemon zest and juice. It's a great way to make a roast chicken dinner stretch into a couple of nights' worth of meals.

¼ cup olive oil

1 yellow onion, finely diced

4 celery stalks, thinly sliced

3 large carrots, thinly sliced

2 large bone-in, skin-on chicken breasts

8 cups chicken broth

1 cup long-grain white rice

Zest of 2 lemons

¼ cup fresh lemon juice (from about 2 lemons)

1 cup fresh flat-leaf parsley, minced

Kosher salt

1 In a large heavy pot, heat the olive oil over medium heat. Add the onion and sauté until soft and tender, 5 to 7 minutes. Add the celery and the carrots and cook for 2 to 3 minutes more.

2 Add the chicken breasts and broth. Cover, reduce the heat to low, and simmer for 30 minutes.

3 Transfer the chicken breasts to a plate and let sit until cool enough to handle. Shred the chicken meat, discarding the bones and skin, and add the meat to the pot along with the rice. Cover and cook over very low heat for 15 minutes, until the rice is tender.

4 Stir in the lemon zest, lemon juice, and parsley and stir well. Season with salt and serve hot.

NOTE: If the soup gets too thick (the rice absorbs the liquid), add some water and add more salt as needed.

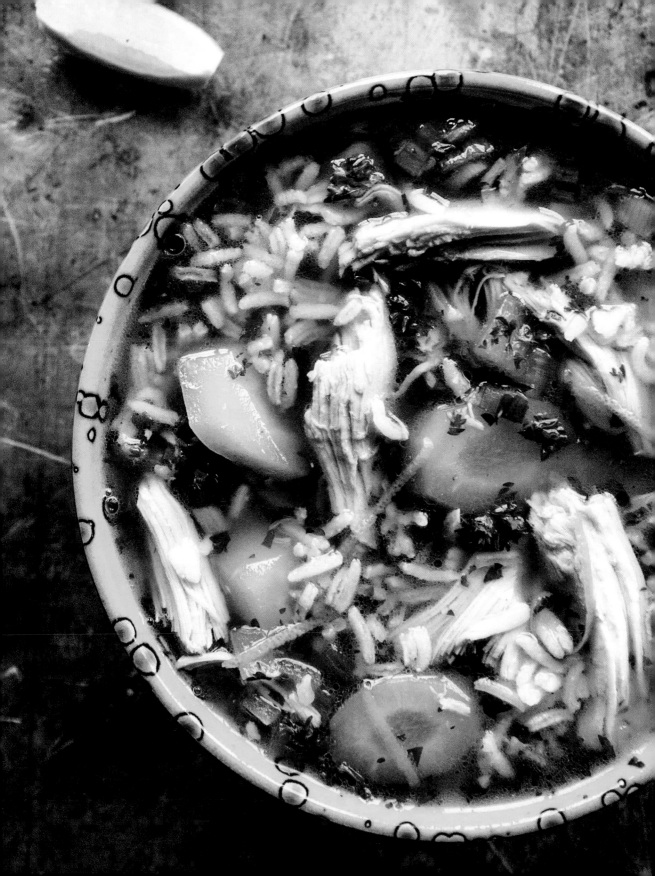

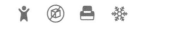

MULLIGATAWNY SOUP

PREPARATION 15 MINUTES **COOK TIME** 45 MINUTES **SERVINGS** 4 TO 6

Remember *Seinfeld* (all these years later, I am still addicted to the reruns) and the Soup Nazi's mulligatawny soup? That's where I first heard about it, but I first *had* mulligatawny when one of my closest friends, Missy, brought me a big vat that she and her mom, Merriann, made for me after I had Coco. I had a toddler and a new baby and it was the dead of winter and I was curled into a sweatpants ball. When they showed up with this fantastic-smelling soup, I clung to it like a life raft. I still remember the way it tasted—absolutely amazing and unlike anything I had ever had before. Merriann gave me her recipe for the soup. Over the years it has morphed into my own allergen-free version, but it still remains one of my favorite soups ever. Thanks, ladies.

2 tablespoons olive oil

½ cup coconut oil

1 tablespoon tomato paste

2 tablespoons all-purpose gluten-free flour

1 yellow onion, cut into small dice

2 carrots, thinly sliced

4 celery stalks, thinly sliced

1 large pear, cut into small dice

2 cups chopped cooked turkey

¼ cup curry powder

2 teaspoons fresh thyme leaves

1½ cups long-grain white rice

8 cups chicken or turkey broth

1 cup unsweetened coconut cream, plus more for serving

Kosher salt

Fresh parsley and pomegranate seeds, for garnish (optional)

1 In a large heavy pot, heat the olive oil and coconut oil over medium heat. Add the tomato paste and flour and stir until smooth. Cook for 2 minutes.

2 Stir the onion into the mixture, then add the carrots and celery and cook for 3 to 4 minutes. Add the pear and cook for 2 to 3 minutes more.

3 Add the turkey, curry powder, and thyme and cook, stirring, for about 2 minutes. Add the rice and broth and stir well. Bring to a light boil, then cover the pot. Reduce the heat to low and simmer for 30 minutes.

4 Stir in the coconut cream. Season with salt and serve hot, with an extra dollop of coconut cream, some fresh parsley, and a sprinkle of pomegranate seeds, if desired.

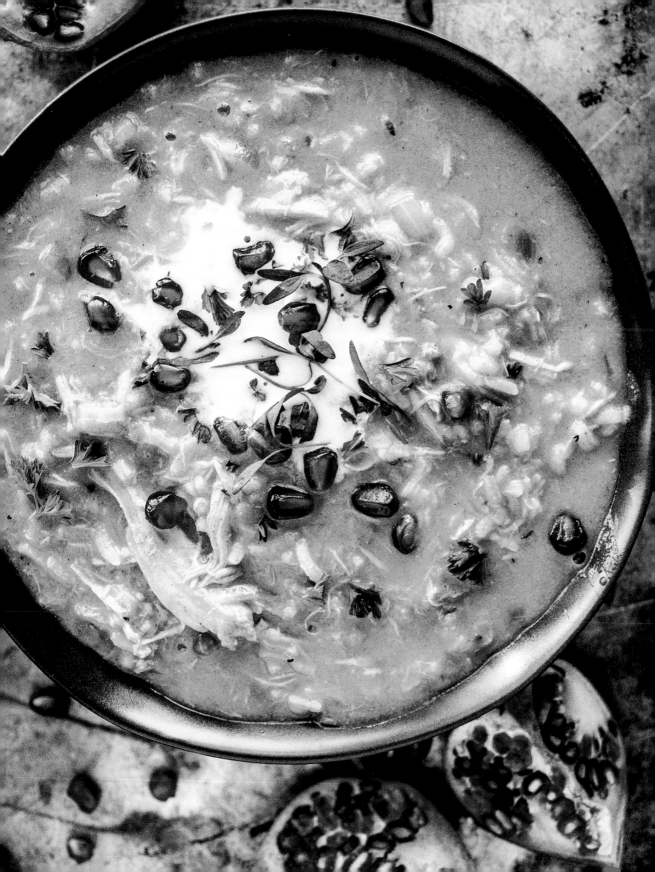

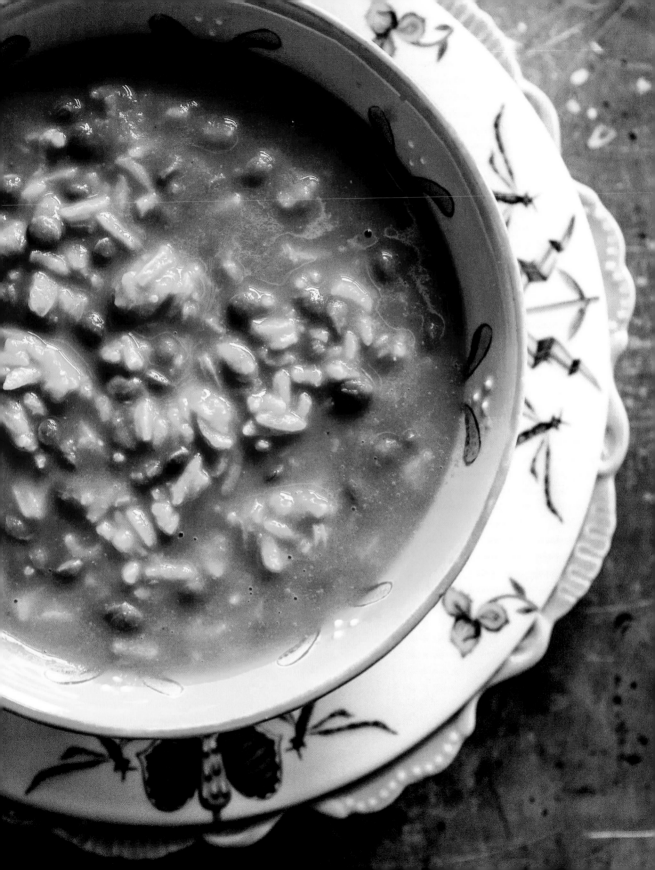

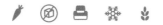

SPICY TOMATO, LENTIL, AND RICE SOUP

PREPARATION 10 MINUTES   **COOK TIME** 40 MINUTES   **SERVINGS** 6

This soup has an unexpected blend of ingredients that creates a surprisingly sweet broth with a nice spicy kick at the end. The addition of lentils and rice makes it really hearty and filling. I have given instructions for cooking dry lentils, but many grocery stores sell plain cooked lentils (check the refrigerated section of the produce aisle), and they are very convenient. As for the rice, we often have leftover rice in our refrigerator and just about any type will do.

3 tablespoons olive oil

1 large yellow onion, coarsely chopped

1 pound cherry tomatoes

4 cups vegetable broth

1 tablespoon soy-free vegan butter

1 garlic clove, minced

½ yellow onion, finely diced

½ teaspoon crushed red pepper flakes

½ cup unsweetened coconut cream

Kosher salt

2 cups cooked lentils (see Note)

1 cup cooked long-grain white rice

1 In a large heavy pot, heat the olive oil over medium heat. Add the onion and cook, stirring occasionally, for 5 minutes, then stir in the tomatoes. Cook until the tomatoes have softened, 2 to 3 minutes more. Add the vegetable broth, cover the pot, and simmer for 15 minutes.

2 Transfer the soup to a blender (you may need to do this in batches) and purée on high until smooth. Set aside in the blender jar.

3 In that same pot, melt the vegan butter over medium heat. Add the garlic, onion, and red pepper flakes and sauté until soft and tender, 5 to 7 minutes.

4 Pour the soup back into the pot with the garlic, onion, and pepper. Stir in the coconut cream and season with salt.

5 Add the cooked lentils and cooked rice and stir to combine. Reheat the soup over low heat and add a bit more salt if needed. Serve hot.

NOTE: To cook dry lentils, rinse and drain 1 cup dry lentils. In a saucepan, combine the lentils and 3 cups water. Bring to a boil over medium-high heat, then reduce the heat to low and simmer for 15 minutes, until the water has cooked off and the lentils are tender.

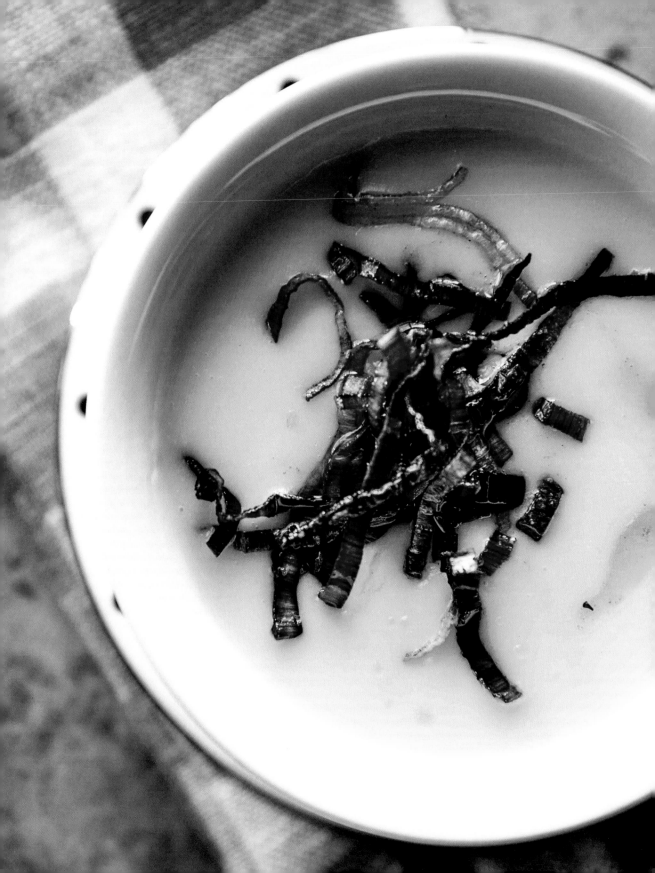

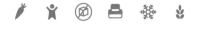

POTATO LEEK SOUP

PREPARATION 15 MINUTES **COOK TIME** 50 MINUTES **SERVINGS** 4 TO 6

This soup reminds me of my sister, since she is how I came to know about potato leek soup. When I was a junior in college, I lived in her basement (glamorous). At the time, I was obsessed with my little tiny nephew and niece, and my sister and cool brother-in-law were so easygoing that it actually turned out to be a really good thing. My sister is a great cook, and I remember how she made soups, including potato leek, for lunch all the time. I always appreciated that cream wasn't necessary to make it creamy; the potato takes care of that all on its own. I do occasionally enjoy the fried leek topping for something a little crispy and special, but I promise this simple, humble soup is just as good unadorned.

SOUP

¼ cup olive oil

2 large leeks, white and tender green parts only, thinly sliced (4 cups)

Kosher salt

½ cup dry white wine

6 cups large-diced peeled Yukon Gold potatoes (about 6 to 8 medium potatoes)

6 cups vegetable or chicken broth

FRIED LEEKS (OPTIONAL)

⅓ cup olive oil

½ cup thinly sliced leeks

Kosher salt

1 In a large heavy pot, heat the olive oil over medium heat. Add the leeks and a sprinkle of salt. Cover, reduce the heat to low, and slowly sweat the leeks, stirring often, until they are very soft and tender, 15 minutes. You don't want the leeks to brown, so if you need to add a little water and stir often, do so.

2 Uncover and raise the heat to medium. Add the white wine and stir well, cooking for 2 to 3 minutes. Add the potatoes and the broth and bring to a simmer. Cover and reduce the heat to low, simmering for 30 minutes.

3 Use an immersion blender to purée the soup directly in the pot until smooth. Season with salt.

4 To make the fried leeks, if desired: In a small pan, heat the olive oil over medium-high heat until a drop of water flicked into the pan splatters. Add a small handful of the leeks and fry just until brown and crisp, about 1 minute. Transfer them immediately to a paper towel and sprinkle them with salt. Repeat until you have fried all the leeks. Reserve the olive oil.

5 If necessary, reheat the soup over low heat. Ladle it into warm bowls and serve topped with some of the fried leeks and a drizzle of the hot leek olive oil.

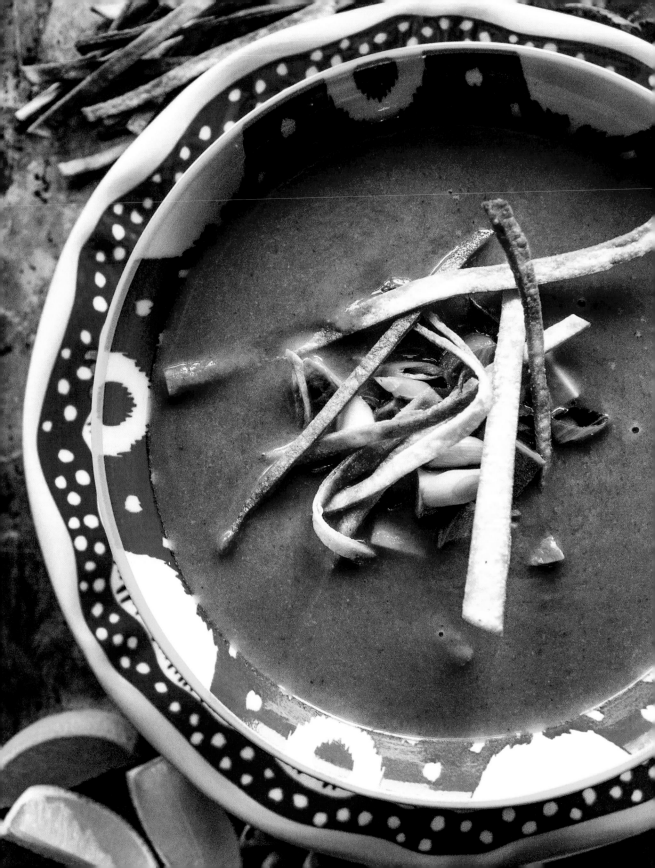

TORTILLA SOUP

PREPARATION 15 MINUTES   **COOK TIME** 1 HOUR 15 MINUTES   **SERVINGS** 6 TO 8

Cabo San Lucas, Mexico, was my family's annual vacation spot growing up, and I still try to get back when I can. I've watched it grow from a tiny fishing village into a huge tourist destination. I remember when Cabo got its first stoplight and, later, its first fast-food restaurants. Fortunately, Pancho's, one of our favorite family restaurants, still exists. And if Pancho's instilled a love of one dish in me from a young age, it would have to be tortilla soup. Oh em gee, how I love tortilla soup. The spicy red broth has so many layers of flavor, it is hard to imagine that it cooks up so quickly. When you add fried tortilla strips, cilantro, green onions, and big, luscious chunks of ripe avocado, it is just off-the-charts great. You could also add shredded cooked chicken.

¼ cup vegetable oil

2 corn tortillas, sliced into skinny strips

1 yellow onion, diced

4 garlic cloves, coarsely chopped

1 jalapeño, coarsely chopped

2 tablespoons Mexican chili powder

1 tablespoon ground cumin

1 (28-ounce) can crushed tomatoes

6 cups chicken broth

1 bay leaf

Kosher salt

1 avocado, pitted, peeled, and chopped

½ cup chopped fresh cilantro

2 green onions, thinly sliced

Lime wedges, for serving

1 In a large pot, heat the oil over medium-high heat. When a drop of water sizzles in the hot oil, add the tortilla strips and fry until golden. Using a slotted spoon, transfer the tortilla strips to paper towel to drain, leaving the oil in the pot.

2 Add the yellow onion to the pot and fry over medium-high heat for 3 to 4 minutes. Add the garlic and jalapeño and cook, stirring often, for 5 minutes more.

3 Add the chili powder and the cumin and cook, stirring, for 2 minutes more. Add the tomatoes and their liquid, the broth, and the bay leaf. Cover, reduce the heat to low, and simmer for 1 hour.

4 Remove from the heat and discard the bay leaf. Working in batches, transfer the soup to a blender and carefully (it's hot!!) purée the soup on high until smooth. Return the puréed soup to the pot and reheat over medium heat. Season with salt.

5 Serve hot, with the avocado, cilantro, onions, lime, and fried tortilla strips sprinkled on top.

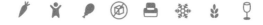

SWEET CORN AND YELLOW TOMATO SOUP

PREPARATION 15 MINUTES   **COOK TIME** 40 MINUTES   **SERVINGS** 4 TO 6

The sweetness of this soup always surprises me. It's easy to forget how naturally sweet corn is, and of all the varieties of tomatoes, I like the yellow ones best. When they are paired with yellow onion and rich coconut cream, the result is a velvety yellow soup with a wonderful, subtle balance of sweet and savory. I like it with a dollop of the brazenly flavored cilantro sauce, which gives it a nice zing and a brilliant color contrast.

SOUP

3 tablespoons olive oil, plus more for garnish

1 large yellow onion, coarsely chopped

Kosher salt

2 pounds sweet corn kernels (frozen is fine!)

4 cups chopped tomatoes, preferably yellow

4 cups vegetable broth

½ cup unsweetened coconut cream

CILANTRO SAUCE

1 cup cilantro

1½ cups tomatillos

2 garlic cloves

Juice of 1 lime

Kosher salt

1 In a large pot, heat the olive oil over medium heat. Add the onion, sprinkle with a little salt, and sweat the onion gently for 5 to 7 minutes, until the onion is soft and translucent. Do not let the onion brown!

2 Add the corn (set a few tablespoons aside for garnish, if desired) and tomatoes and stir. Add the broth and bring to a simmer, then reduce the heat to low and cover the pot. Simmer for 25 to 30 minutes.

3 Working in batches, transfer the soup to a blender and purée on high until the soup is fairly smooth. Return the puréed soup to the pot and reheat over medium heat. Stir in the coconut cream and season with salt.

4 To make the cilantro sauce: In a blender, combine the cilantro, tomatillos, garlic, and lime juice. Purée on high until you have a somewhat smooth, thick sauce. Season to taste with kosher salt.

5 Serve hot, topped with a drizzle of cilantro sauce, the reserved corn kernels (if using), and a drizzle of olive oil.

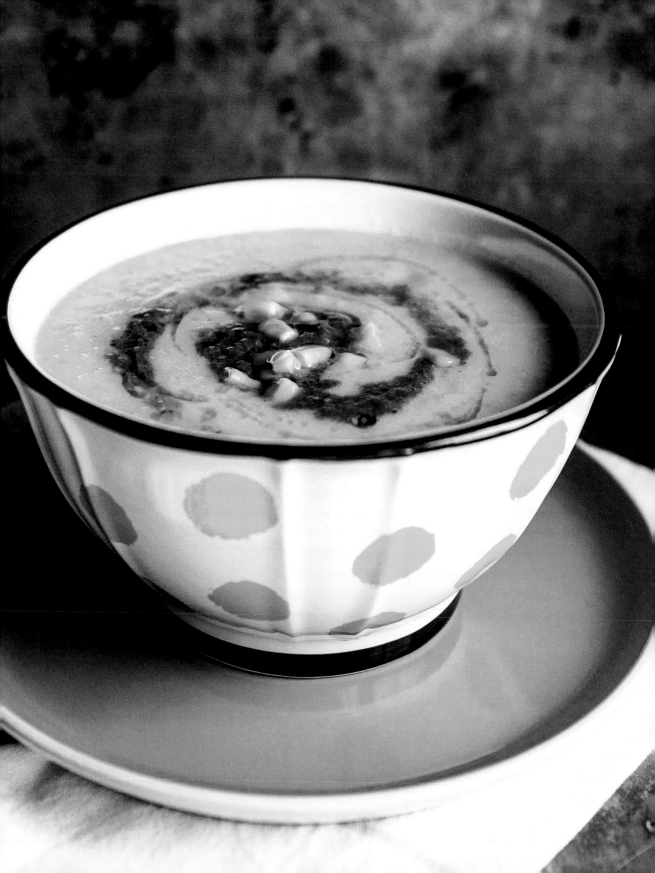

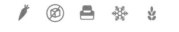

SPRING MINESTRONE

PREPARATION 15 MINUTES **COOK TIME** 30 MINUTES **SERVINGS** 4 TO 6

You'll often find minestrone simmering on my stovetop in the colder months. Come spring though, I am always looking for way to lighten things up and take advantage of the just-emerging fresh produce that makes it feel like warmer weather is just around the corner. My solution takes the form of a clear broth instead of a tomato-based one, plus quinoa in place of pasta and generous amounts of fresh green vegetables. The best part, though, is what happens when you add a nice big dollop of electric-green arugula pesto. Both the color and flavor add quite a lot to this lovely bowl of soup.

ARUGULA PESTO

2 garlic cloves

4 cups lightly packed fresh arugula

¼ cup olive oil

2 tablespoons fresh lemon juice

Kosher salt

SOUP

¼ cup olive oil

1 yellow onion, diced

4 celery stalks, finely diced

2 carrots (I use yellow carrots), finely diced

½ cup white wine

1 cup shelled green peas (about 1 pound in the pod) or frozen peas

½ cup white quinoa, rinsed and drained

2 (15-ounce) cans cannellini beans, drained and rinsed

4 cups vegetable broth

Kosher salt

1 cup packed fresh baby spinach leaves

1 To make the arugula pesto: In a blender, combine the garlic, arugula, olive oil, and lemon juice. Purée until smooth and then season with salt. Set aside.

2 To make the soup: In a large heavy pot, heat the olive oil over medium heat. Add the onion, celery, and carrots and sweat until tender, 5 to 7 minutes.

3 Add the wine, stir well, and cook for 2 minutes. Add the peas, quinoa, white beans, and broth. Cover and simmer over low heat until the quinoa is cooked, 20 minutes. Season with salt. Right before serving, stir the spinach into the hot soup and ladle into serving bowls. Add a dollop of the pesto to each bowl and serve.

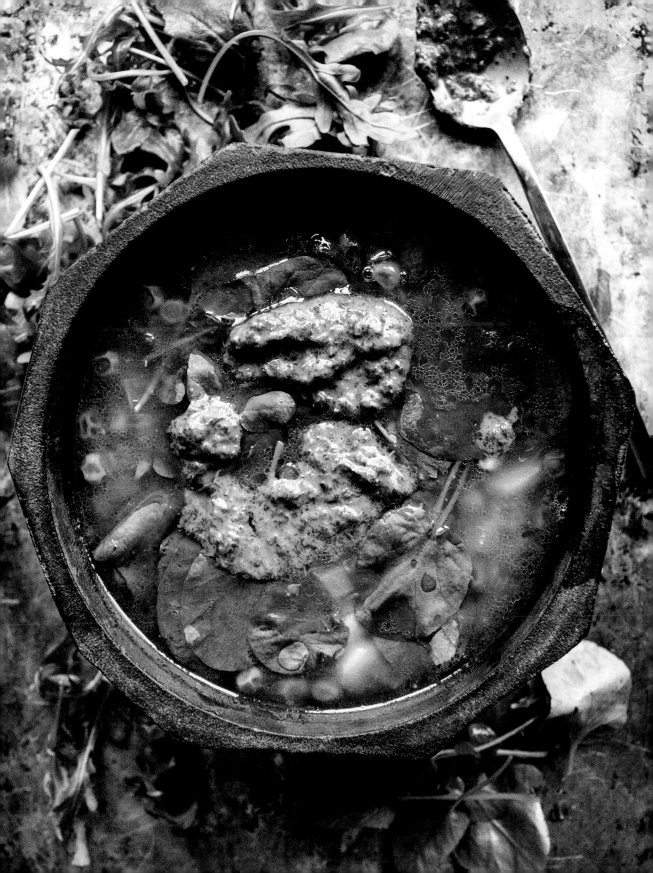

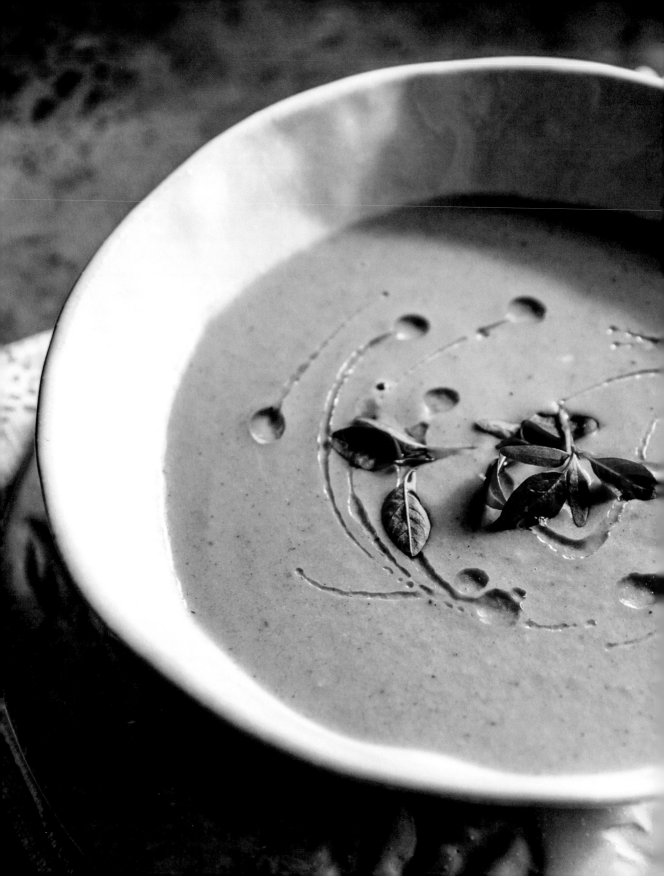

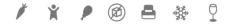

CREAMY MUSHROOM BISQUE

PREPARATION 15 MINUTES   **COOK TIME** 40 MINUTES   **SERVINGS** 4 TO 6

A traditional French bisque is made with serious amounts of heavy cream, but in this version, finely puréed and well-seasoned onions and mushrooms are finished off with a generous amount of coconut cream for practically the same silky, decadent experience. It's indulgent and perfect for a cold autumn or winter day. Add a drizzle of olive oil, or truffle oil if you have it, for a little extra depth of flavor.

¼ cup olive oil

1 yellow onion, coarsely chopped

Kosher salt

1½ pounds cremini mushrooms

½ cup dry sherry

4 cups mushroom or chicken broth

1 cup unsweetened coconut cream

Pinch of ground nutmeg

Microgreens or a bit of snipped fresh chives or parsley, for garnish

Truffle oil or olive oil, for garnish (optional)

1 In a large pot, heat the olive oil over high heat. Add the onion, sprinkle with a little salt, and cook, stirring occasionally, until tender and browned, 5 to 7 minutes.

2 Meanwhile, brush any dirt off of the mushrooms and cut each mushroom in half. Add the mushrooms to the pot and sprinkle with a little salt. Cook, stirring occasionally, for 5 minutes. The pot will be getting brown on the bottom and the mushrooms will make a squeaky noise as they cook.

3 Add the sherry and stir well, scraping up any browned bits from the bottom of the pot. Cook for 5 minutes more.

4 Add the broth and reduce the heat to low. Cover and simmer for 20 minutes.

5 Working in batches, transfer the soup to a blender and purée on high until smooth. Return the soup to the pot and stir in the coconut cream and the nutmeg. Season with salt and bring the soup to a simmer.

6 Serve hot, with a sprinkle of microgreens and a drizzle of truffle oil, if desired.

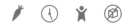

SPICY THAI CURRY NOODLE SOUP

PREPARATION 10 MINUTES   **COOK TIME** 17 MINUTES   **SERVINGS** 4 TO 6

If I had to name the most-viewed (and most-cooked) recipe on my blog over the last nine years, I'm pretty sure it would be this one. A lack of time and a desperate need for immediate gratification is what led me to this recipe. And that is what this soup will give you. In fifteen minutes, you have a broth with a depth of flavor that will convince you it's been simmering all day, and the instant-cook rice noodles have the most wonderful texture ever. The pile of fresh toppings cuts through the rich broth and makes the whole soup sing. You could certainly add some shredded chicken for the last two minutes of cooking to make it even more hearty.

8 ounces rice stick noodles (very fine rice noodles)

3 garlic cloves, minced

2 tablespoons minced fresh ginger

2 tablespoons red curry paste

2 tablespoons coconut oil

4 cups vegetable or chicken broth

3 cups unsweetened coconut milk

Chopped fresh cilantro and Thai basil, for garnish (optional)

Sliced red Fresno chiles and green onions, for garnish (optional)

1 Bring a large pot of water to a boil. Add the rice stick noodles and boil for 3 minutes. Drain in a colander, then rinse with cold water until cool. Set aside.

2 Combine the garlic, ginger, and curry paste in a small food processor or mince and mash together in a small bowl. Add the coconut oil and combine well.

3 In a large pot, heat the curry-coconut paste over medium heat, frying the paste gently for 1 to 2 minutes.

4 Add the broth and deglaze the pot. Add the coconut milk and bring the mixture to a boil. Season with salt.

5 Add the drained noodles and let them cook and soak up the hot broth for 2 minutes.

6 Divide the soup among serving bowls and serve garnished with cilantro, Thai basil, red Fresno chiles, and green onions, if desired.

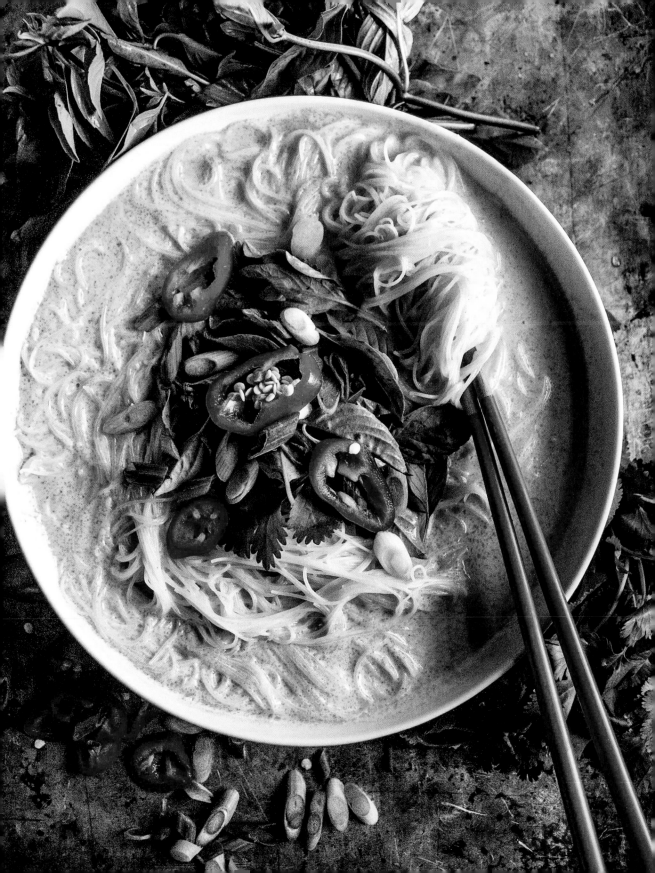

ASIAN VEGETABLE NOODLE SOUP

PREPARATION 10 MINUTES   **COOK TIME** 30 MINUTES   **SERVINGS** 4

When I was a kid (and even a few years past that), I loved the kind of ramen that came in little packages. My mom only let us have them once in a while, but oh boy, slurping up those salty noodles was a great joy. When I was really little, I would doctor up my ramen with chopped celery and carrots (which I would cut with a butter knife), and my little brother would add a ton of chile-garlic sauce to his. We would eat our noodles with chopsticks, thinking we were very sophisticated. My grown-up version is a lot less salty, but has much more flavor and the same satisfying slurpability. It even has little chunks of celery and carrots, a nod to my seven-year-old self (photograph on page 58).

¼ cup vegetable oil

1 yellow onion, finely diced

1 (2-inch) piece fresh ginger, peeled and sliced into coins

2 garlic cloves, minced

3 carrots, thinly sliced on an angle

3 celery stalks, thinly sliced on an angle

8 cups chicken broth

12 ounces rice noodles

Juice of 1 lime

2 teaspoons sesame oil

Kosher salt

1 cup thinly sliced green onions, white and green parts

½ cup chopped fresh cilantro

1 In a large pot, heat the vegetable oil over medium heat. Add the yellow onion and sauté until tender, 3 minutes, then add the ginger and garlic. Reduce the heat to medium-low and cook for 5 minutes. Add the carrots and celery and cook for 3 minutes more.

2 Add the broth and bring to a boil over medium-high heat, then reduce the heat to medium-low and simmer for 15 minutes. Add the rice noodles and cook for 5 minutes, or until the noodles are soft. Stir in the lime juice and sesame oil and season with salt. Sprinkle with the green onions and cilantro and serve hot.

SPICY WHITE BEAN, CHICKEN SAUSAGE, AND TOMATO STEW

PREPARATION 15 MINUTES   **COOK TIME** 1 HOUR 5 MINUTES   **SERVINGS** 6

This stew is the real deal. Incredibly easy and mostly a dump-and-stir type of recipe, it will absolutely knock your socks off. In about an hour, you will be attracting people off the streets with the smell coming from your kitchen.

¼ cup olive oil

1 yellow onion, cut into small dice

½ teaspoon crushed red pepper flakes

¾ pound mild or spicy chicken sausage, casings removed

½ cup dry white wine

3 (15-ounce) cans cannellini beans, drained and rinsed

1 (28-ounce) can crushed tomatoes

4 cups chicken broth

3 teaspoons fresh thyme leaves

Kosher salt

1 In a large heavy pot, heat the olive oil over medium heat. Add the onion and red pepper flakes and cook until the onion is soft and translucent, 5 to 7 minutes.

2 Crumble the sausage into the pan in very small pieces. Stir the sausage into the onions and cook until lightly browned, 4 to 5 minutes. Add the wine and deglaze the pan, scraping up any browned bits from the bottom of the pot.

3 Add the white beans, tomatoes, broth, and 2 teaspoons of the thyme.

4 Bring the stew to a gentle boil, then reduce the heat to low, cover, and simmer for 30 minutes.

5 Uncover and simmer for 20 minutes more, or until the stew thickens. Season with salt and stir in the remaining 1 teaspoon thyme. Serve hot.

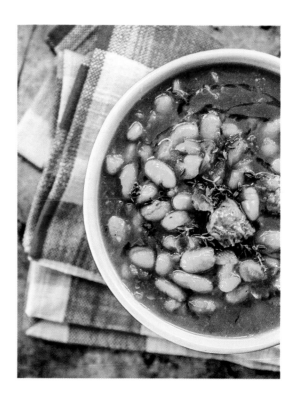

CLASSIC BEEF CHILI

PREPARATION 10 MINUTES   COOK TIME 1 HOUR   SERVINGS 8

Beef chili is the kind of staple you can make over and over and over again when it's as good as this one. Ancho chile powder, unsweetened chocolate, and honey are the secret ingredients that give it such rich flavor—for maximum deliciousness, don't skip any of them!

4 tablespoons vegetable oil

2 pounds 80% lean ground beef

1 (12-ounce) bottle gluten-free beer

2 red onions, cut into small dice

2 jalapeños, seeded and minced

3 tablespoons ground cumin

3 tablespoons ancho chile powder

3 tablespoons chili powder

4 cups chicken broth

2 (15-ounce) cans pinto beans, drained and rinsed

2 (15-ounce) cans kidney beans, drained and rinsed

2 ounces unsweetened chocolate

2 tablespoons honey

Kosher salt

FOR GARNISH

Faux Sour Cream (page 87)

Avocado cubes

Fresh cilantro

Sliced green onions

1 In a large heavy pan, heat 2 tablespoons of the vegetable oil over high heat. Add the beef and cook, breaking up the meat up with a wooden spoon, until the meat is almost cooked through, about 10 minutes.

2 Drain off any liquid and return the pan to high heat. Cook for 5 minutes more to brown the beef. Add the beer and scrape up any browned bits from the bottom of the pan. Cook until the liquid has cooked off, about 5 minutes. Transfer the meat to a bowl and return the pan to the stove.

3 Add the remaining 2 tablespoons vegetable oil and reduce the heat to medium. Add the onions, stir, and cook for 5 minutes.

4 Add the jalapeños, cumin, ancho chile powder, and chili powder and stir. Cook for 5 minutes more.

5 Add the broth, cover the pot, and let the mixture simmer for 20 minutes.

6 Use an immersion blender (or blend in batches in a blender) to purée the sauce until smooth. Return the meat to the pan and add the beans, as well as the unsweetened chocolate and the honey. Mix well. Season with salt.

7 Partially cover the pot, and simmer over very low heat for 30 minutes. (If you want the chili to be thicker, cook with the lid off.)

8 Serve with the garnishes of your choice.

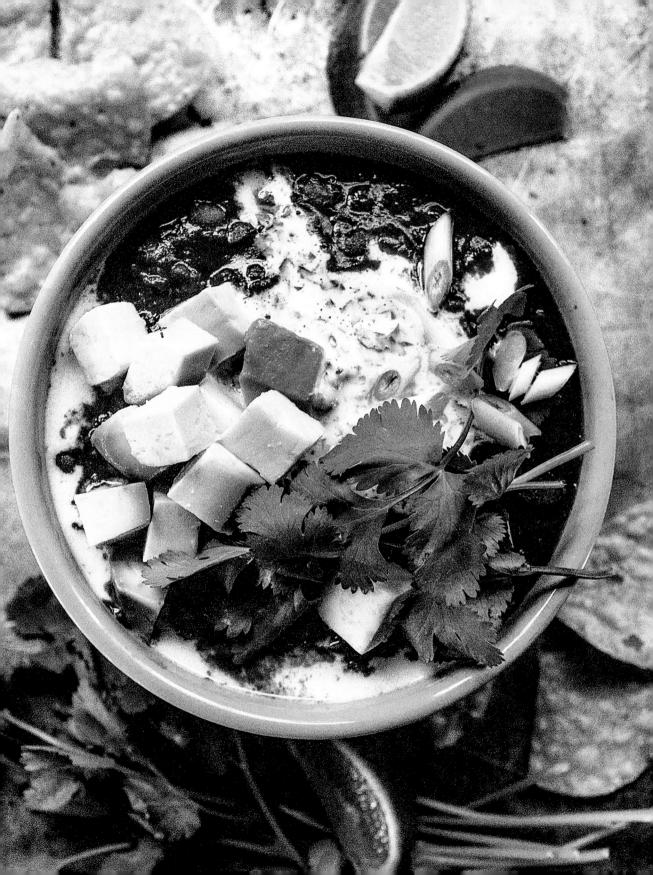

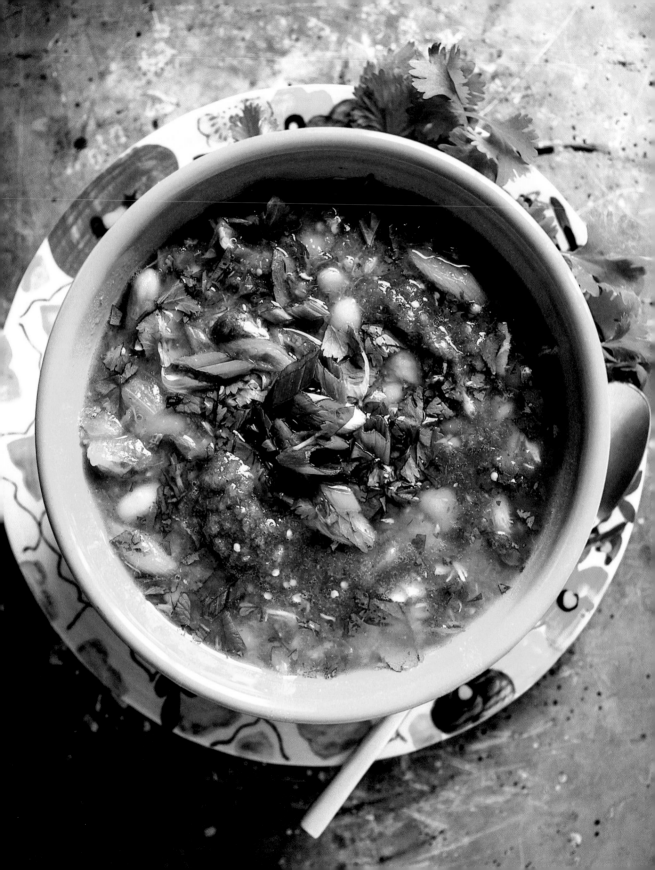

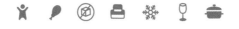

CHICKEN CHILI VERDE

PREPARATION 15 MINUTES   **COOK TIME** 1 HOUR 45 MINUTES   **SERVINGS** 6 TO 8

I have big love for chili—there are three versions of it in this book (and many more on my blog). It is hard not to sing the praises of such a nutritious and complete meal, especially when it is this delicious. This is a lighter and less spicy chili, with a focus on the shredded chicken, white beans, and intensely flavorful greens. I serve this with Sweet Potato Green Onion Biscuits (page 182).

CHILI

¼ cup vegetable oil

1 yellow onion, cut into small dice

1 jalapeño, seeded and minced

3 (15-ounce) cans cannellini beans, drained and rinsed

4 cups shredded cooked chicken

8 cups chicken broth

2 teaspoons ground cumin

GREEN SAUCE

3 cups chopped tomatillos

1 jalapeño, seeded and chopped

2 garlic cloves

½ yellow onion, roughly chopped

1 cup fresh cilantro, stems and leaves

• • •

Kosher salt

Thinly sliced green onions and coarsely chopped fresh cilantro, for garnish

1 In a large pot, heat the vegetable oil over medium heat. Add the onion and jalapeño and cook, stirring occasionally, until tender, 5 to 7 minutes.

2 Add the beans and chicken, then add the chicken broth and cumin. Simmer over medium heat while you prepare the sauce.

3 To make the green sauce: In a blender, combine the tomatillos, jalapeño, garlic, onion, and cilantro. Purée on high until well combined.

4 Stir the green sauce into the chili. Cover the pot, reduce the heat to low, and gently simmer the chili for 1 hour. Remove the lid and simmer for 30 minutes more. Season with salt and serve garnished with generous amounts of green onions and fresh cilantro.

NOTE: An extra dollop of Cilantro Sauce (page 72) or Faux Sour Cream (page 87) is also a delicious addition.

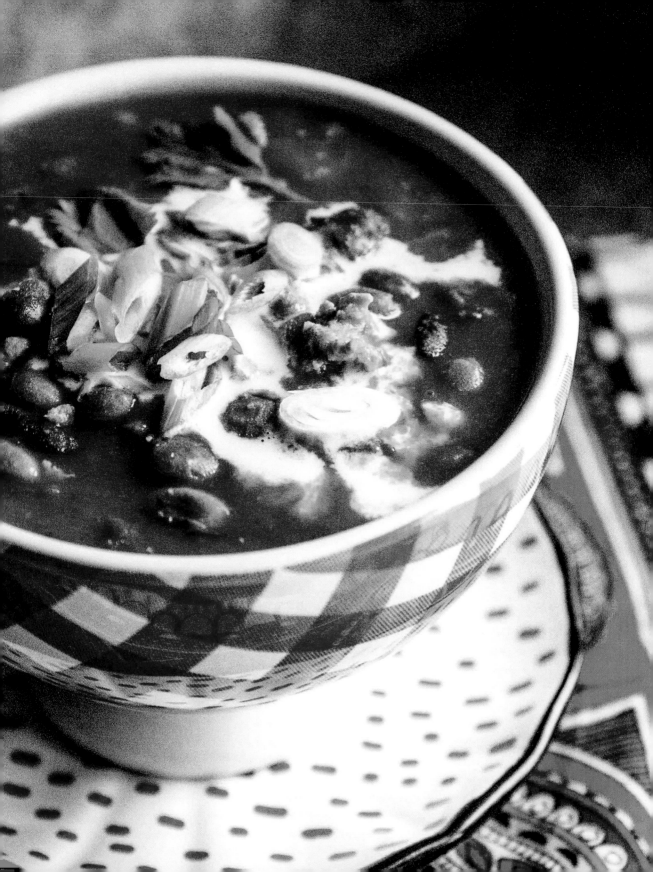

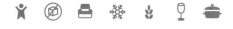

SPICY CHIPOTLE TURKEY CHILI

PREPARATION 15 MINUTES   **COOK TIME** 60 MINUTES   **SERVINGS** 6 TO 8

I am sure that my affinity for chili is clear by now, but the roundup would not be complete without a turkey version—a leaner, lighter take with unique spicy flavors. The chipotle gives some smoky dimension to the spice that is a welcome addition. Add a big dollop of Faux Sour Cream and a football game, and I'm in heaven.

CHILI

¼ cup olive oil

1 large yellow onion, finely diced

1 jalapeño, seeded and diced

1 (28-ounce) can tomato purée

4 ounces canned chipotle chile in adobo sauce

1 pound ground turkey

3 (15-ounce) cans pinto beans, drained and rinsed

2 (15-ounce) cans kidney beans, drained and rinsed

4 cups chicken broth

Kosher salt

FAUX SOUR CREAM

1 cup chilled coconut cream

2 garlic cloves, minced

¼ cup minced cilantro

Zest of 2 limes

2 tablespoons lime juice

Kosher salt

• • •

Thinly sliced green onions and chopped fresh cilantro, for garnish

1 In a large heavy pot, heat 3 tablespoons of the olive oil over medium heat. Add the yellow onion and jalapeño and cook, stirring often, for 5 to 7 minutes. Transfer the onion, jalapeño, and oil to a blender and add the tomato purée and chipotle in adobo sauce. Purée on high until smooth. Set aside.

2 In the same pot in which you cooked the onion and jalapeño, heat the remaining 1 tablespoon olive oil over medium heat. Add the turkey and cook, breaking up the turkey with a wooden spoon, until the turkey is mostly cooked through, about 5 minutes.

3 Add the chipotle sauce, beans, and broth. Stir well to combine. Cover the pot, reduce the heat to low, and simmer for at least 45 minutes.

4 To make the faux sour cream: Combine the ingredients in a bowl and whisk until smooth. Season with salt.

5 Season the chili with salt and serve hot, garnished with the faux sour cream, green onions, and cilantro.

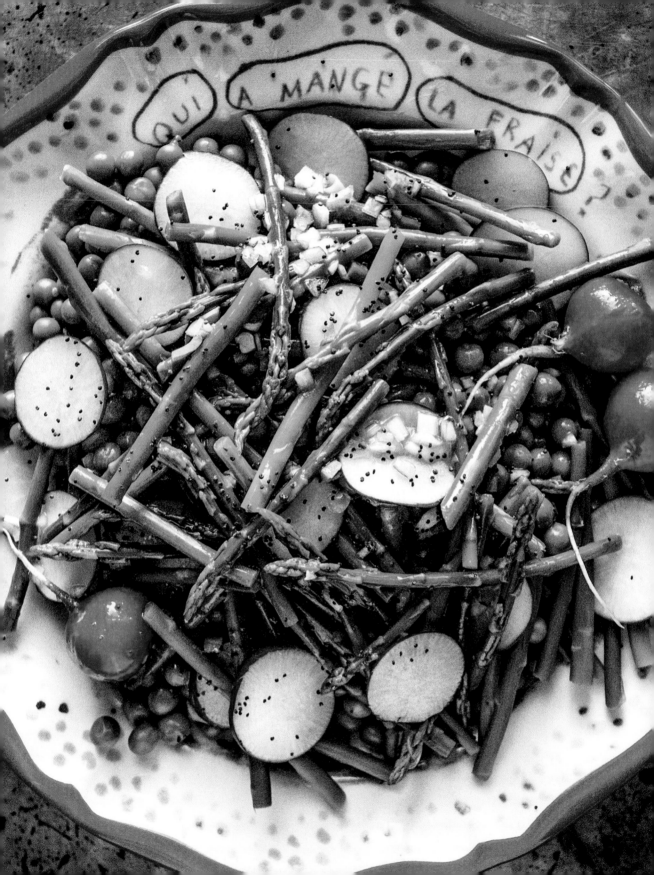

salads

My love of salad is a far cry from my childhood days when "Would you like salad?" wasn't my mom asking a real question, but just a formality before a big helping was dropped on my plate. Salad every night, no matter what. I remember all the different ways I devised to get rid of it without her seeing, including feeding it to the dog, hiding it in my napkin, and, in the summer when we would eat outside, scraping it directly into the garden beds.

I would like to think that my own children don't feel quite as vehemently averse to salad as I once did. In fact, Pia loves any type of raw kale salad, and will sample most other varieties. Coco? Well, she would probably rather send it to the backyard perennial beds like her mom did, but I have faith that she will come around.

The salads I like best are those you can make a real meal of. Even skeptics like my husband, who would never agree that a salad qualifies as a "meal," have come around to salads like the Crunchy Taco Salad and the Asian Chicken Salad. These are hearty, filling, salad-for-dinner kinds of dishes. My aim is to bring both intense and subtle flavors to these salads, with very distinctive seasonings and an emphasis on fresh ingredients. I'm betting they will create some converts in your house, too.

◄ Asparagus and Pea Salad with Honey-Shallot Vinaigrette (page 115)

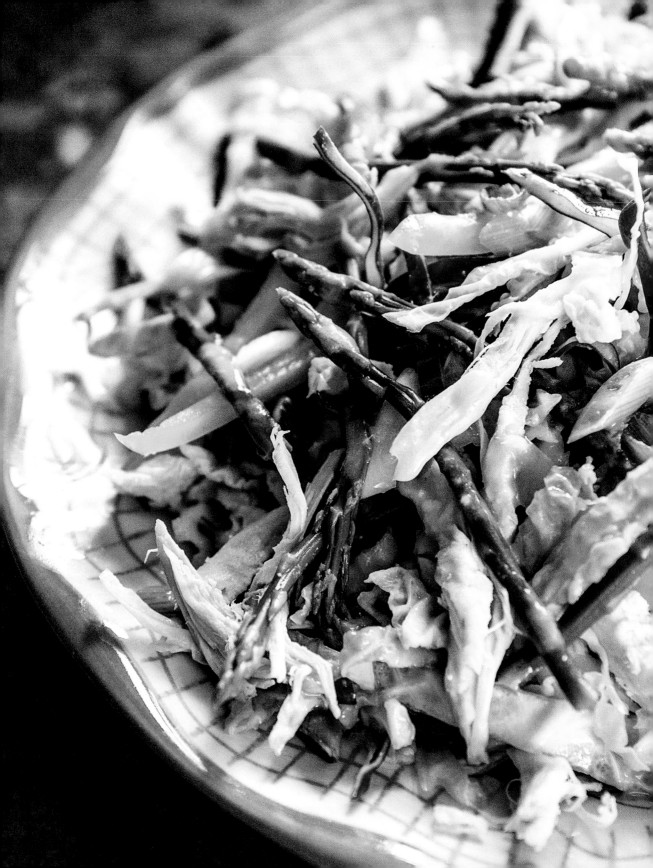

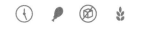

ASIAN CHICKEN SALAD
WITH GINGER VINAIGRETTE

PREPARATION 10 MINUTES   **COOK TIME** 5 MINUTES   **SERVINGS** 4

Talk about a good dish gone bad. Too many cloying versions at "fast casual" restaurants have given Asian chicken salads a bad rap, but I'm determined to rehabilitate that reputation with this more refined, non-clichéd version. The dressing has a kick from all the fresh ginger and garlic, but none of the sweetness of a traditional Asian-style dressing. It's perfect paired with the crunchy cabbage and delicate sweetness of the yellow peppers and asparagus.

ASPARAGUS

Kosher salt

½ pound asparagus, trimmed

GINGER VINAIGRETTE

1 garlic clove

2 tablespoons thinly sliced fresh ginger

¼ cup rice vinegar

3 tablespoons sesame oil

2 tablespoons vegetable oil

Kosher salt

SALAD

6 cups thinly shredded savoy cabbage

2 cups thinly shredded purple cabbage

1 yellow bell pepper, seeded and thinly sliced

3 green onions, thinly sliced

2 cups shredded cooked chicken breast

1 Bring a large saucepan of salted water to a boil. Fill a large bowl with ice and water.

2 Slice the asparagus stalks in half lengthwise. Add the asparagus to the boiling water and simmer for about 2 minutes, or until just tender. Immediately remove them from the simmering water and plunge them into the ice water to stop the cooking. Let the asparagus cool and then drain it and set it on a kitchen towel to dry.

3 To make the ginger vinaigrette: In a blender, combine the garlic, ginger, vinegar, sesame oil, and vegetable oil. Purée on high until you have a smooth, creamy dressing. Season with salt.

4 In a large bowl, combine the asparagus, cabbages, bell pepper, green onions, and chicken. Add the dressing and toss gently. Season with salt, if necessary. Serve immediately.

ROSEMARY CHICKEN SALAD WITH AVOCADO AND BACON

PREPARATION 10 MINUTES   COOK TIME 15 MINUTES   SERVINGS 2

I once got trapped at the Regency Hotel in New York by a snowstorm, and when I couldn't fly home (or even brave the cold outside) I ate this salad three times a day for more than a week. Clearly the obsession lingers. The salty bacon and pungent rosemary make the chicken and greens shine, and the little burst of juicy cherry tomatoes and chunks of creamy avocado add so much flavor.

SALAD

4 thick-cut uncured bacon slices, diced

Kosher salt

2 boneless chicken thighs, skin on

1 tablespoon olive oil

2 tablespoons minced fresh rosemary

1 head romaine, chopped into bite-size pieces

1 bunch watercress

1 cup cherry tomatoes, halved

¼ red onion, thinly sliced

1 large avocado

ROSEMARY VINAIGRETTE

2 teaspoons Dijon mustard

¼ cup olive oil

¼ cup red wine vinegar

1 teaspoon minced fresh rosemary

Kosher salt

1 In a heavy skillet, cook the bacon over medium heat until crispy, about 7 minutes. Transfer the bacon to a paper towel to drain and set aside.

2 Salt the chicken thighs. Add the olive oil to the bacon fat in the pan and heat over medium-high heat. Add the rosemary and the chicken thighs, skin-side down, and cook until the chicken is golden and crisp. Flip the chicken and cook until the thighs are cooked through, about 10 minutes.

3 Make a bed of the romaine and watercress in a serving bowl or on a platter. Scatter the cherry tomatoes, red onion, and bacon pieces on top.

4 Slice the avocado, sprinkle the slices with salt, and arrange them on the salad. Slice the chicken and add it to the salad.

5 To make the rosemary vinaigrette: In a small bowl, whisk together the mustard, olive oil, vinegar, and rosemary until smooth. Season with salt.

6 Gently toss the salad with the vinaigrette and serve immediately.

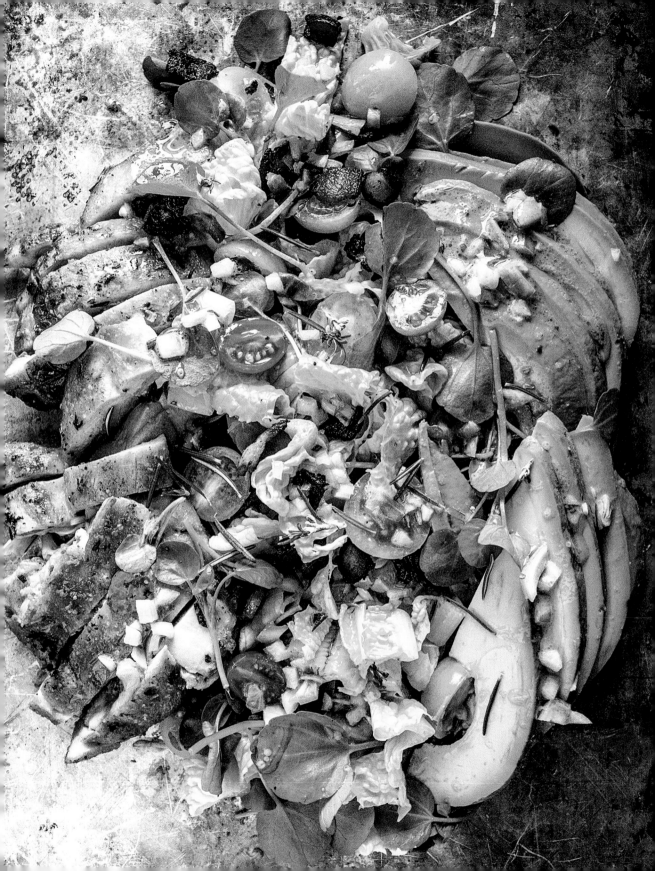

BÁNH MÌ SALAD
WITH SRIRACHA VINAIGRETTE

PREPARATION 25 MINUTES **COOK TIME** 3 MINUTES **SERVINGS** 4

I'm kind of obsessed with the flavors of Vietnamese bánh mì sandwiches. Asian Pulled Pork is the base, allowing one batch to serve as the centerpiece of two very different meals! I serve the pulled pork as is for dinner one night and then enjoy the leftovers in this gorgeous and delicious salad the next day.

SWEET AND SPICY PICKLED ONIONS

1 large red onion, thinly sliced

1 jalapeño, thinly sliced, with seeds

1 cup rice vinegar

½ cup granulated beet sugar

½ teaspoon kosher salt

SRIRACHA VINAIGRETTE

1 garlic clove

2 tablespoons Sriracha

¼ cup rice vinegar

¼ cup vegetable oil

2 tablespoons honey

Kosher salt

SALAD

6 cups mixed greens

½ cup lightly packed fresh mint leaves

½ cup lightly packed fresh cilantro leaves

1 cup carrot ribbons (made with a peeler)

1 cup thin bell pepper strips

2 cups Asian Pulled Pork (page 245)

1 To make the pickled onions: Place the onion and jalapeño slices in a heatproof medium bowl.

2 In a small pot, combine the vinegar, sugar, and salt. Bring to a simmer over medium heat and cook, stirring, until the sugar has dissolved, about 2 minutes.

3 Pour the vinegar mixture over the onion and jalapeño slices. Cover the bowl with plastic wrap and set aside for at least 25 minutes. (These can be kept in the refrigerator for up to 5 days.)

4 To make the Sriracha vinaigrette: In a blender, combine the garlic, Sriracha, vinegar, vegetable oil, and honey. Purée until smooth and then season with salt. Set aside.

5 In a large bowl or on a platter, combine the mixed greens, mint, cilantro, carrots, and bell pepper. Drizzle the salad with the vinaigrette and toss until well coated and combined.

6 Top with the pulled pork and sprinkle with the pickled onions. Serve immediately.

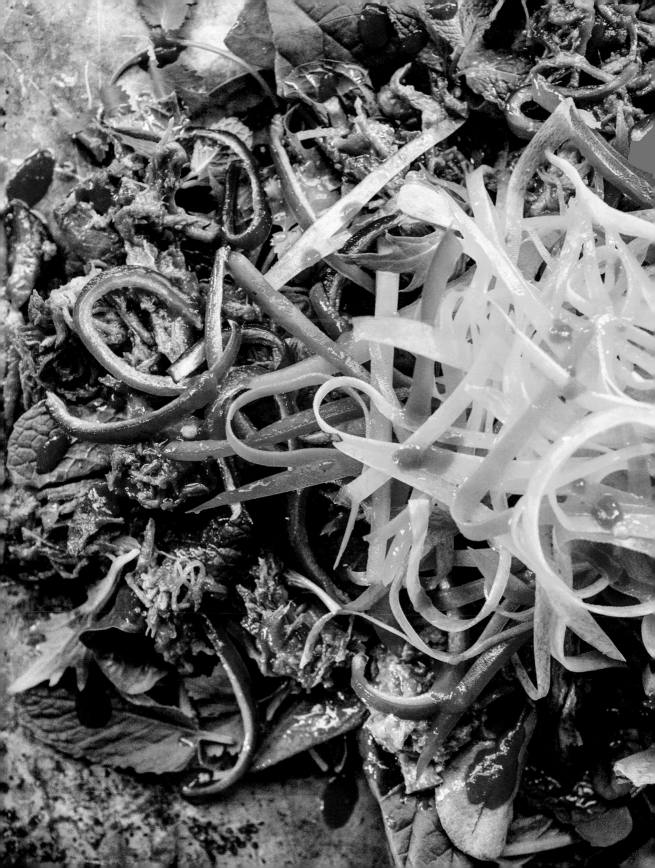

CRUNCHY TACO SALAD WITH SPICED GROUND TURKEY AND CILANTRO-LIME VINAIGRETTE

PREPARATION 15 MINUTES **COOK TIME** 15 MINUTES **SERVINGS** 4

If Pete had to choose a go-to salad, this would be it—probably because it's so loaded with meat and "toppings" that you can just barely call it a salad at all! When you crumble tortilla chips on top, he likes it even better. But he does have a point about how good it is. The cilantro-lime vinaigrette takes it over the top.

CILANTRO-LIME VINAIGRETTE

1 cup packed fresh cilantro stems and leaves

1 garlic clove, coarsely chopped

2 tablespoons agave

¼ cup fresh lime juice (from 1 to 2 limes)

¼ cup vegetable oil

SALAD

Kosher salt

3 tablespoons vegetable oil

½ red onion, finely diced

1 pound ground turkey

1 tablespoon chili powder

1 tablespoon ground cumin

1 teaspoon kosher salt

4 cups finely shredded red cabbage

4 cups chopped romaine hearts

1 cup julienned peeled jicama

6 radishes, finely sliced

½ cup lightly packed fresh cilantro leaves

1 red Fresno chile, thinly sliced

1 To make the cilantro-lime vinaigrette: In a blender, combine the cilantro, garlic, agave, lime juice, and vegetable oil. Purée on high until smooth and season with salt. Set aside.

2 In a large heavy pan, heat the oil over medium heat. Add the red onion and sweat for 5 to 7 minutes. Add the turkey and cook, breaking it up with a wooden spoon, until cooked through, about 3 minutes. Stir in the chili powder, cumin, and salt. Add ⅓ cup water, stir, and cook until the turkey is completely cooked through and the water has cooked off, 3 minutes more. Remove from the heat.

3 Arrange the cabbage and romaine hearts on a large serving platter or on individual plates. Top with the jicama, radishes, cilantro, and chile. Spoon the ground turkey on top and drizzle the salad with a generous amount of the vinaigrette.

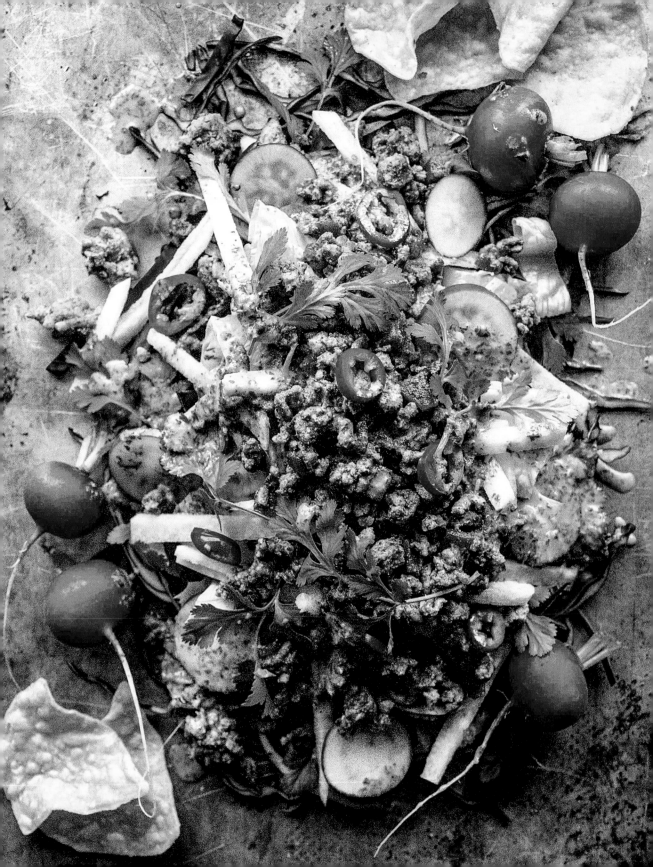

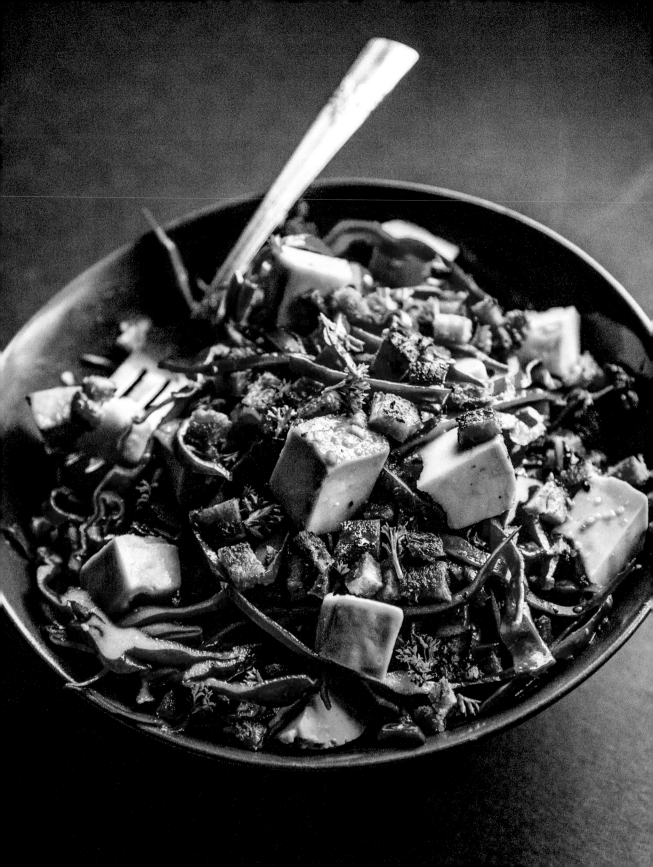

RED CABBAGE, BACON, AND AVOCADO SLAW WITH BALSAMIC VINAIGRETTE

PREPARATION 15 MINUTES   **COOK TIME** N/A   **SERVINGS** 6

This crunchy, sweet, and salty combination is a fresh take on slaw to serve with anything grilled or piled on a burger. Because cabbage stands up so well to dressing, this is an excellent dish to make ahead or bring to a party—just add the avocado at the last minute.

BALSAMIC VINAIGRETTE

2 garlic cloves, minced

1 tablespoon Dijon mustard

1 tablespoon honey

¼ cup balsamic vinegar

⅓ cup olive oil

Kosher salt

SALAD

1 small head red cabbage, cored and thinly sliced

4 uncured bacon slices, cooked until crisp, drained and chopped

½ cup chopped fresh flat-leaf parsley

4 large radishes, thinly sliced

3 green onions, thinly sliced

Kosher salt

1 large avocado, pitted, peeled, and cut into chunks

1 To make the balsamic vinaigrette: In a blender, combine the garlic, mustard, honey, vinegar, and olive oil. Blend until smooth and creamy. Season with salt and set aside.

2 In a large bowl, combine the cabbage, bacon, and parsley. Drizzle with a few tablespoons of the vinaigrette to start (you can always add more!) and toss to coat.

3 Add the radishes and green onion and toss again. Season with salt.

4 Transfer to a serving platter and top with the avocado.

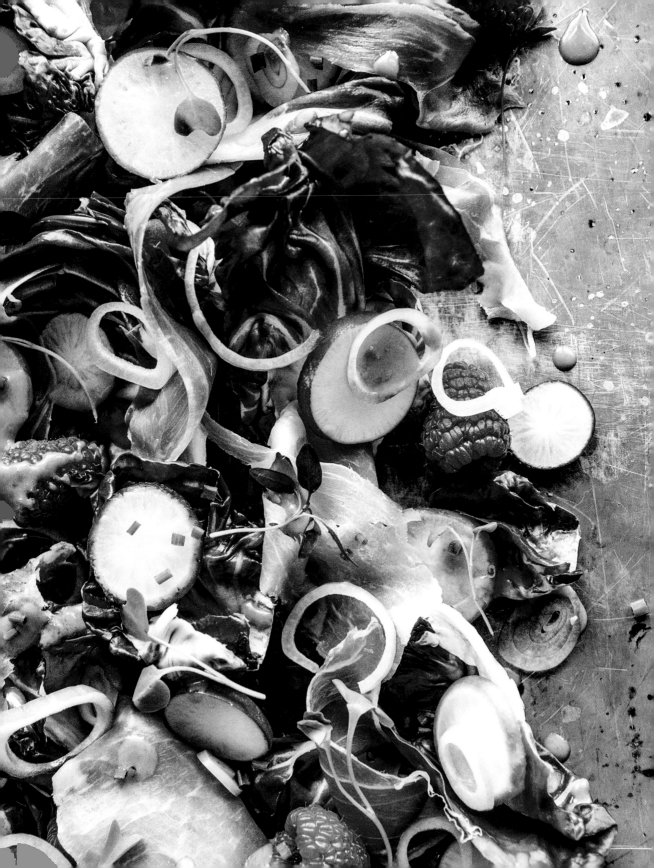

RADICCHIO SALAD WITH RASPBERRIES, RADISHES, PROSCIUTTO, AND RASPBERRY CHAMPAGNE VINAIGRETTE

PREPARATION 10 MINUTES   COOK TIME N/A   SERVINGS 2 TO 4

The sweet raspberry champagne vinaigrette adds a retro pink touch to the colors and textures of this beautiful salad. The bitter radicchio and sweet raspberries contrast with the peppery radishes and salty prosciutto for a really dynamic flavor combination.

SALAD

4 cups radicchio (approximately 2 heads) torn into bite-size pieces

4 ounces prosciutto, thinly sliced

6 radishes, thinly sliced

1 cup fresh raspberries

1 shallot, thinly sliced

RASPBERRY CHAMPAGNE VINAIGRETTE

¼ cup fresh or frozen raspberries

2 garlic cloves, coarsely chopped

2 tablespoons honey

¼ cup Champagne vinegar

¼ cup olive oil

Kosher salt

1 On a platter or in a serving bowl, combine the radicchio, prosciutto, radishes, raspberries, and shallot. Set aside.

2 To make the raspberry champagne vinaigrette: In a blender, combine the vinaigrette ingredients and purée until smooth.

3 Drizzle the salad with the vinaigrette and gently toss to coat. Serve immediately.

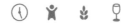

HOT SPINACH, STRAWBERRY, AND BACON SALAD

PREPARATION 5 MINUTES   **COOK TIME** 10 MINUTES   **SERVINGS** 4

At my first restaurant job, when I wasn't doing things like cleaning out the deep-fat fryer, I got to make the salads. I loved making those salads, which seemed like a treat after all my other duties. I often made hot spinach and bacon salad, a heavy affair traditionally garnished with crumbled eggs, mushrooms, red onions, and mustard vinaigrette. This is my lighter, fresher version—the strawberries add a bright, sweet juiciness. It makes for a beautiful dish and has become a regular when I am entertaining.

5 uncured bacon slices

1 large shallot, minced

Kosher salt

2 tablespoons olive oil

2 tablespoons balsamic vinegar

1 tablespoon honey

1 (6-ounce) bag baby spinach (see Note)

1 cup thinly sliced strawberries

1 In a skillet or heavy pan, cook the bacon until crispy on both sides. Transfer the bacon to a paper towel to drain, leaving the rendered fat in the pan.

2 Add the shallot and a sprinkle of salt to the bacon fat and cook over low heat, stirring often, until the shallot is soft, about 5 minutes. Add the oil, vinegar, and honey and stir. Cook for 5 minutes more.

3 Remove the dressing from the heat and add the spinach, strawberries, and crumbled bacon to the pan. Toss the salad well to coat the leaves (they will wilt slightly) and season with salt. Transfer to a platter and serve immediately.

NOTE: If possible, try using one of the beautiful artisanal spinaches available seasonally, like the red spinach in the photo.

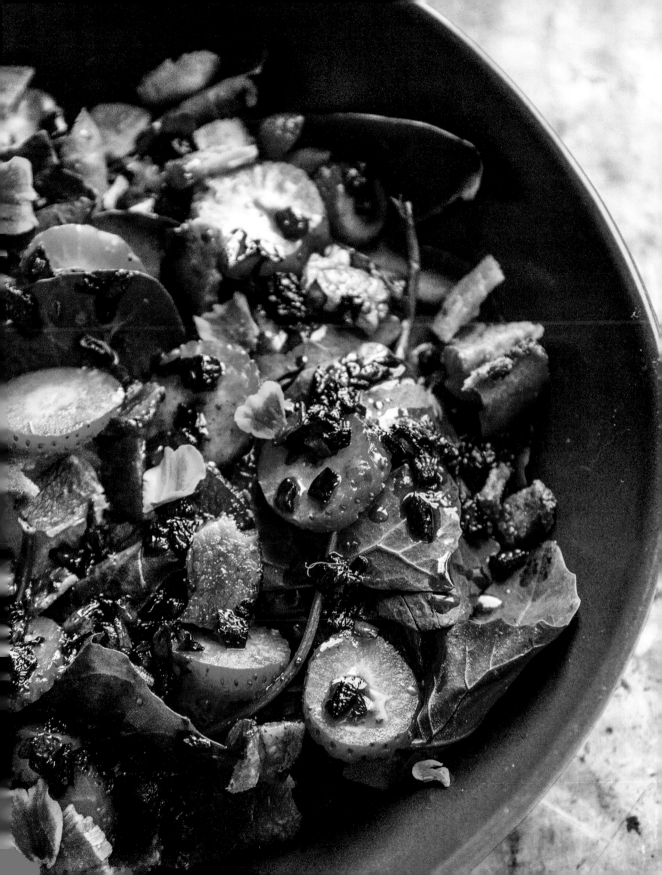

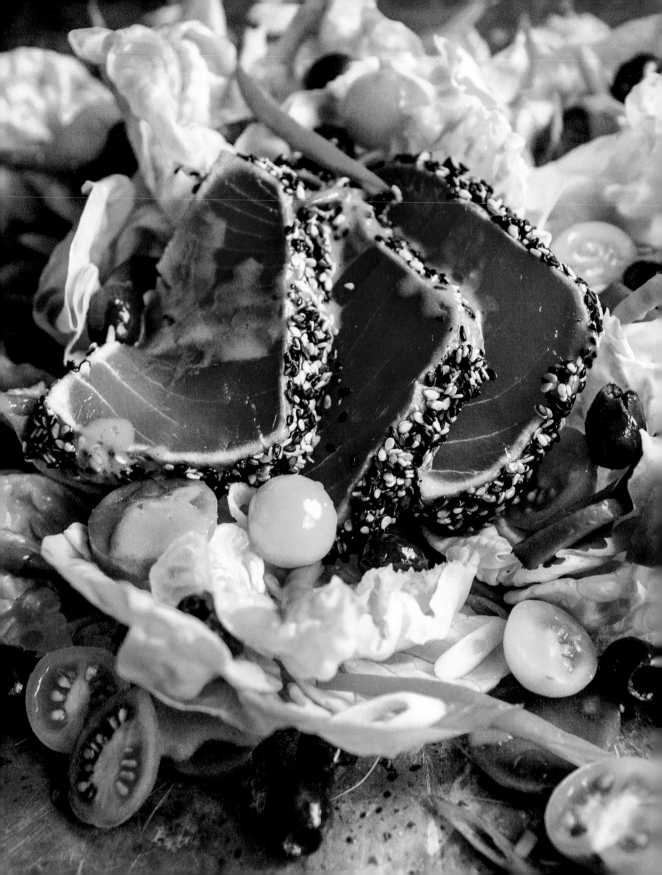

NIÇOISE SALAD WITH
SESAME-CRUSTED TUNA

PREPARATION 10 MINUTES   **COOK TIME** 30 MINUTES   **SERVINGS** 4

This is not only one of the prettiest plates of food you will ever have, it's also one of the most delicious. It's a truly elegant celebration of color, flavor, and texture, a play on traditional Niçoise salad that you won't forget.

SALAD

1 pound tuna steaks

Kosher salt

¼ cup toasted sesame seeds

24 green beans

1 pound small waxy potatoes (I like to use purple and red potatoes)

1 tablespoon olive oil

2 heads butter or Bibb lettuce

1 cup halved cherry tomatoes

½ cup pitted Niçoise olives

ROASTED RED PEPPER VINAIGRETTE

1 garlic clove, minced

⅓ cup roasted red pepper pieces (packed in water), drained

2 tablespoons red wine vinegar

¼ cup olive oil

Kosher salt

1 Season the tuna with salt and then press the sesame seeds in a thick layer onto all sides of the fish. Set aside.

2 Bring a medium pot of salted water to a boil. Fill a large bowl with ice and water. Blanch the green beans for about 2 minutes. Use a spider strainer or tongs to transfer the beans to the ice water to stop the cooking. Drain the beans and set aside.

3 Bring the water back to a boil and cook the potatoes until tender, 15 to 20 minutes. Drain well. Slice the potatoes and set aside.

4 Place a nonstick pan over medium-high heat. Add the olive oil and sear the tuna, 30 seconds

to 1 minute on each side, depending on how well cooked you like it. Cut the tuna into ¼-inch-thick slices and set aside.

5 Arrange the lettuce leaves on a platter and arrange the beans, potatoes, tomatoes, and olives on top.

6 To make the roasted red pepper vinaigrette: In a blender, combine the garlic, red pepper, vinegar, and olive oil and purée until smooth and creamy. Season with salt.

7 Top the salad with the seared tuna slices and drizzle everything with the vinaigrette. Serve immediately.

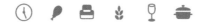

ROASTED SQUASH AND ARUGULA SALAD WITH MAPLE-MUSTARD VINAIGRETTE

PREPARATION 10 MINUTES **COOK TIME** 20 MINUTES **SERVINGS** 4 TO 6

The flavors of peppery arugula and sweet, earthy roasted squash come to life when tossed with a sweet-and-savory viniagrette. While this salad is probably best suited to autumn, when acorn squash are freshly harvested, you can often find them well into the spring at most grocery stores, and they are still wonderful.

SQUASH

1 (2-pound) acorn squash

2 tablespoons olive oil

Kosher salt

MAPLE-MUSTARD VINAIGRETTE

2 tablespoons whole-grain mustard

2 tablespoons pure maple syrup

¼ cup red wine vinegar

¼ cup olive oil

Kosher salt

SALAD

8 cups baby arugula

½ red onion, thinly sliced

3 uncured bacon slices, cooked crisp and crumbled

1 Preheat the oven to 425°F.

2 Split the squash in half. Scoop out and reserve the seeds. Cut the squash into slices 1½ to 2 inches thick.

3 Spread the squash slices on a rimmed baking sheet. Toss them with 1½ tablespoons of the olive oil and sprinkle them with salt. Roast the squash for about 20 minutes, until golden and tender. Remove and set aside to cool.

4 On a separate baking sheet, toss the squash seeds with the remaining ½ tablespoon olive oil and a little salt. Roast the seeds for about 7 minutes, or until golden. Remove and set aside to cool.

5 To make the maple-mustard vinaigrette: In a small bowl, whisk together the mustard, maple syrup, vinegar, and olive oil. Season with salt.

6 Arrange the arugula and squash on a serving platter and top with the red onion and bacon. Sprinkle with the squash seeds and drizzle with the vinaigrette. Season with salt and serve.

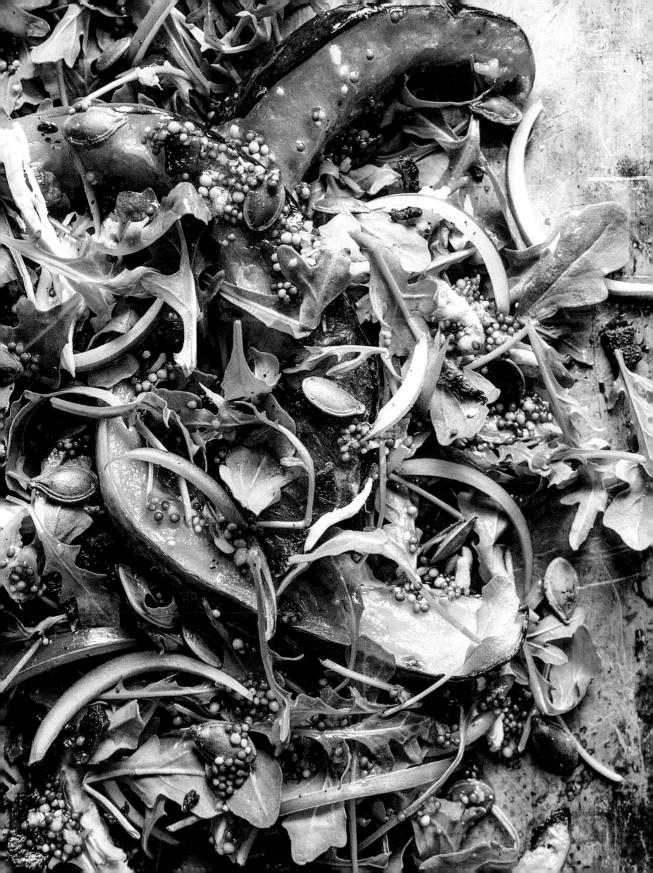

KALE POWER SALAD WITH
GARLIC HONEY SESAME DRESSING

PREPARATION 15 MINUTES   COOK TIME N/A   SERVINGS 4

I call this a "power salad" because it is so jam-packed with superfoods like raw kale, peppers, peas, and fresh ginger and garlic. It is intensely flavorful and really bright and colorful. It's plenty satisfying on its own but would also be an excellent base on which to serve grilled meat or fish. You could also add shredded chicken or even a scoop of quinoa.

GARLIC HONEY SESAME DRESSING

2 garlic cloves

3 tablespoons sesame oil

1 tablespoon vegetable oil

⅓ cup rice vinegar

3 tablespoons honey

Kosher salt

SALAD

6 cups very thinly shredded curly kale

1 yellow bell pepper, seeded and thinly sliced

1 red bell pepper, seeded and thinly sliced

4 green onions, thinly sliced

1 cup green peas, blanched (see Note)

½ cup fresh cilantro leaves

1 tablespoon toasted sesame seeds

1 To make the garlic honey sesame dressing: In a blender, combine the garlic, sesame oil, vegetable oil, vinegar, and honey. Purée until smooth, then season with salt.

2 In a large bowl, combine the kale, bell peppers, green onions, peas, and cilantro. Toss the vegetables gently with the dressing and then sprinkle with the sesame seeds. Serve immediately.

NOTE: To blanch the peas, prepare an ice bath and bring a small pot of water to a simmer. Add the peas to the simmering water and cook for 4 to 5 minutes, until the peas float to the top of the pot and are bright green. Drain them and plunge into the ice bath to cool them completely. Drain the peas and set aside to dry.

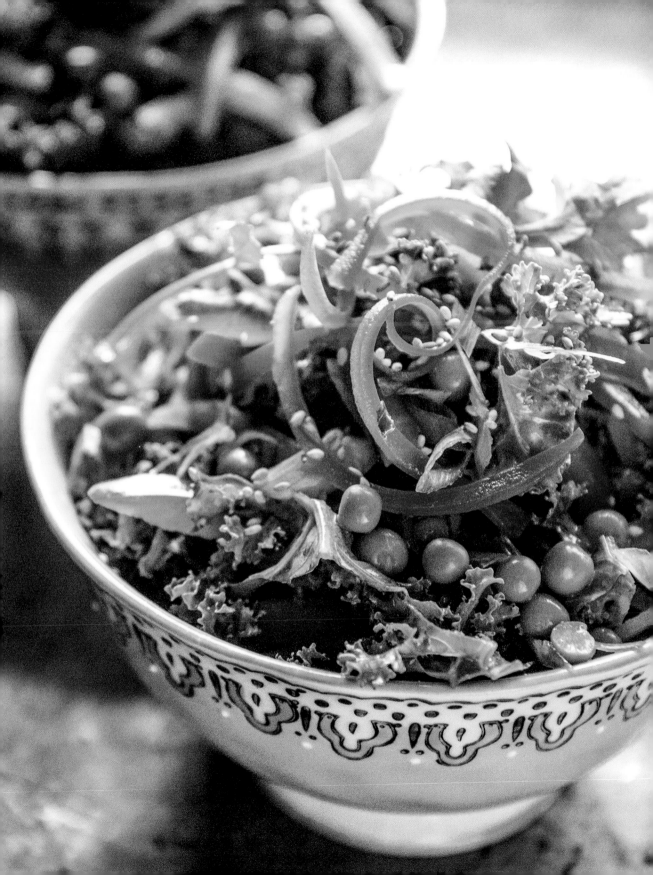

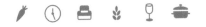

WINTER FRUIT AND KALE SALAD
WITH CRANBERRY VINAIGRETTE

PREPARATION 20 MINUTES   **COOK TIME** N/A   **SERVINGS** 4

Earthy Tuscan kale is a great match for the vivid, sweet-and-tart flavors of winter fruits, such as pomegranate and cranberries. We sometimes call this Christmas Salad, as the colors and textures lend themselves to celebration, and the ingredients are certainly in season during the winter months.

SALAD

8 cups finely chopped curly kale leaves

1 orange, sectioned

1 ripe pear, cored and thinly sliced

½ cup pomegranate seeds

½ cup unsweetened dried cranberries

1 cup thinly sliced green onions

CRANBERRY VINAIGRETTE

1 shallot, minced

2 tablespoons agave

2 tablespoons unsweetened cranberry juice

2 tablespoons red wine vinegar

¼ cup olive oil

Kosher salt

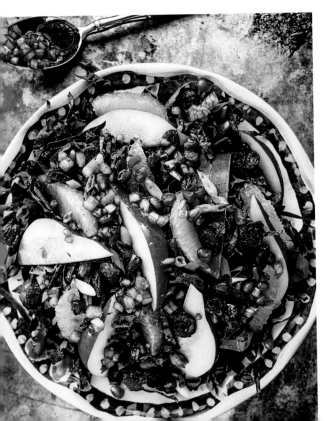

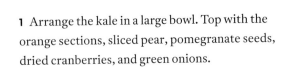

1 Arrange the kale in a large bowl. Top with the orange sections, sliced pear, pomegranate seeds, dried cranberries, and green onions.

2 Whisk the cranberry vinaigrette ingredients together in a small bowl and season with salt.

3 Drizzle the vinaigrette over the salad and toss gently to combine. Season with salt, if needed.

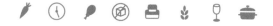

BROCCOLI CHOPPED SALAD
WITH TAHINI VINAIGRETTE

PREPARATION 20 MINUTES COOK TIME:N/A **SERVINGS** 4 TO 6

Of all the recipes in this book, this one may have been the biggest surprise to me. When I made it, I was just playing around with textures and flavors, but the result was so good, I couldn't believe it. When I threw in some gorgeous pomegranate seeds I had sitting in my fridge, the salad just exploded. I can't even count how many times I have made and enjoyed it since. Another perk is that it can be made way ahead, since the broccoli really holds up.

4 cups finely chopped broccoli stems and florets

½ cup finely diced red onion

½ cup pomegranate seeds

2 tablespoons tahini

1 garlic clove

⅓ cup olive oil

¼ cup red wine vinegar

1 tablespoon fresh lemon juice

Kosher salt

1 tablespoon toasted sesame seeds

1 In a large bowl, toss together the broccoli, red onion, and pomegranate seeds.

2 In the blender, combine the tahini, garlic, olive oil, vinegar, and lemon juice. Purée until smooth and then season with salt.

3 Pour the tahini dressing over the salad and toss to coat. Season with salt and sprinkle the salad with the toasted sesame seeds. Serve at room temperature or chilled.

BROCCOLI has really high amounts of vitamins K and C, as well as a good amount of vitamin A. It is also high in fiber.

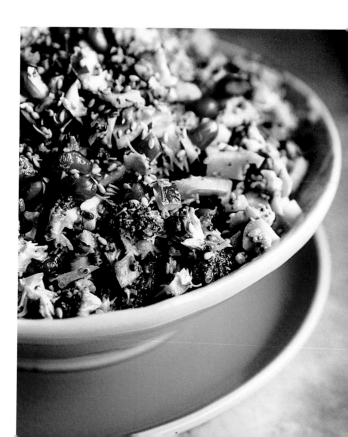

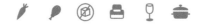

BEET SALAD WITH PARSLEY–PUMPKIN SEED PESTO AND FRESH MINT

PREPARATION 15 MINUTES   **COOK TIME** 30 MINUTES   **SERVINGS** 4 TO 6

I find the sweet, earthy flavor of beets is well complemented by this fresh herbal pesto, highlighted with fresh mint and thickened with pumpkin seeds. It's a full-flavored salad with ravishing colors that's right at home on a fall table.

BEETS

6 large beets, tops trimmed

Kosher salt

PARSLEY–PUMPKIN SEED PESTO

3 garlic cloves, minced

2 cups packed fresh flat-leaf parsley

¼ cup packed fresh mint leaves

¼ cup pepitas, toasted

¼ cup olive oil

Juice of 1 lemon

Kosher salt

TO SERVE

Kosher salt

2 tablespoons olive oil

3 tablespoons loosely packed fresh mint leaves

1 tablespoon fresh flat-leaf parsley leaves

1 Bring a medium pot of water to a boil. Salt the water, then add the beets and simmer for 25 to 30 minutes, or until fork-tender.

2 Drain the beets and rinse under cold water, using your fingers to rub off the skins off—they should come off quite easily. Set the beets aside.

3 To make the parsley–pumpkin seed pesto: In a food processor, combine the garlic, parsley, mint, pepitas, olive oil, and lemon juice. Pulse until very well combined. Season with salt.

4 Place the beets on a serving platter and sprinkle lightly with salt. Drizzle with the pesto and the olive oil, then sprinkle with the mint and parsley leaves. Serve immediately or refrigerate and serve chilled.

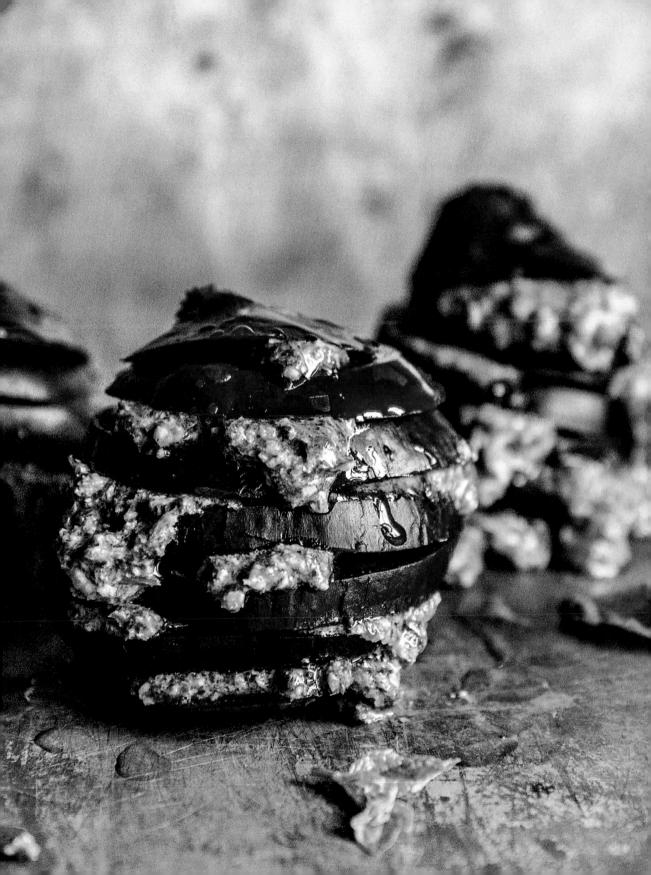

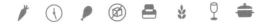

FRESH TOMATO SALAD
WITH BASIL-MINT VINAIGRETTE

PREPARATION 15 MINUTES   **COOK TIME** N/A   **SERVINGS** 4 TO 6

You just can't overrate a good tomato salad. This one, with a kiss of basil-mint vinaigrette, may replace your standard caprese salad. It's best made with heirloom tomatoes for their sweet intense flavor and their beautiful and diverse colors. This is a great dish for parties or potlucks since it can sit out at room temperature for several hours.

4 to 6 large tomatoes (preferably heirloom), cut into thick slices

Kosher salt

BASIL-MINT VINAIGRETTE

2 garlic cloves

1 cup lightly packed fresh basil leaves

¼ cup lightly packed fresh mint leaves

¼ cup olive oil

¼ cup red wine vinegar

Kosher salt

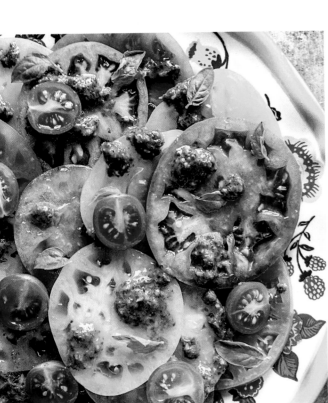

1 Arrange the tomato slices on a serving platter and sprinkle with salt.

2 To make the basil-mint vinaigrette: In a food processor, combine the garlic, basil, mint, olive oil, and vinegar. Pulse until you have a somewhat smooth sauce. Season with salt.

3 Drizzle the vinaigrette over the tomatoes and serve at room temperature.

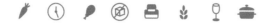

ASPARAGUS AND PEA SALAD WITH HONEY-SHALLOT VINAIGRETTE

PREPARATION 15 MINUTES   **COOK TIME** 10 MINUTES   **SERVINGS** 2 TO 4

This is the kind of salad I enjoy serving family-style as an addition to a light dinner, or even at brunch. The fresh, tender, crisp vegetables have delicate flavor, and the honey-shallot vinaigrette adds just enough subtle sweetness to complement but not overwhelm the rest of the salad. Using fresh peas is an integral and delicious part of the dish. If you don't want to shell your own, they are really easy to find already shelled at the grocery store. Trader Joe's carries them year-round. (Photograph on page 88.)

HONEY-SHALLOT VINAIGRETTE

2 tablespoons minced shallot

2 tablespoons honey

2 tablespoons rice vinegar

2 tablespoons vegetable oil

Kosher salt

SALAD

Kosher salt

1 pound asparagus, tough ends trimmed

1½ cups shelled green peas (about 1¼ pounds in the pod)

6 radishes, thinly sliced

Kosher salt

½ teaspoon poppy seeds

1 To make the honey-shallot vinaigrette: In a small bowl, whisk together the shallot, honey, vinegar, and vegetable oil. Season with salt.

2 Bring a large saucepan of salted water to a boil. Fill a large bowl with ice and water.

3 Slice the asparagus stalks into thirds lengthwise. Add half at a time to the boiling water and simmer them for about 2 minutes or until just tender. Immediately remove them from the simmering water and plunge them into the ice water to stop the cooking. Drain well. Repeat with the remaining asparagus.

4 Return the water to a boil and add the peas. Cook until they are bright green and float to the top, about 2 minutes.

5 Meanwhile, remove the asparagus from the ice water and set on a kitchen towel to dry.

6 Drain the peas and transfer them to the ice water. Let them cool, then drain the peas.

7 Gently toss the peas, asparagus, and radishes with the vinaigrette. Season the salad with salt and sprinkle with the poppy seeds.

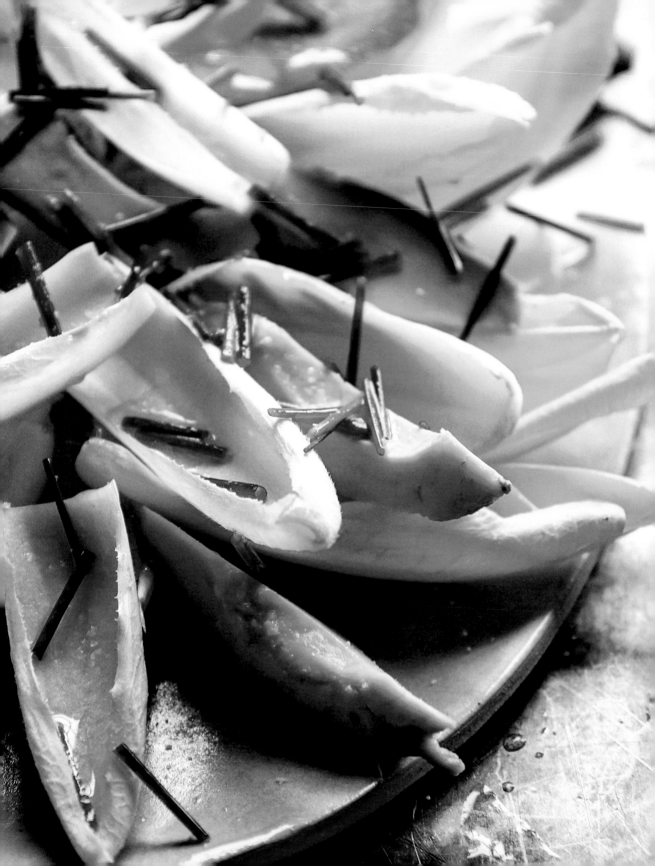

ENDIVE AVOCADO SALAD WITH LEMON, HONEY, AND CHIVE VINAIGRETTE

PREPARATION 15 MINUTES   COOK TIME N/A   SERVINGS 2 TO 4

Of all the complex and unusual salads in this book, this incredibly simple one is my mom's favorite. It's a sophisticated blend of crisp, slightly bitter endive and creamy, rich avocado. Fragrant chives and a lemony vinaigrette are the perfect complements. You can taste every component, and it is so fresh and light that it pairs well with just about anything.

SALAD

4 heads Belgian endive

2 ripe but firm avocados

Kosher salt

LEMON, HONEY, AND CHIVE VINAIGRETTE

¼ cup fresh lemon juice (from about 2 lemons)

¼ cup olive oil

2 tablespoons honey

⅓ cup 1-inch pieces fresh chives

½ teaspoon kosher salt

1 Separate the endives into individual leaves and place them in a large bowl.

2 Pit and peel the avocados and cut them lengthwise into eighths. Set the avocado slices on a plate and sprinkle with salt. Set aside.

3 To make the lemon, honey, and chive vinaigrette: In a small bowl, whisk together the lemon juice, olive oil, honey, and chives. Season with salt.

4 Very gently toss the endive with some of the vinaigrette. Transfer to a serving platter and add the avocado slices. Drizzle with more vinaigrette as desired and serve immediately.

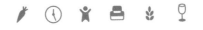

CARROT SALAD WITH CHILE-SESAME VINAIGRETTE

PREPARATION 20 MINUTES   COOK TIME N/A   SERVINGS 4 TO 6

This salad is so simple, but sometimes the simple things are the best. Like how the bright fresh flavors, colors, and textures of this salad just make me happy!

CHILE-SESAME VINAIGRETTE

1 red Fresno chile, minced

2 garlic cloves, minced

1 tablespoon agave or honey

3 tablespoons sesame oil

⅓ cup rice vinegar

Kosher salt

SALAD

2 pounds carrots, grated

Kosher salt

Toasted sesame seeds

Fresh chives, minced

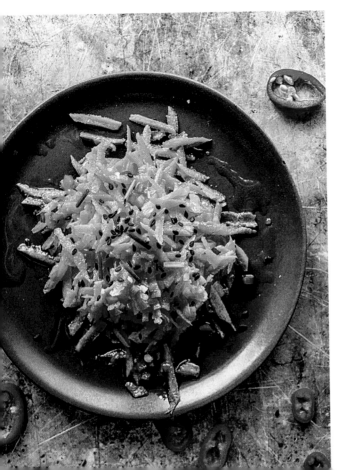

1 To make the chile-sesame vinaigrette: In a large bowl, whisk together the chile, garlic, agave, sesame oil, and vinegar. Season with salt.

2 Add the shredded carrots and toss to combine. Season with salt and serve sprinkled with sesame seeds and chives.

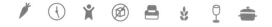

FRESH CORN AND MANGO SALAD

PREPARATION 10 MINUTES   **COOK TIME** N/A   **SERVINGS** 4 TO 6

The first time I ate raw corn, I was shocked at how sweet and delicious it was. The little kernels burst in my mouth with a perfect little *pop*! When you pair raw corn with sweet mango and lots of fresh herbs, sharp red onion, and spicy chile, you get a salad that is absolutely perfect as a side dish or topping for any kind of protein. Frankly, I could just eat this whole bowl with a spoon.

2 ears fresh corn, husked

2 fresh mangoes, peeled, pitted, and diced

½ yellow bell pepper, cut into small dice

½ orange bell pepper, cut into small dice

1 cup cherry tomatoes, halved

1 red chile, minced

½ red onion, cut into small dice

½ cup minced fresh cilantro

2 tablespoons rice vinegar

Grated zest of 2 limes

2 tablespoons fresh lime juice

1 tablespoon avocado oil or olive oil

Kosher salt

1 Use a sharp knife to cut the corn kernels from the cobs. Place in a large bowl.

2 Add the remaining ingredients to the bowl and mix well. Serve immediately or cover and refrigerate until ready to serve, up to 2 days.

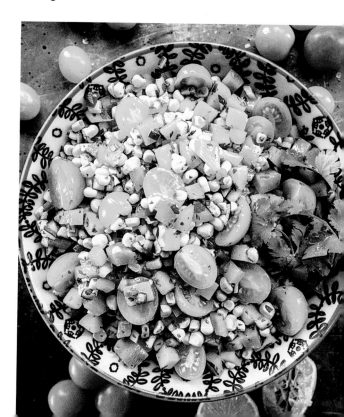

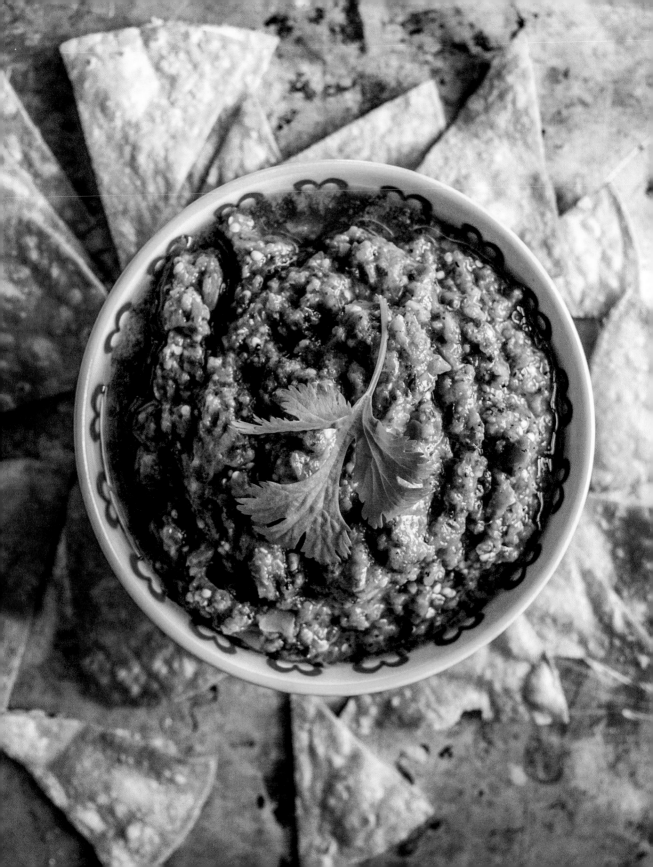

appetizers

....

The former caterer in me is fascinated by appetizers. And when you cook for guests, it's nice to put in some extra effort. In fact, I think I would take a whole dinner made up of appetizers over anything traditional on any given night. I like to set the mood with the appetizers by serving something that hints at the meal to come. That said, the portions should be small and light, so guests will have plenty of room for the delicious dinner ahead of them. And sometimes it's fun just to go for a big spread of appetizers, served up with cocktails.

Some of the recipes in this chapter could easily do double-duty as a light lunch, like the Steak Lettuce Tacos with Mango Cilantro Ginger Sauce or Mini Crispy Salmon Corn Cakes. And then there are the dips and the fresh summer rolls, all of which are snack staples in my refrigerator and keep me from going off the rails when I am starving.

◄ Oven-Roasted Spicy Green Salsa with Fried Tortilla Chips (page 131)

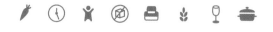

BEET HUMMUS

PREPARATION 10 MINUTES · **COOK TIME** N/A · **SERVINGS** 8

This hummus has all of the delicious versatility of the classic hummus, but it is so much more fun! It stops traffic both in looks and flavor. You would be amazed how many people who think they don't like hummus will try it (and love it) because it's pink (ahem, kids), or who think they don't like beets but will try it because it is hummus (ahem, sisters).

1 beet, boiled until fork-tender, peeled, and chopped

2 garlic cloves, minced

2 tablespoons tahini

1½ cups canned garbanzo beans, drained and rinsed

⅓ cup fresh lemon juice (from about 2 lemons)

½ cup olive oil, plus more for serving

Kosher salt

1 In a food processor, combine the beet, garlic, tahini, and garbanzo beans and pulse until the beans are well broken up.

2 Add the lemon juice. With the processor running, add the olive oil in a thin stream. Continue to run the food processor until the hummus is very smooth and creamy. Season with salt.

3 Transfer the hummus to a bowl and drizzle with olive oil. Serve immediately or refrigerate for up to 5 days.

BEETS are incredibly high in nutrients like potassium, magnesium, fiber, phosphorus, iron, and folic acid, as well as vitamins A, B, and C. They are also beneficial for liver health and have been known to help lower blood pressure. Also, beets can help you test your stomach acid levels (I find this fascinating!): If you pee pink after eating beets, your stomach acid levels are low and healthy.

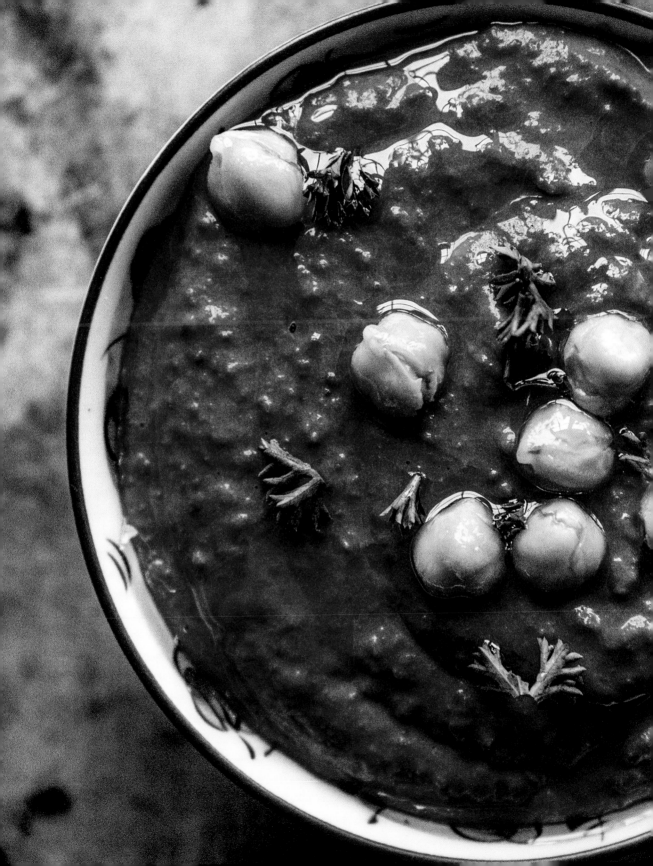

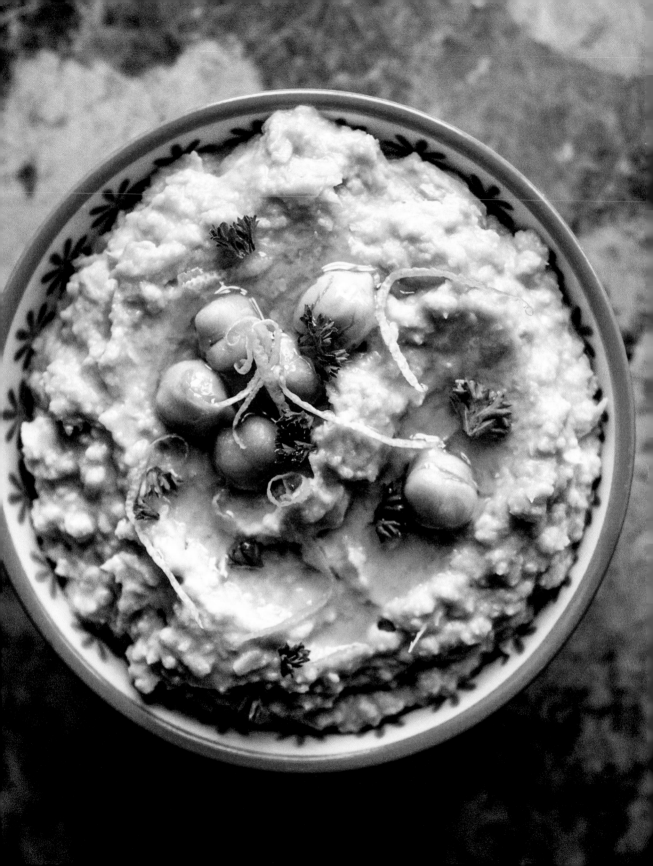

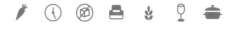

LEMON-ARTICHOKE HUMMUS

PREPARATION 10 MINUTES   COOK TIME N/A   SERVINGS 6

Big chunks of artichoke heart and fresh lemon contribute extra texture and zing to the classic hummus. Not only is it a great dip for fresh veggies, but I also really like it with falafel and slathered on Everything Crackers (page 187).

2 garlic cloves, minced

2 tablespoons tahini

1½ cups canned garbanzo beans, drained and rinsed

⅓ cup fresh lemon juice (from about 2 lemons)

½ cup olive oil, plus more for serving

1 cup frozen artichoke hearts, thawed, rinsed, and drained

Zest of 2 lemons

Kosher salt

1 In a food processor, combine the garlic, tahini, and garbanzo beans and pulse until the beans are well broken up.

2 Add the lemon juice. With the processor running, add the olive oil in a thin stream and continue to run the food processor until the hummus is very smooth and creamy. Add the artichoke hearts and lemon zest and pulse until chunky. Season to taste with salt.

3 Transfer the hummus to a bowl and drizzle with olive oil. Serve immediately or refrigerate for up to 5 days.

ARTICHOKES are good sources of fiber, folate, and vitamins C and K. Artichokes are number seven on the USDA's top-twenty list of antioxidant-rich foods!

GARBANZO BEANS, or chickpeas, are super high in fiber. Two cups of garbanzo beans fulfill your entire day's requirement of fiber and are a great source of many nutrients, like manganese, folate, and copper, as well as protein. They promote colon health and have the power to help regulate blood sugar.

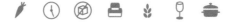

SMOKY RED PEPPER CHICKPEA DIP

PREPARATION 10 MINUTES   **COOK TIME** N/A   **SERVINGS** 6 TO 8

And yet another riff on hummus, this one packed with ultra-flavorful smoked paprika, sweet roasted red peppers, and a touch of zesty red wine vinegar. I could eat this with flatbread (page 184) for days and never get bored. (Photograph on page 7.)

2 garlic cloves, minced

2 tablespoons tahini

1½ cups canned garbanzo beans, drained and rinsed

¼ cup roasted red pepper pieces (packed in water), drained

1 teaspoon smoked paprika

¼ cup fresh lemon juice (from about 2 lemons)

1 tablespoon red wine vinegar

½ cup olive oil, plus more for serving

Kosher salt

1 In a food processor, combine the garlic, tahini, garbanzo beans, red pepper, and paprika and pulse until the beans and pepper are well broken up.

2 Add the lemon juice and vinegar. With the processor running, add the olive oil in a thin stream and continue to run the food processor until the hummus is very smooth and creamy. Season with salt.

3 Transfer the hummus to a bowl and drizzle with olive oil. Serve immediately or refrigerate for up to 5 days.

RED BELL PEPPERS are a major source of the antioxidant vitamin C, and good sources of vitamins B, A, and E, as well as fiber.

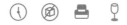

SALMON CEVICHE

PREPARATION 10 MINUTES   **COOK TIME** N/A   **SERVINGS** 2 TO 4

In Seattle, where I live, salmon is a mainstay, so I am constantly thinking up new ways to enjoy this amazing rich fish. In warmer weather, ceviche is one of the best and most versatile ways to eat it. I will make this and enjoy it for lunch (all by myself), but more often I serve it as an appetizer. Freshly sliced cucumbers and fried tortilla chips (page 131) both make nice accompaniments, but I have been known to pile it into tortillas for tacos, too.

8 ounces sashimi-quality raw salmon fillet

Zest of 2 limes

Juice of 1 lime

1 red Fresno chile, minced

⅓ cup small diced yellow bell pepper

⅓ cup small diced orange bell pepper

⅔ cup small diced ripe mango

½ cup finely chopped fresh cilantro

Kosher salt

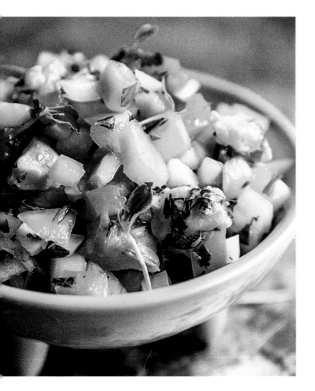

1 Remove the skin from the salmon and use pliers or your fingers to remove any bones. Cut the fish into small cubes. Place in a medium bowl.

2 Add the lime zest and juice, the chile, bell peppers, mango, and cilantro to the bowl with the salmon and toss gently to combine. Season with salt.

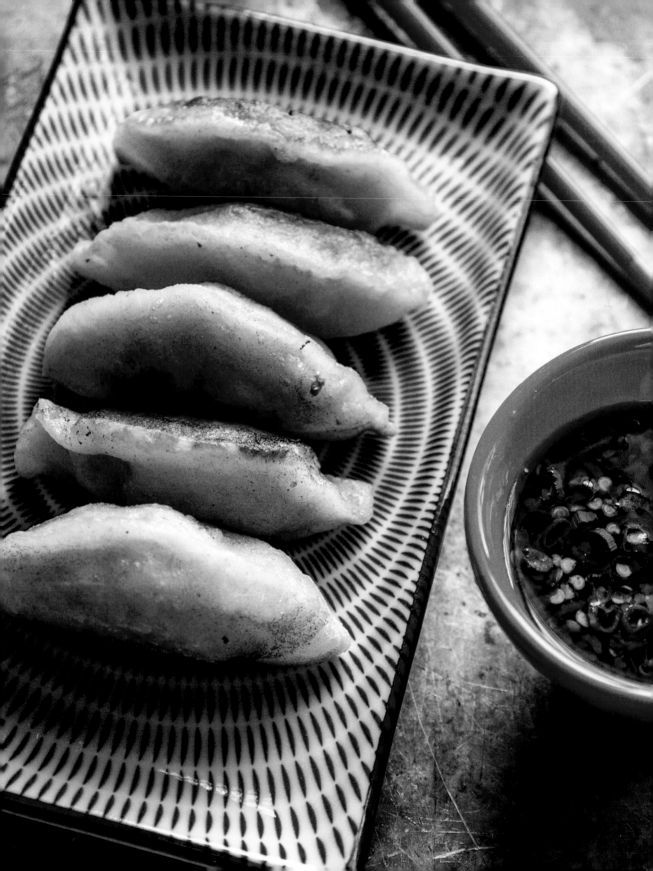

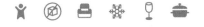

PAN-FRIED PORK POTSTICKERS WITH SWEET GINGER DIPPING SAUCE

PREPARATION 30 MINUTES   **COOK TIME** 20 MINUTES
SERVINGS 30 TO 40 POTSTICKERS; 6 TO 8 PER SERVING

When my daughter Coco first learned about her allergies, the foods she shed tears over were potstickers and doughnuts. I felt determined to find a way that she could still enjoy them. I'm not going to lie: these are labor intensive, but the results are wonderful. The dough is delicate, with a slight chewiness, and develops a wonderful seared crust when pan-fried. They are a great substitute for the wheat-based wonton wrappers that you find at the store. I always make a ton at once and freeze them for later use. We love these fried until crispy and dipped generously in the lightly sweet spiced dipping sauce. You can also add them to broth and vegetable-based soups for homemade wonton soup.

WRAPPER DOUGH

1¾ cups sweet white rice flour

½ cup tapioca flour

¼ cup potato starch

1 teaspoon xanthan gum (see page 34)

1 teaspoon kosher salt

1 cup boiling water

2 tablespoons vegetable oil

PORK FILLING

½ pound ground pork

1 (¾-inch) piece fresh ginger, peeled and minced

½ red Fresno chile, minced

2 garlic cloves, minced

1 green onion, minced

1 tablespoon coconut amino acids

1 tablespoon sesame oil

½ teaspoon kosher salt

1 tablespoon minced fresh cilantro

DIPPING SAUCE

2 tablespoons coconut amino acids

2 tablespoons rice vinegar

1 tablespoon sesame oil

2 teaspoons honey

¼ teaspoon crushed red pepper flakes

1 tablespoon finely minced green onions

• • •

¼ cup vegetable oil, for frying

1 To make the wrapper dough: In a food processor, combine the rice flour, tapioca flour, potato starch, xanthan gum, and salt and pulse to combine. Add the boiling water in a thin stream, then add the vegetable oil to make a wet dough.

2 Transfer the dough to a large resealable plastic bag. Press out the air and seal the bag. Set aside.

(recipe continues)

3 To make the pork filling: Rinse out the food processor bowl and add the filling ingredients. Pulse to make a well-mixed pastelike mixture.

4 Lightly flour your counter and a rolling pin with rice flour. Pinch off a small ball of dough, about half the size of a golf ball, and immediately seal the bag to keep the rest of the dough moist. Roll the dough into a ball with your palms and then use the rolling pin to roll the dough into a thin round. Use a 3-inch round cookie cutter to cut out a perfect dough circle.

5 Place a rounded teaspoon of filling in the center of the circle and fold the dough in half to enclose the filling. The filling should be neatly contained. Use a little water to adhere the edges of the dough, if necessary, then press with the tines of a fork to seal. Arrange the potstickers upright on a baking sheet to create a flat bottom with the sealed edge on top. Cover them with a damp cloth so the dough doesn't dry out and crack as you continue to roll and fill the dough. (At this point, the potstickers can be frozen for later use. I put them in resealable plastic bags with a sheet of wax paper or parchment paper between layers.)

NOTE: You may find it helpful to keep a small spray bottle of water handy to mist the dough and keep it moist while you are working with it. When it dries out, it tears easily.

6 To make the dipping sauce: Combine all the dipping sauce ingredients in a small bowl. Set aside.

7 In a heavy skillet or nonstick pan, heat 2 tablespoons of the vegetable oil over medium-high heat. When hot, add 5 or 6 of the potstickers.

(If you have a large pan, you can cook 8 to 10 at a time.) Fry the flat bottom for about 2 minutes, until they have a golden crust on the bottom, then add ¼ cup water to the pan. Immediately cover the pan and steam the potstickers for 2 to 3 minutes. Serve immediately with the dipping sauce or transfer to a warm oven while you fry additional batches, using the remaining 2 tablespoons of oil.

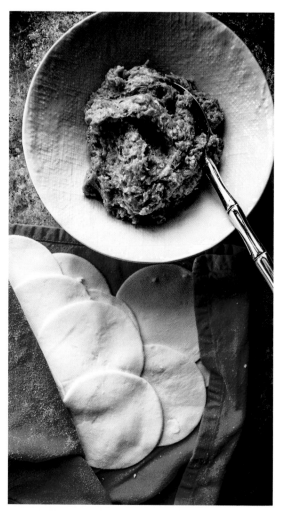

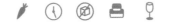

OVEN-ROASTED SPICY GREEN SALSA
WITH FRIED TORTILLA CHIPS

PREPARATION 10 MINUTES   **COOK TIME** 20 MINUTES   **SERVINGS** 4

As die-hard Seahawks fans, my husband, Pete, and I invite friends over for every football game during the season. Chips and salsa are a game-day staple. Homemade tortilla chips are always a hit, and when I fry them myself I know exactly what goes into them; many store-bought chips are not gluten-free. There are a few prepared salsas that I like, but I always make my green salsa from scratch—you just can't get anything like it. Seriously, *everyone* asks where I got it because it is just so good. It's really spicy; if you need it toned down, just use one jalapeño and seed your chiles. The seeds make the salsa spicier, so I leave them in. (Photograph on page 120.)

2 jalapeños, split lengthwise

2 Anaheim chiles, split lengthwise

1 poblano chile, split lengthwise

1 yellow onion, coarsely chopped

2 garlic cloves

3 cups quartered tomatillos

2 tablespoons vegetable oil, plus more for frying

1 cup packed fresh cilantro leaves and stems

Juice of 1 lime

Kosher salt

8 gluten-free corn tortillas, cut into eighths

1 Preheat the oven to 400°F.

2 On a rimmed baking pan, place the jalapeños, Anaheim chiles, poblano chile, onion, garlic, and tomatillos. Toss gently with the vegetable oil and roast for 25 minutes.

3 Transfer the roasted vegetables to a food processor and add the cilantro and lime juice. Purée on high until fairly smooth. Season with salt. Set aside or chill until ready to use. You can make this a day or two ahead of time, if desired, and refrigerate in an airtight container until ready to serve.

4 While the vegetables are roasting, in a heavy pot or skillet, heat 1 inch of vegetable oil until it registers 350°F to 375°F on a candy or deep-fry thermometer clipped to the side of the pot. Fry the tortillas, 8 pieces or so at a time, until they are golden brown and crisp. Transfer to a bowl and toss each batch with a little salt.

5 Serve the salsa with the hot chips.

STEAK LETTUCE TACOS WITH MANGO CILANTRO GINGER SAUCE

PREPARATION 20 MINUTES, PLUS 4 TO 8 HOURS MARINATING TIME

COOK TIME 8 MINUTES   SERVINGS 10

Few appetizers at my recent parties have received a warmer reception than this one. Many years of entertaining, both professionally and personally, have taught me that people love "do it yourself" anything. So with groups that know one another well, I like to serve this quite casually, with a big platter of fresh veggies and lettuce leaves next to the sliced steak and a bowl of sauce so people can just dig in and build their own tacos. If your group is a little less well acquainted or you are looking to make these more formal, you can certainly assemble them yourself and serve them premade on platters.

MARINADE

¼ cup coconut amino acids

2 tablespoons balsamic vinegar

2 tablespoons rice vinegar

3 tablespoons vegetable oil

¼ cup honey

4 garlic cloves, grated

2 teaspoons sambal oelek (Asian red chili garlic sauce)

2 tablespoons grated fresh ginger

1½ pounds flank steak

MANGO CILANTRO GINGER SAUCE

1 (2-inch) piece fresh ginger, peeled and thinly sliced

1 garlic clove

1 red Fresno chile, thinly sliced, with seeds

½ cup loosely packed fresh cilantro, leaves and stems

½ cup diced mango

3 tablespoons olive oil

3 tablespoons rice vinegar

Kosher salt

TO SERVE

10 large butter or bibb lettuce leaves

1 red bell pepper, seeded and julienned

2 carrots, julienned

2 green onions, julienned

1 red Fresno chile, seeded and thinly sliced

1 cup lightly packed fresh cilantro leaves and stems

½ cup lightly packed fresh mint leaves

1 In a bowl, whisk together the coconut aminos, vinegars, oil, honey, garlic, sambal, and ginger. Place the steak in a large resealable plastic bag, pour in the marinade, and seal. Refrigerate for at least a few hours and up to overnight.

2 Thirty minutes before you want to cook the steak, take it out of the fridge and let it come to room temperature.

3 Preheat the broiler. Line a rimmed baking sheet with aluminum foil and place the steak on the pan.

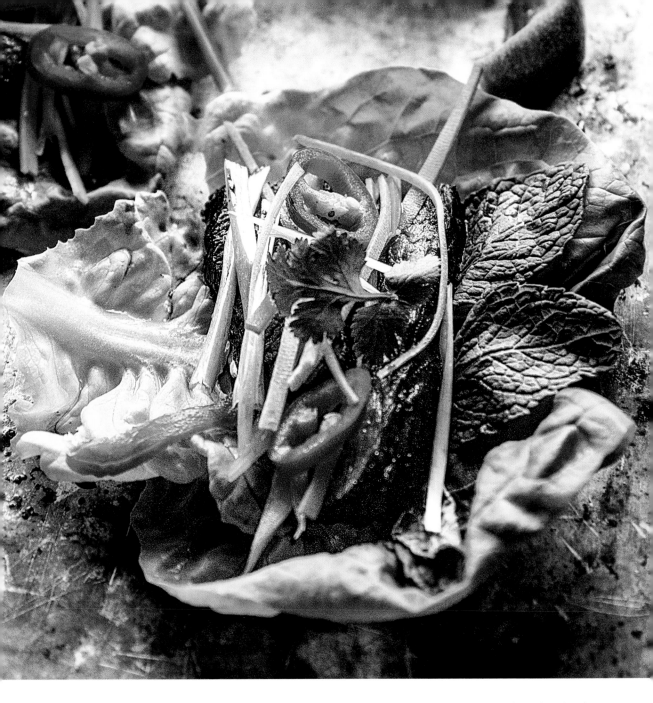

Broil the steak for 3 to 4 minutes on each side, then let the steak rest for at least 5 minutes.

4 To make the mango cilantro ginger sauce: Combine all the sauce ingredients in a blender and purée on high until smooth. Season with salt.

(You can make this sauce up to two days ahead and refrigerate until ready to use.)

5 Slice the steak across the grain. Pile some steak and condiments into each lettuce leaf like a taco and serve immediately.

SWEET AND SPICY APRICOT CHICKEN WINGS

PREPARATION 10 MINUTES   COOK TIME 15 MINUTES   SERVINGS 4 TO 6

These made several showings at our football tailgates this year, and I was told more than once that they were the best wings *ever*. The fried wings are crisp and juicy, and the sweet, sour, and spicy glaze is absolutely finger-licking good. Literally.

2½ pounds chicken wings (with tips)

1 cup all-purpose gluten-free flour

1 tablespoon kosher salt

Vegetable oil, for frying

SPICY APRICOT GLAZE

1 cup apricot preserves

¼ cup sambal oelek (Asian red chili garlic sauce)

¼ cup Dijon mustard

3 tablespoons red wine vinegar

• • •

1 red Fresno chile, thinly sliced, for garnish

1 Rinse the chicken wings with cold water and pat dry. Toss the flour and salt together on a plate or baking dish.

2 In a large heavy pot, heat several inches of vegetable oil until it registers 375°F on a candy or deep-fry thermometer clipped to the side of the pot.

3 While you are waiting for the oil to come to temperature, toss the chicken wings lightly in the flour and salt mixture to coat. You will probably have to do this in two or three batches.

4 When the oil is hot, carefully add the chicken wings, frying one-third of the wings at a time. Fry, stirring and flipping occasionally, for about 12 minutes, or until crisp and a deep golden

brown. Set aside to drain on a baking sheet covered with paper towels. (If you want to serve the wings all at once, you can keep the cooked wings hot in a 250°F oven.)

5 To make the spicy apricot glaze: In a medium saucepan, whisk together the apricot preserves, sambal, mustard, and vinegar until smooth. Cook gently over low heat until the jam has melted into the sauce, about 5 minutes. Season with salt, then transfer one-third of the sauce to a bowl and toss with the first batch of chicken wings until well coated. Repeat with the rest of the sauce and remaining batches of wings.

6 Sprinkle the wings with fresh red chiles. Serve immediately.

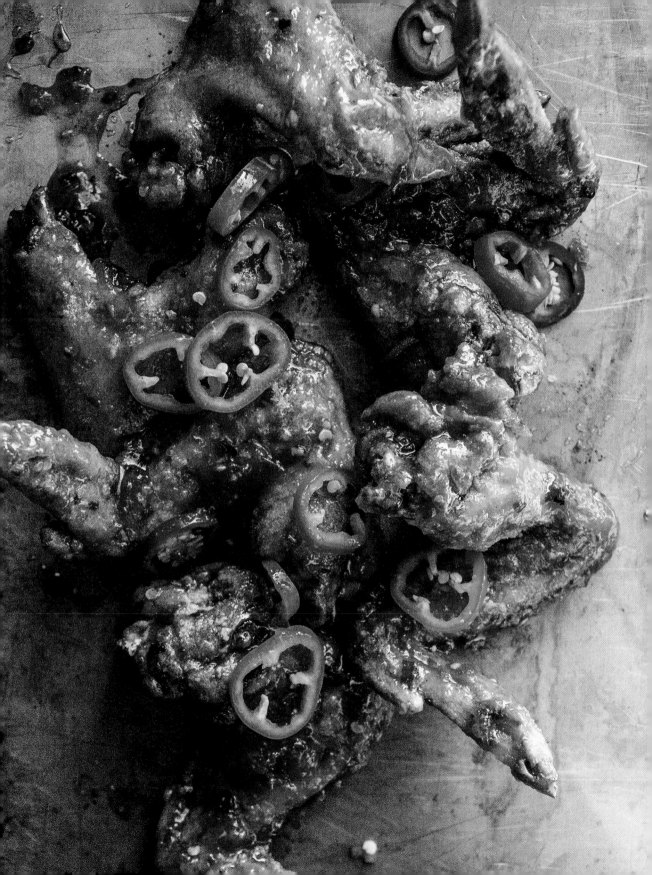

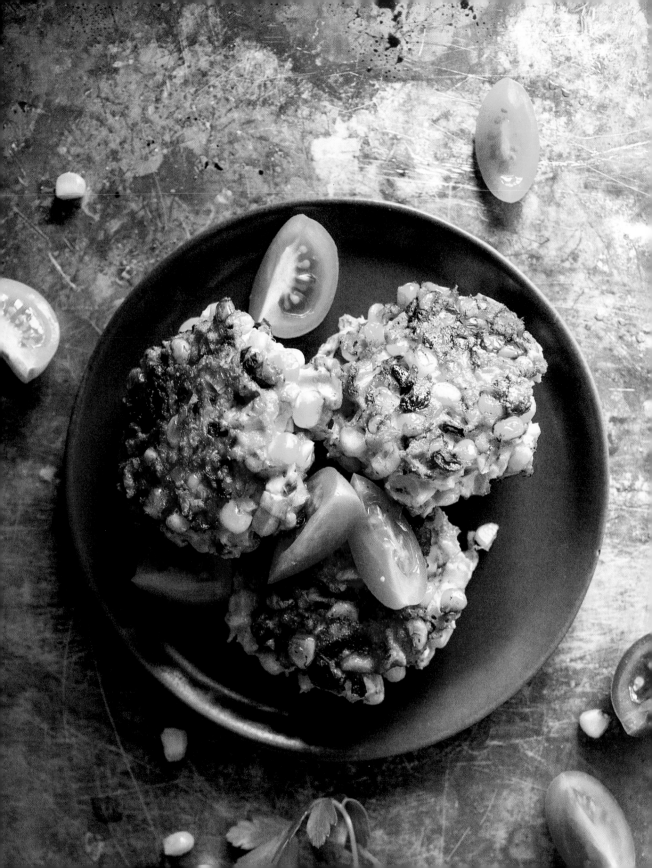

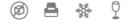

CRISPY SALMON CORN CAKES

PREPARATION 25 MINUTES **COOK TIME** 10 MINUTES **SERVINGS** 10 CAKES

The combination of fresh corn and salmon has always been a great one, but here they come together in a less traditional way—as little crispy cakes! The salmon blends beautifully with the green onions, garlic, and jalapeño for a little spicy kick, and then you also get wonderful little bursts of sweet, juicy corn. These make a great first course or light dinner over a bed of greens, but are also fantastic in miniature, passed as a hot appetizer.

1 pound salmon fillet, skinned and deboned

Zest of 2 lemons

Kernels from 2 ears corn

3 green onions, thinly sliced

½ jalapeño, seeded and minced

1 garlic clove, minced

2 tablespoons minced fresh flat-leaf parsley

½ teaspoon kosher salt

Vegetable oil, for frying

Mango Cilantro Ginger Sauce (page 132), for serving (optional)

Fresh tomatoes, for serving

1 Preheat the oven to 200°F.

2 In a food processor, combine the salmon and the zest of 1 lemon and pulse to make a paste. Transfer the salmon paste to a large bowl and add the remaining lemon zest, the corn kernels, green onions, jalapeño, garlic, parsley, and salt. Mix well. Using clean hands, form the mixture into 10 small patties.

3 In a large sauté pan, heat a thin layer of vegetable oil over medium heat. Add a few of the salmon cakes and cook for about 2 minutes, until the bottoms are golden and crispy. Flip the cakes and cook for a few minutes more, until the second side is also golden and crispy and the cakes are opaque in the center.

4 Keep the finished cakes warm in the oven while you fry the remaining cakes, but if you are planning to keep them warm in the oven before serving, then cook them for a few minutes less, as they can easily overcook.

5 Serve the salmon cakes warm with mango cilantro ginger sauce and a few fresh tomatoes on the side.

NOTE: Watch the cooking time carefully—it is easy to overcook the salmon!

ZUCCHINI CHICKPEA FRITTERS WITH RED ONION MARMALADE

PREPARATION 20 MINUTES **COOK TIME** 30 MINUTES **SERVINGS** 10

These soft and golden cakes are jam-packed with shredded zucchini and chickpeas, which makes them not only seriously tasty, but full of fiber and nutrients. But I have to say that the red onion marmalade is what makes these totally irresistible. The sweet and savory play on caramelized onions is just too good, and I find myself piling it on these cakes as high as possible!

RED ONION MARMALADE

1 tablespoon olive oil

1 large red onion, thinly sliced

Kosher salt

2 tablespoons red wine vinegar

2 tablespoons granulated beet sugar

ZUCCHINI CHICKPEA FRITTERS

1 (15-ounce) can garbanzo beans, drained and rinsed

½ yellow onion, finely diced

3 cups shredded zucchini

½ cup garbanzo bean flour

½ teaspoon kosher salt

Vegetable oil, for frying

1 To make the red onion marmalade: In a nonstick pan or heavy skillet, heat the olive oil over medium heat. Add the onion and sprinkle with salt. Stir and cook until tender and translucent, 5 to 7 minutes. Add 1 cup water and cook for 10 minutes more, until the onion is very soft and the water has cooked off. Add the vinegar and sprinkle the onions with the sugar. Stir well and cook for 2 to 3 minutes more, until the vinegar has cooked off completely. Season with salt and set aside.

2 To make the zucchini chickpea fritters: Preheat the oven to 375°F.

3 To a food processor, add the chickpeas and pulse until they are a thick paste. Transfer the beans to a large bowl and add the onion and zucchini. Use clean hands to mix well, then form the mixture into 10 cakes. Set aside.

4 On a plate, combine the garbanzo bean flour and the salt. Gently dredge each cake in the flour, patting it onto all sides of the cake.

5 In a heavy pan or skillet, over medium-high heat add enough vegetable oil to cover the bottom of the pan. Add 3 or 4 cakes at a time and cook for 2 to 3 minutes on each side, until the cakes are golden. Transfer the cakes to a rimmed baking sheet and bake for 10 to 15 minutes, until hot and a deeper golden color.

6 Serve hot, with the red onion marmalade.

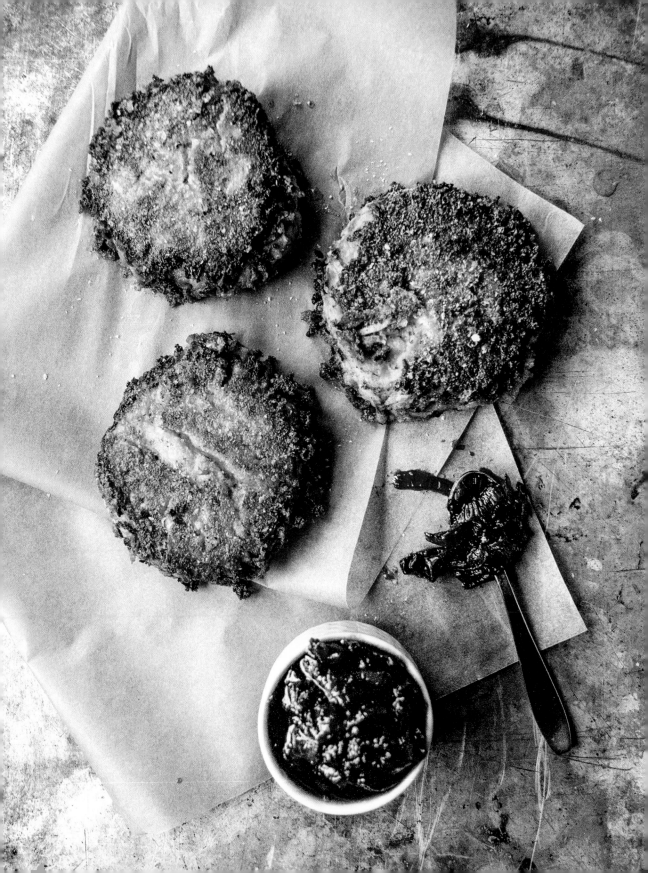

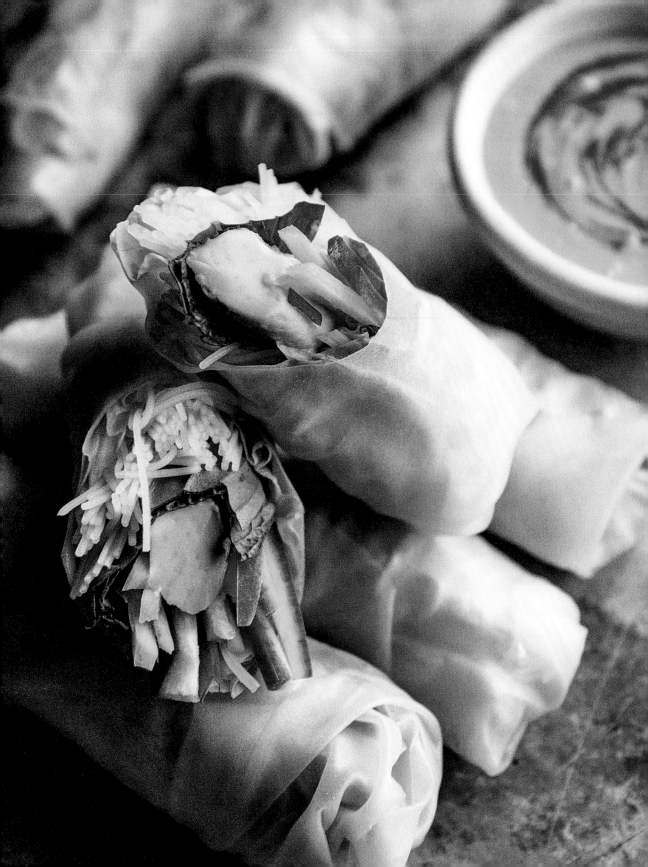

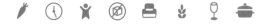

VEGGIE SUMMER ROLLS WITH SPICY SUNFLOWER BUTTER DIPPING SAUCE

PREPARATION 30 MINUTES   **COOK TIME** N/A   **SERVINGS** 12

These right here are Pia's most-requested snack. I guess I should feel lucky that she had an old favorite that missed the allergy boat—fresh summer rolls. She will order a dozen of these for herself at a Thai restaurant and swat other peoples' hands away, and does the same thing at home. But I love to make her happy with a big batch of these, and I also find them an easy and healthy "eat on the go" snack for me as well. If I keep a bunch in the refrigerator, I can grab one of these when I might be tempted to grab a cookie, and it takes the edge off my hunger.

SPICY SUNFLOWER BUTTER DIPPING SAUCE

1 red Fresno chile, minced, with seeds

2 garlic cloves, finely minced

2 tablespoons finely minced or grated fresh ginger

2 tablespoons thinly sliced green onion

2 tablespoons rice vinegar

2 tablespoons coconut amino acids

2 tablespoons sunflower butter

2 tablespoons Sriracha, plus more as needed

1 tablespoon sesame oil

½ cup unsweetened coconut milk

• • •

12 spring roll wrappers (Rose brand is easy to find and is made with rice and tapioca flour)

FILLINGS

3 cups cooked rice stick noodles

1 large avocado, sliced

½ cup julienned cucumber

½ cup julienned carrots

4 julienned green onions

2 red Fresno chiles, seeded and thinly sliced

½ cup loosely packed fresh Thai basil leaves

½ cup loosely packed fresh mint leaves

½ cup loosely packed fresh cilantro leaves and stems

1 To make the spicy sunflower butter dipping sauce: In a blender, combine all the sauce ingredients and purée on high until you have a smooth sauce. Season with extra Sriracha, if desired. Refrigerate until ready to use or for up to 3 days.

2 Fill a pie plate with hot water, put a rice paper wrapper in the water, and soak for 20 to 30 seconds, until soft and pliable.

(recipe continues)

3 Gently lay the wrapper on a work surface. In the center of the wrapper, place a smallish pile of the fillings of your choice.

4 Carefully fold the sides over toward the center of the filling so they cover half of your little pile on each side, then begin to roll the wrapper around the filling into a cigar shape. Pile the rolls on a platter as you finish them.

5 Serve immediately with the dipping sauce, or wrap the platter in plastic wrap up and refrigerate for up 24 hours.

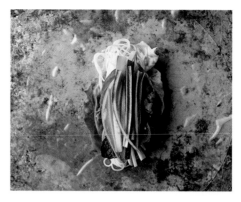

....

SUNFLOWER SEEDS have amazing levels of vitamin E, which is a major player in fighting inflammation and reducing the symptoms of asthma and arthritis. A quarter cup of sunflower seeds gives you 82 percent of your recommended daily vitamin E.

....

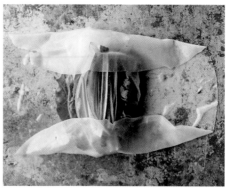

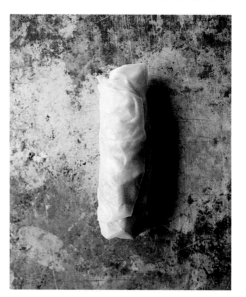

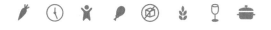

CASTELVETRANO OLIVE TAPENADE

PREPARATION 5 MINUTES   **COOK TIME** N/A   **SERVINGS** 6

I have always loved olive tapenade, but had never really strayed from a pretty traditional black olive version until my friend Betsy brought this beautiful green version to Thanksgiving dinner. It was such a simple change, but so amazing! Castelvetrano olives are my favorite olives by far—they are just so rich and buttery. Here they are combined with fresh garlic, red pepper flakes, and fragrant thyme, and the combination is absolutely fantastic.

3 garlic cloves

¼ teaspoon crushed red pepper flakes

¼ cup olive oil

2 cups Castelvetrano olives, pitted

½ teaspoon fresh thyme leaves

Place the garlic cloves and red pepper flakes in the bowl of a food processor. Pulse until the garlic is minced. Add the olive oil, olives, and thyme and pulse until the tapenade is well combined but still chunky. Transfer to a bowl and refrigerate until ready to serve.

CASTELVETRANO OLIVE extracts are known to have antihistamine effects and overall anti-inflammatory qualities.

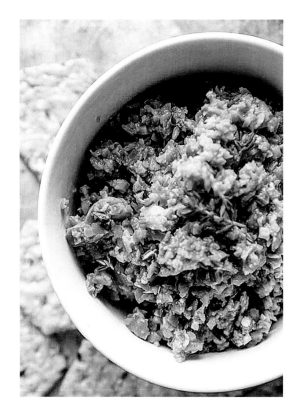

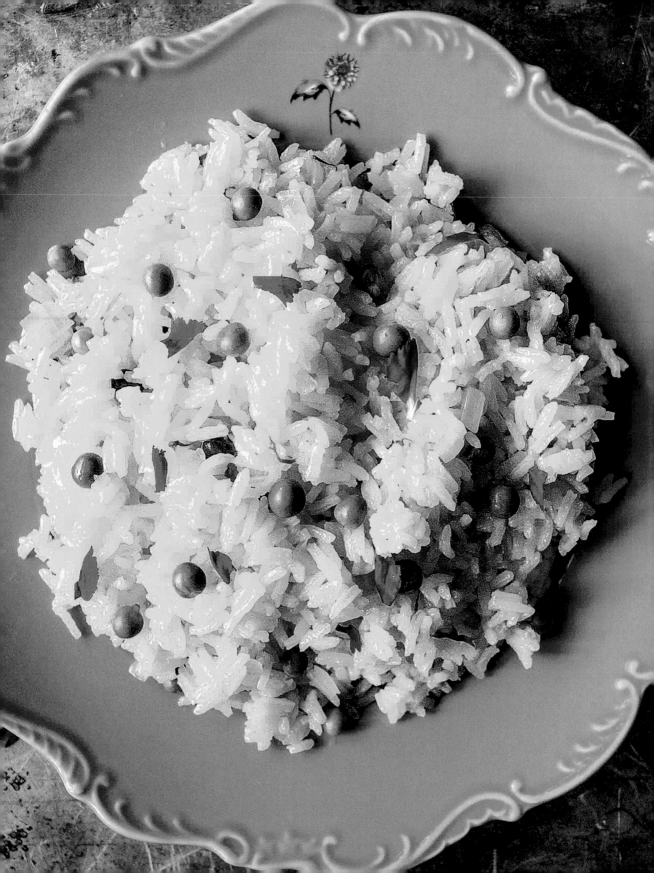

sides

....

Sides, in my opinion, are what *make* a meal come together. At restaurants I more often base my decision on which side dishes will be served with an entrée than on the entrée itself—there is so much personality and variety in these accompaniments that they help define the meal.

So with all these side dishes, I have kept the greater picture of a whole meal in mind. Each recipe, from Ginger Sunflower Butter Buckwheat Noodles to Mustard-Crusted Potatoes, notes which other dishes it pairs well with.

I think you will find everything delicious, from the "traditionals" (Creamy Mashed Potatoes) to the unusual (Gigantes, Greek-style white beans). There are new twists on classics, like Sweet Potato Salad with Bacon, and advice and recipes for how to make your own crispy french fries and authentic black beans. Enjoy the variety in dishes and flavors that will build the foundation for your meal.

◄ Saffron Rice with Peas (page 167)

ROASTED HONEY, HARISSA, AND BACON CARROTS

PREPARATION 10 MINUTES   COOK TIME 27 MINUTES   SERVINGS 4 TO 6

I love this dish so much. I am not usually the biggest fan of cooked carrots, but this totally changed my mind. I mean, when you are dealing with crispy bacon and spicy harissa paste mixed with sweet honey, it's hard to complain. And the beautiful colors of these rainbow carrots just made it all the more exciting to "eat with my eyes." A lovely side dish at any meal, and a great way to get people excited about eating their veggies!

3 bunches whole carrots
(I use rainbow carrots)

4 thick-cut uncured bacon
slices, finely chopped

2 tablespoons olive oil

1 garlic clove, minced

3 tablespoons harissa

3 tablespoons honey

Kosher salt

1 Preheat the oven to 400°F. Arrange the carrots on a rimmed baking sheet in a single layer and set aside.

2 In a heavy pan, cook the bacon over medium heat until the bacon is crispy and the fat has rendered, 5 to 7 minutes. Transfer the bacon to a bowl, leaving the rendered fat in the pan.

3 Add the olive oil, garlic, harissa, and honey to the pan with the bacon fat and whisk over medium heat to create a thick sauce, simmering for just 1 minute.

4 Pour the sauce over the carrots on the baking sheet. Toss the carrots to coat and then sprinkle with salt.

5 Roast the carrots for 20 minutes. Transfer to a serving platter and top them with all the sauce and little cooked bits still on the baking sheet. Sprinkle the carrots with the crispy bacon pieces and serve immediately.

GARLIC is not only highly nutritious, supplying us with great amounts of manganese, vitamin B6, C, and selenium, but it is also known to boost our immune system and have positive effects on blood pressure and high LDL cholesterol.

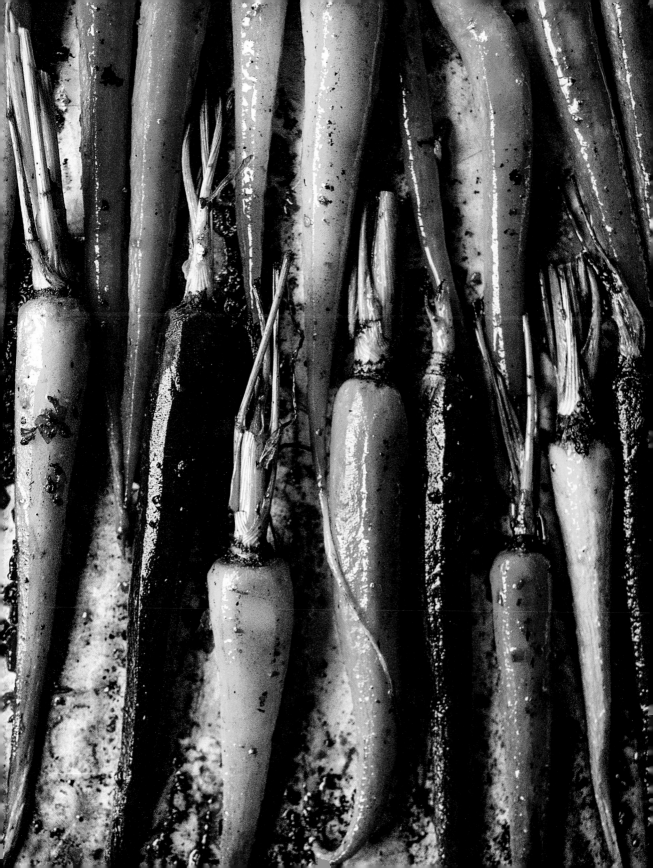

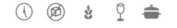

BRUSSELS SPROUTS WITH BACON, RED ONION, AND AVOCADO

PREPARATION 10 MINUTES   **COOK TIME** 20 MINUTES   **SERVINGS** 6

This has been a family favorite for years now, and it graces every cold weather holiday table as well as lots of Sunday dinners. It is an awesome twist on standard Brussels sprouts and bacon, if I do say so myself. I love the bite of the red onions and the creamy richness from the avocado, all drizzled with that sweet-sour balsamic vinaigrette. A must-try.

4 thick-cut uncured bacon slices

½ red onion, thinly sliced

Kosher salt

2 tablespoons plus 2 teaspoons olive oil

1 pound Brussels sprouts, trimmed and halved

¾ cup chicken broth

1 medium avocado, pitted, peeled, and cut into chunks

2 tablespoons balsamic vinegar

1 In a large nonstick saucepan, cook the bacon over medium heat until the bacon is crisp and the fat has rendered, 5 to 7 minutes. Drain the bacon on paper towels, leaving the rendered fat in the pan.

2 Add the red onion to the bacon fat and sprinkle with salt. Cook, stirring, until the onions are golden brown, about 5 minutes. Transfer to a small bowl.

3 To the same pan, add 2 teaspoons of the olive oil and the Brussels sprouts. Raise the heat to high and cook the sprouts for about 2 minutes, or until they are starting to brown and the pan looks dry. Add the broth and sauté the Brussels sprouts, uncovered, stirring often, until just tender and the broth has cooked off, about 5 minutes. Stir in the onions and season with salt.

4 Stir the bacon into the Brussels sprouts and then transfer to a serving dish. Arrange the chunks of avocado on top of the sprouts.

5 Mix the remaining 2 tablespoons olive oil and the vinegar together and drizzle over the dish. Serve warm.

BRUSSELS SPROUTS. All cruciferous vegetables contain glucosinolates, which offer cancer protection, but Brussels sprouts have the highest levels of all vegetables. They also have outstanding amounts of vitamin C, with just 1 cup providing 129 percent of your recommended daily value.

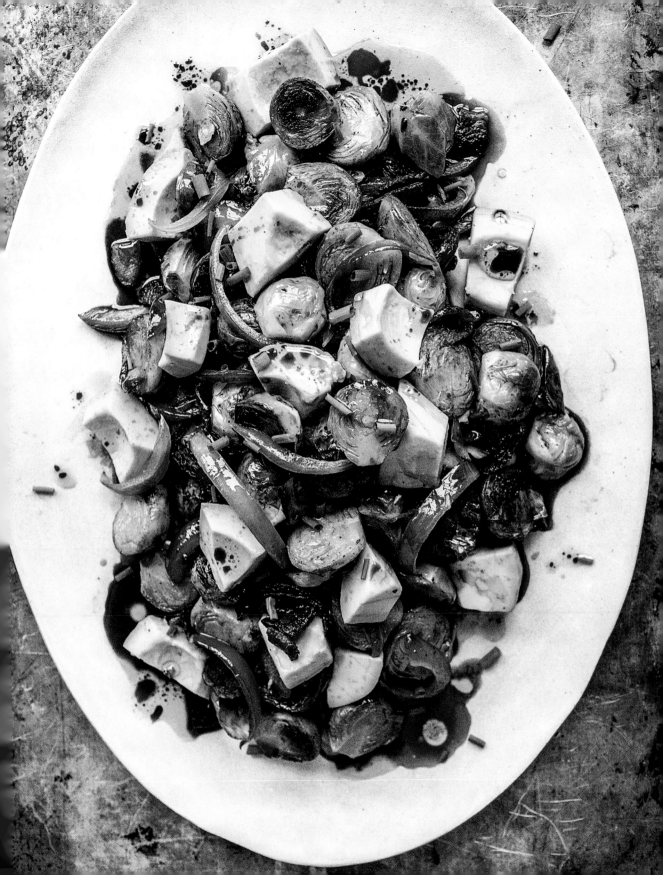

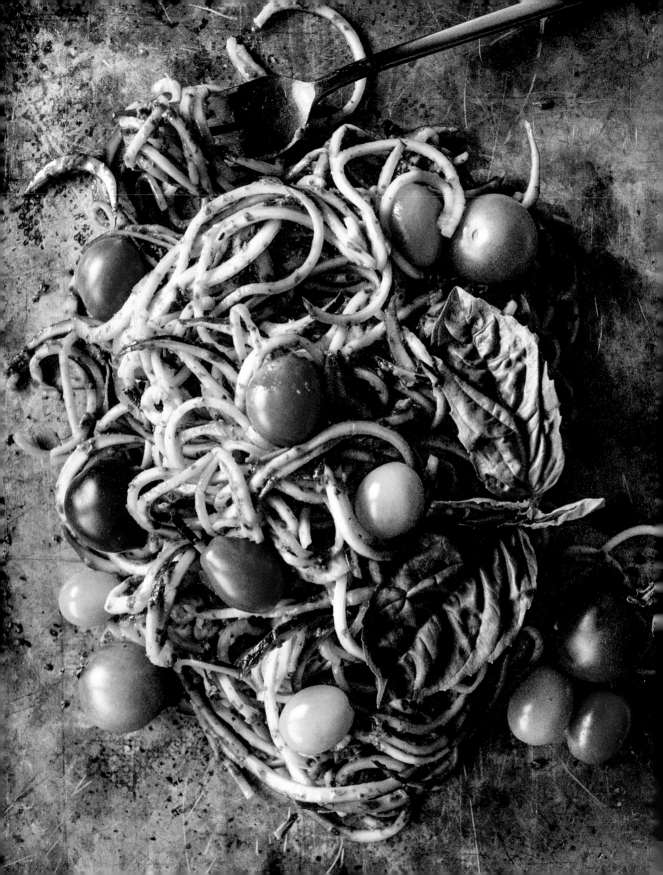

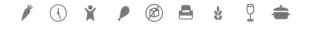

ZUCCHINI NOODLES WITH BASIL–PUMPKIN SEED PESTO

PREPARATION 20 MINUTES   **COOK TIME** N/A   **SERVINGS** 4

A few years ago I purchased a vegetable spiralizer that allows me to turn raw zucchini into noodles. It's incredible! Raw vegetable noodles that somehow manage to mimic the texture of real pasta and are essentially calorie-free are right up my alley. Aren't they up everyone's alley? And because you will be too busy digging in for second and third helpings based purely on the taste, you won't even think about the fact that you are consuming a raw, vegan dinner. When you add a handful of the sweet cherry tomatoes that will burst in your mouth with a bite of garlicky pesto noodles, you kind of have magic on your hands.

BASIL–PUMPKIN SEED PESTO

½ yellow onion, diced

1 garlic clove, thinly sliced

2 cups packed fresh basil leaves

½ cup pepitas, toasted

⅓ cup olive oil

2 teaspoons red wine vinegar

Pinch of crushed red pepper flakes

Kosher salt

ZUCCHINI NOODLES

3 large zucchini

Kosher salt

1 pint cherry tomatoes

Fresh basil leaves, for garnish

1 In a food processor, combine the onion, garlic, basil, pepitas, olive oil, vinegar, and red pepper flakes. Pulse until smooth and season with salt.

2 Run the zucchini through a vegetable spiralizer (or grate the zucchini the long way to make strands) and place the "noodles" in a large bowl. Toss the zucchini with the pesto until well coated. Season with salt.

3 Transfer to a platter and sprinkle with the cherry tomatoes. Tuck the fresh basil into the corners to garnish.

PUMPKIN SEEDS One quarter-cup of pumpkin seeds contains nearly half your daily amount of magnesium. They are also rich in zinc, which is important for your immune system health as well as helping to regulate your sleep, moods, and blood sugar. They are also thought to be one of the best plant-based sources for omega-3 fatty acids.

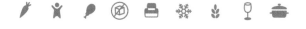

RED WINE MUSHROOMS

PREPARATION 10 MINUTES   **COOK TIME** 45 MINUTES   **SERVINGS** 4 TO 6

Mushrooms are one of the few vegetables that my children will eat happily. I'm not really sure how that happened, since they were an acquired taste for me, but I am not arguing. Instead, I try to find lots of ways to use them. This is a vegan play on one of our old favorite mushroom dishes, and it has a richness that lands it on our holiday tables these days. A touch of vegan butter gives the mushrooms a nice sweetness that complements the flavor of the red wine.

¼ cup olive oil

½ yellow onion, minced

8 cups quartered assorted mushrooms (I use cremini and chanterelle)

2 cups dry red wine

2 sprigs fresh thyme

2 tablespoons soy-free vegan butter

Kosher salt

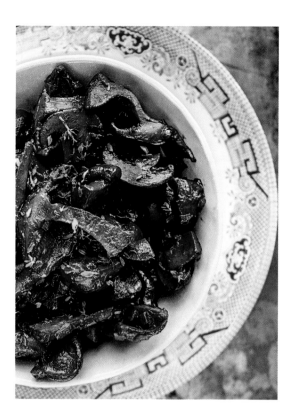

1 In a large heavy pan, heat the olive oil over medium heat. Add the onion and sauté until tender, 5 to 7 minutes. Add the mushrooms and stir well. Cook until the mushrooms are soft and tender, another 5 to 7 minutes.

2 Add the wine and deglaze the pan, scraping up any browned bits off the bottom of the pan. Add 1 thyme sprig and reduce the heat to low. Simmer, stirring often, until most of the liquid has cooked off, about 30 minutes.

3 Stir in the vegan butter and cook for 2 minutes more. Season with salt, then transfer to a serving bowl. Garnish with the leaves from the remaining sprig of thyme.

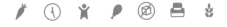

PAN-SEARED BROCCOLI WITH LEMON, CHILE, AND TOASTED GARLIC

PREPARATION 10 MINUTES   **COOK TIME** 7 TO 8 MINUTES   **SERVINGS** 4

Sometimes a really easy, basic recipe just happens to be incredibly delicious. This is one of those gems. When the flavor of toasted garlic teams up with broccoli hitting a seriously hot pan, you get a seared, slightly charred flavor that goes well with just about anything.

3 tablespoons olive oil

4 garlic cloves, thinly sliced

1 red Fresno chile, thinly sliced

6 cups broccoli florets

Zest and juice of 2 lemons

Kosher salt

1 In a large heavy pan or skillet, heat the olive oil over medium-high heat. Add the garlic and let it toast until the garlic slices are light golden (not dark or burning!), about 2 minutes. Use a slotted spoon to transfer the garlic to a plate, then raise the heat to high. When the pan is really hot, add the chile, broccoli, and lemon zest.

2 Cook the broccoli over high heat for 4 minutes. Add the lemon juice and toasted garlic, stir well, and cook for another minute, or until the broccoli is tender and slightly browned. Season with salt and serve hot.

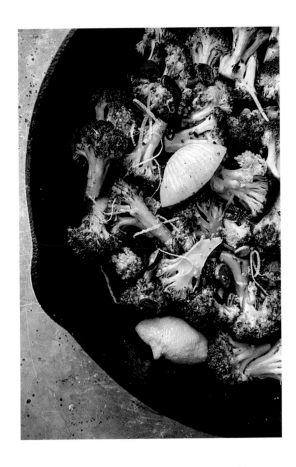

CREAMY MASHED POTATOES

PREPARATION 25 MINUTES   **COOK TIME** 15 MINUTES   **SERVINGS** 4 TO 6

The secret to making truly decadent mashed potatoes without dairy is coconut milk. Don't worry, these don't taste "coconutty" at all—they just have a wonderful rich and creamy texture. Plus, the Yukon Gold potatoes already have a buttery flavor, which is just enhanced by the coconut milk. I made these gloriously creamy, super-rich, and velvety mashed potatoes for my whole big family (who are sticklers for good mashed potatoes, by the way), and they had no idea that they were chowing down on "vegan" mashed potatoes. It was deeply satisfying to see the looks on their faces when I told them.

2¾ cups unsweetened coconut milk

2 pounds Yukon Gold potatoes, peeled and cut into bite-size pieces

2 garlic cloves, minced

1 teaspoon kosher salt, plus more as needed

5 tablespoons soy-free vegan butter, cut in large chunks, plus more for serving

Snipped fresh chives, for garnish (optional)

1 In a large pot, combine 2 cups of the coconut milk, the potatoes, garlic, and salt and bring to a simmer over medium heat. Reduce the heat to very low, cover the pot, and simmer for 15 minutes. The liquid should be almost completely absorbed into the potatoes.

2 Transfer the potatoes to the bowl of a stand mixer fitted with the paddle attachment and add the vegan butter and remaining ¾ cup coconut milk. Beat until light and fluffy. Season with salt. Garnish with more vegan butter and chives, if desired.

NOTE: I usually make these potatoes a day ahead of time and then store them in a baking dish. Cover the dish with aluminum foil and warm them in a 350°F oven for 20 minutes to reheat.

YUKON GOLD POTATOES One serving of these mashed potatoes has enough vitamin C for your whole day, twice as much vitamin C as regular russet potatoes. Yukon Golds are also a great source of potassium.

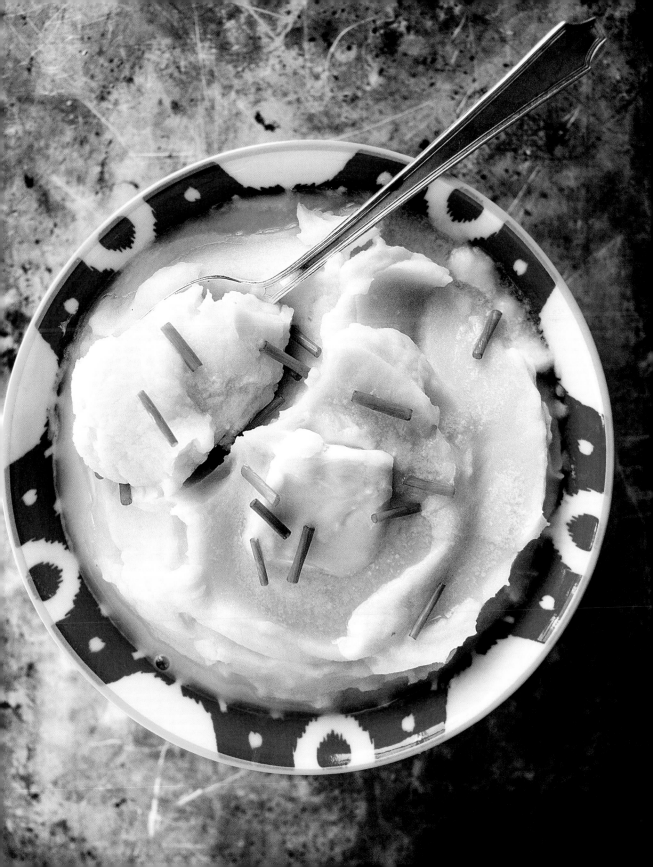

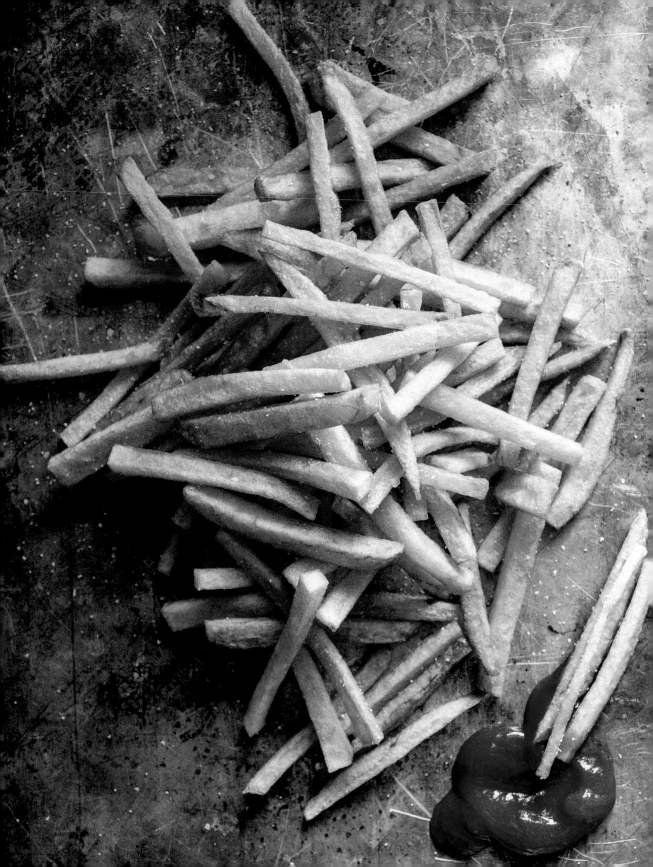

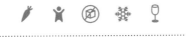

FRENCH FRIES

PREPARATION 30 MINUTES   **COOK TIME** 20 MINUTES   **SERVINGS** 4 TO 6

....

What can I say? French fries are a real problem for me. By which I mean, once I start eating them, it's hard for me to stop. When I realized how many food vices I had to swear off after discovering my allergies, my obsession with the remaining few seemed to become stronger than ever. French fries definitely fall into that category, and none are better than the ones I makes at home. I love skinny fries best, but occasionally I will thick-cut them (like when we make fish and chips, page 269). Either way, they are generally devoured straight from the fryer around here.

¼ cup distilled white vinegar

2 tablespoons kosher salt, plus more as needed

3 pounds russet potatoes

2 quarts canola oil

1 Fill a pot with 2 quarts water and add the vinegar and salt.

2 Peel the potatoes and place them in a bowl of water to keep them from browning. Slice the potatoes into thin or thick fries, as you prefer, dropping the fries directly into the pot as you cut them. Bring the water to a boil over high heat. Boil for 6 minutes; the potatoes should be tender, but not falling apart.

3 Drain the fries and spread them on a paper towel–lined rimmed baking sheet. Allow them to dry for at least 5 minutes and blot them with a paper towel to make sure they are really quite dry before they are fried.

4 In a 5-quart Dutch oven, heat the oil until it registers 400°F on a candy or deep-fry thermometer clipped to the side of the pot.

5 When the oil is hot, add a quarter of the fries to the pot. The oil temperature should not drop below 350°F, so adjust the heat as needed until it returns to 400°F. Cook for 60 to 90 seconds, until light golden brown, stirring occasionally with a spider strainer or slotted spoon. Transfer to a dry paper towel–lined rimmed baking sheet.

6 Cook the remaining potatoes in three more batches, making sure the oil returns to 400°F after each addition. Allow the potatoes to cool to room temperature, about 15 minutes.

7 Return the oil to 400°F over high heat. Working in batches, fry the fries a second time until crisp and light golden brown, 2 to 3 minutes, adjusting the heat to keep the temperature around 350°F to 375°F. Transfer to a bowl lined with paper towels and season immediately with salt. The cooked fries can be kept hot and crisp on a wire rack set on a baking sheet in a 200°F oven. Serve immediately.

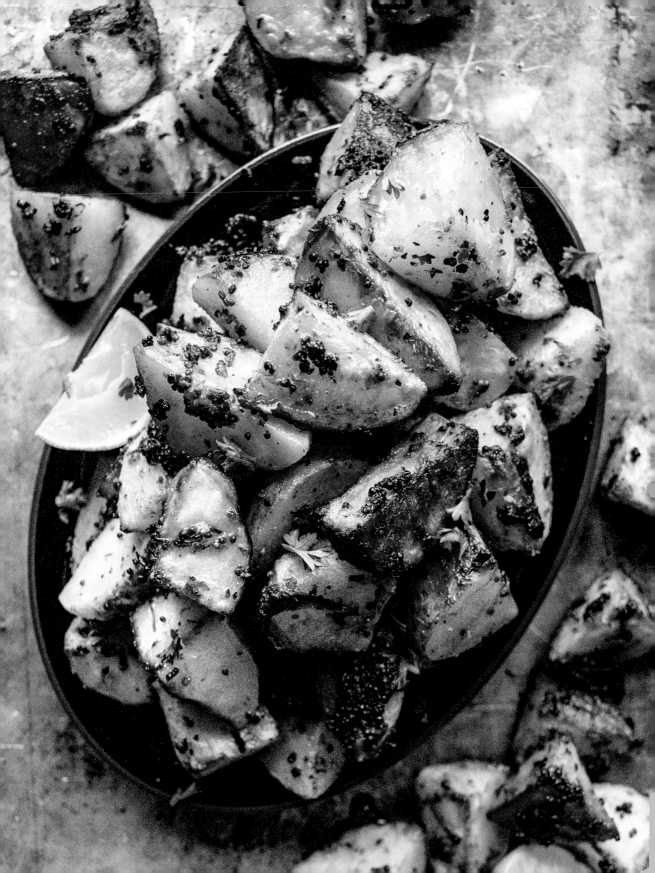

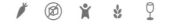

MUSTARD-CRUSTED POTATOES

PREPARATION 20 MINUTES   **COOK TIME** 45 MINUTES   **SERVINGS** 4 TO 6

This is a great side dish for a couple of reasons: it's the perfect match for just about any type of protein, and it is so easy to make. You just toss the potatoes with the super-strong mustard sauce and throw it in the oven, then worry about the rest of dinner for 30 minutes. After a quick shake, they are back in for another 15 minutes to roast to a gorgeous golden brown—just enough time to enjoy a glass of wine and get the rest of the dinner on the table.

⅓ cup olive oil

⅓ cup Dijon mustard

⅓ cup whole-grain mustard

Grated zest and juice of 2 lemons

4 garlic cloves, minced

6 Yukon Gold potatoes, peeled and quartered (about 6 cups)

Kosher salt

½ fresh lemon, cut into wedges

Minced fresh flat-leaf parsley, for garnish

1 Preheat the oven to 400°F.

2 In a large bowl, whisk together the olive oil, mustards, lemon zest, lemon juice, and garlic. Add the potatoes and toss to coat with the mixture.

3 Spread the potatoes on a rimmed baking sheet and sprinkle generously with salt.

4 Bake for 30 minutes. Toss the potatoes, return to the oven, and bake for 15 minutes more, or until the potatoes are a deep golden brown and fork-tender.

5 Transfer the potatoes to a serving platter, squeeze the fresh lemon wedges over them, and sprinkle with parsley. Serve hot.

MUSTARD SEEDS are extremely high in selenium and magnesium, both of which have strong anti-inflammatory properties and are known to help with everything from muscle and arthritis inflammation to asthma and chest colds. They are also high in vitamins A, C, and K, and niacin, thiamine, and folates, which are supposed to really rev up the metabolism!

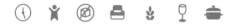

SWEET POTATO SALAD WITH BACON

PREPARATION 15 MINUTES   **COOK TIME** 15 MINUTES   **SERVINGS** 4 TO 6

I love potato salad, but I hate mayonnaise—even before I found out I was allergic to it—so I've always gravitated toward German-style potato salads with a mustardy dressing. This one gets gorgeous color and crunch from sweet potatoes, celery, and a bit of bacon. Serve this at your next backyard BBQ and *no one* will be missing the goopy white old-fashioned potato salad.

SALAD

Kosher salt

3 large sweet potatoes, peeled and cut into chunks

4 uncured bacon slices

1 cup thinly sliced celery hearts

1 cup thinly sliced green onions

MUSTARD VINAIGRETTE

1 red Fresno chile, seeded and minced

2 tablespoons whole-grain mustard

2 garlic cloves, minced

¼ cup rice vinegar

¼ cup olive oil

Kosher salt

1 Bring a medium-large pot of salted water to a boil. Add the sweet potatoes and simmer until just fork-tender, about 15 minutes. Drain the potatoes and briefly and gently rinse them with cold water. Set aside.

2 Cook the bacon slices until crisp. Drain on paper towels then crumble into a large bowl. Add the celery and green onions.

3 To make the mustard vinaigrette: In a small bowl, whisk together the chile, mustard, garlic, vinegar, and olive oil. Season with salt.

4 Add the sweet potatoes to the bacon, celery, and green onions and toss with the mustard vinaigrette. Season with salt. Serve warm or at room temperature, or refrigerate and serve chilled.

SWEET POTATOES are one of nature's best sources of vitamin A and a great source of vitamin C. One 8-ounce sweet potato will give you 100 percent of your recommended daily vitamin A. If you consume a little fat with the sweet potatoes (like the olive oil in the recipe here), it helps your body utilize all the vitamin A even more efficiently.

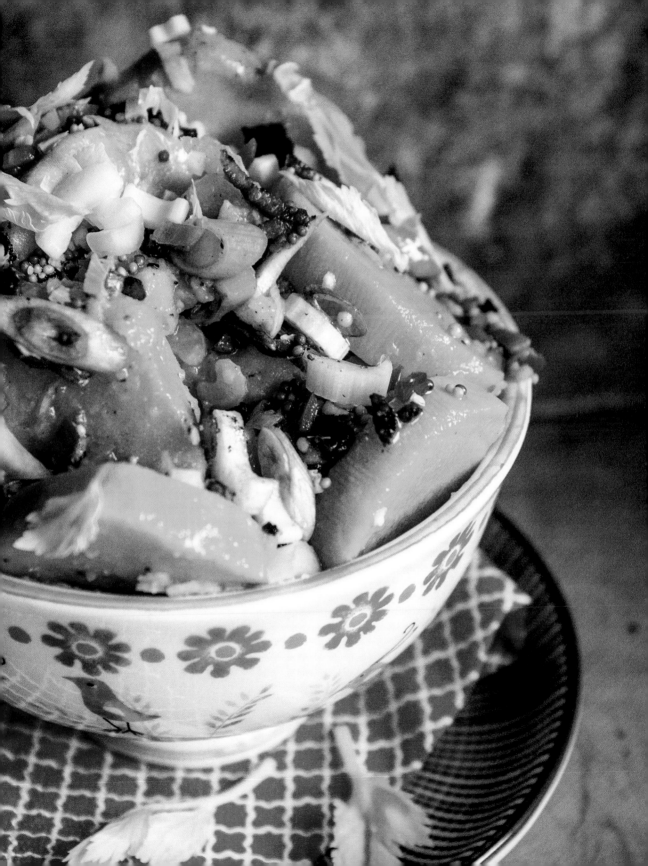

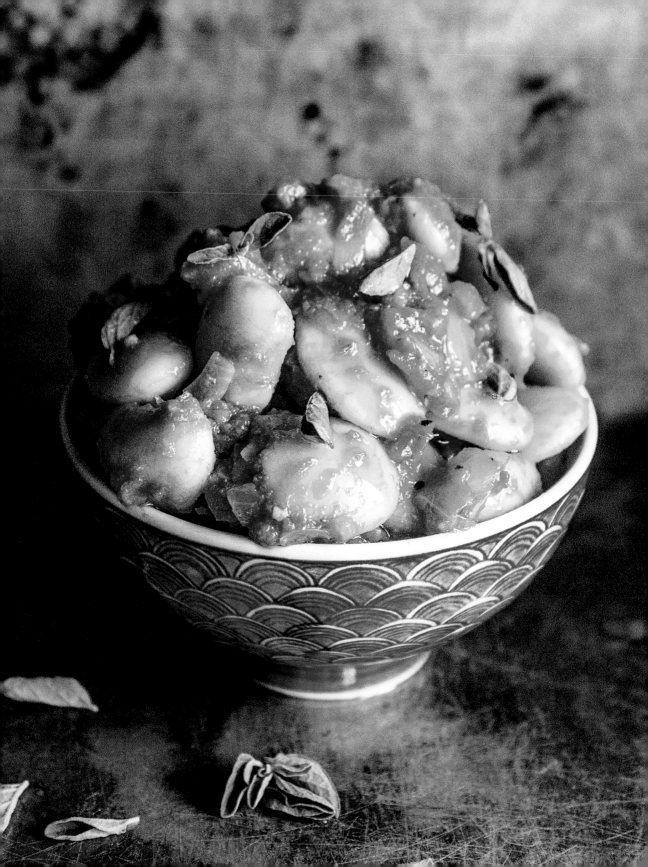

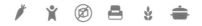

GIGANTES (GREEK-STYLE WHITE BEANS)

PREPARATION 15 MINUTES   **COOK TIME** 6 HOURS   **SERVINGS** 4 TO 6

My mother-in-law, Tula, has introduced me to so much amazing Greek food over the years, and one dish I absolutely adore is *gigantes*, so named for the giant white beans that are the main ingredient. As with all good Greek food, the dish features an abundance of olive oil, garlic, and intense flavor! It's definitely an all-day project, but luckily, you just check on the beans from time to time to make sure they don't need more water added (you don't want them to get dry!). When you finally take them from the oven, the beans will be tender and the sauce will reflect the savory goodness of slow cooking.

1 pound dried gigante or corona beans

½ cup olive oil, plus more for drizzling

1 yellow onion, cut into small dice

4 garlic cloves, minced

1½ cups very finely chopped carrots (you can do this in the food processor)

1 (28-ounce) can crushed tomatoes

2 teaspoons dried oregano

¼ teaspoon crushed red pepper flakes

Kosher salt

1 Preheat the oven to 350°F.

2 Put the dried beans in a medium pot and add water to cover. Bring to a boil over medium-high heat. Reduce the heat to medium and boil the beans for 30 minutes.

3 While the beans are cooking, in a heavy saucepan, heat the olive oil over medium heat. Add the onion and sauté until tender, 5 to 7 minutes. Add the garlic and carrots and sweat for a few minutes more.

4 Add the tomatoes, oregano, and red pepper flakes and stir to combine. Simmer the sauce over low heat for 20 minutes. Season with salt.

5 Drain the beans and rinse with cool water. Add them to the sauce. Gently fold the beans into the sauce, transfer the mixture to a 9 × 13-inch baking dish, and add 1 cup water. Place the dish on a rimmed baking sheet and cover the dish with aluminum foil.

6 Bake the beans for 1 hour, then carefully remove the baking dish from the oven, uncover, and add another cup of water. Stir the beans, replace the foil, and bake for 2 hours more. Repeat the process, adding another cup of water, stir and recovering, and cook for 2 hours more, for 5 hours in total.

7 Season the beans with salt, drizzle with olive oil, and serve hot.

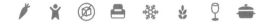

RESTAURANT-STYLE BLACK BEANS

PREPARATION 5 MINUTES   **COOK TIME** 4 HOURS   **SERVINGS** 10 TO 12

I had tried many times to make black beans the "real" way (that is, not simply opening a can), but they always turned out hard and somehow not quite right. Then my Oaxacan friend Lilly showed me the right techniques, including the correct amount of salt, the addition of the fried onion, and the proper cooking time. Now they are a weekday staple. Homemade beans are significantly more delicious than the canned variety, and are also a gateway drug to lots of tasty dishes like Shredded Beef Tostadas (page 255), which will be even better when you include these beans! This recipe makes a huge batch, but you can freeze any leftovers. However, you may be be shocked by how quickly these beans go.

2 pounds dried black beans

4 teaspoons kosher salt, plus more as needed

¼ cup vegetable oil

½ yellow onion, minced

1 Pick through the beans (sometimes there are rocks in there!), then rinse and drain them. Put the beans in a large heavy pot and add enough water to cover them by a couple of inches. Add the salt, cover the pot, and turn the heat to medium-low.

2 After 40 minutes, add 3 cups water, or enough to bring the water back to its original level, covering the beans by about 2 inches. Cook for 2 hours more, then add another cup of water and reduce the heat to low. Cook for 60 to 90 minutes more. The beans should simmer for about 4 hours total.

3 When the beans have been cooking for about 3 hours, heat the vegetable oil in a small pan over medium-high heat. Add the onion and cook until golden and translucent, 5 to 7 minutes. Stir the onion and the oil into the beans, cover, and keep simmering to the 4-hour mark. They should be a little "soupy" and tender. Season with salt and serve hot.

MEXICAN RICE

PREPARATION 5 MINUTES **COOK TIME** 35 MINUTES **SERVINGS** 4 TO 6

My kids would happily live on beans and rice, so I really wanted to get this right. To keep the rice from becoming gummy, the key is using enough oil and not too much liquid. Serve this with homemade black beans (page 164) and Chicken Tacos with Cilantro Pesto (page 244) or Spicy Roasted Vegetable Enchiladas (page 272).

¼ cup vegetable oil

1 onion, finely diced

3 teaspoons kosher salt, plus more as needed

1 jalapeño, seeded and minced (optional)

3 garlic cloves, minced

2 cups basmati or other long-grain white rice

3 cups vegetable or chicken broth

½ cup canned tomato purée

1 In a large sauté pan, heat the vegetable oil over medium heat. Add the onion and a ½ teaspoon of the salt and sauté, stirring often, for 5 minutes. Add the jalapeño and garlic and sauté until the onion is very soft and the garlic is tender, 5 minutes more.

2 Add the rice and the remaining 2½ teaspoons salt and stir well. Cook for 1 minute. Add the chicken broth and the tomato purée, stir well, and cook for another minute. Cover the pan, reduce the heat to low, and simmer for 15 minutes. Remove the pot from the heat and let the rice stand, covered, for 5 minutes. Uncover the rice and fluff with a fork. Season with salt.

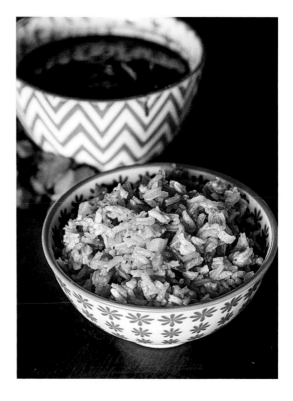

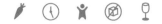

COCONUT-CILANTRO RICE

PREPARATION 2 MINUTES   COOK TIME 17 MINUTES   SERVINGS 4 TO 6

A triple shot of coconut—coconut oil, shredded coconut, and coconut milk—amps up the flavor and texture of basic white rice to make it more complex and delicious. The green onions and generous amounts of cilantro are not only flavorful but create an interesting mix of sweet and savory. It's best served with a spicy dish like a chicken or vegetable curry or Asian Pulled Pork (page 245).

¼ cup coconut oil

1 yellow onion, cut into small dice

2 cups jasmine rice

⅔ cup unsweetened shredded coconut

2½ cups unsweetened coconut milk

1 tablespoon kosher salt

1 finely chopped green onion

⅔ cup finely chopped fresh cilantro stems and leaves

Zest of 3 limes

Toasted unsweetened coconut flakes, for garnish (see Note)

1 In a large sauté pan, melt the coconut oil over medium heat. Add the onion and sauté for 5 minutes, until the onion is tender and soft but not browned. Add the rice and shredded coconut and stir for 1 minute.

2 Add the coconut milk and salt and bring to a simmer. Cover the pan and reduce the heat to low. Simmer the rice for 15 minutes. Remove from the heat and add the green onion, cilantro, and lime zest; fluff the rice with a fork. Serve hot, garnished with toasted coconut flakes.

NOTE: To toast the coconut flakes, preheat the oven to 350°F. Spread the coconut on a rimmed baking sheet and bake for 7 to 8 minutes, or until lightly golden.

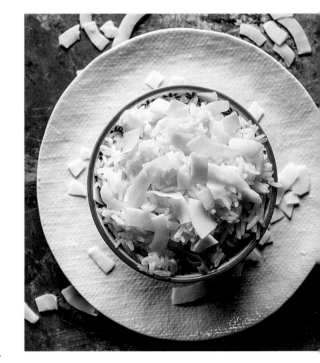

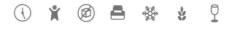

SAFFRON RICE WITH PEAS

PREPARATION 5 MINUTES   **COOK TIME** 25 MINUTES   **SERVINGS** 4 TO 6

Sometimes you just want a more flavorful (and in this case, visually exciting) bowl of rice! The gorgeous color *and* a bit of Spanish flair come from just a pinch of saffron and some green peas. Serve big scoops of this with anything from Ginger-Maple Roasted Pork Tenderloin with Mango Chutney (page 248) to Beef Stew (page 258).

4 cups chicken broth

Large pinch of saffron threads

5 tablespoons olive oil

½ yellow onion, finely diced

2 cups long-grain white rice

2 teaspoons kosher salt, plus more as needed

½ cup shelled green peas (about ¾ pound in the pod)

1 In a saucepan, combine the chicken broth and saffron and bring to a simmer over medium heat. Remove from the heat and set aside.

2 In a large sauté pan, heat 4 tablespoons of the olive oil over medium heat. Add the onion and cook until soft and translucent, about 5 minutes.

3 Add the rice and salt and stir. Add the saffron-infused broth and stir to combine. Cover the

pan and cook the rice for 15 minutes. Add the peas, cover the pot, and cook for 5 minutes more. Remove from the heat and let stand, covered, for 5 minutes.

4 Drizzle the rice with the remaining 1 tablespoon olive oil and fluff with a fork. Season with salt and serve immediately.

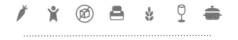

QUINOA TABBOULEH

PREPARATION 10 MINUTES   **COOK TIME** 30 MINUTES   **SERVINGS** 4 TO 6

Mamnoon is one of our favorite restaurants in Seattle. It serves amazing Lebanese food and is incredibly conscientious about food allergies. Mamnoon was the first place I tasted tabbouleh made with quinoa instead of bulgur wheat, and it was love at first bite. I've since re-created it at home, and we enjoy it often. It also happens to be the perfect side to make ahead of time for a party—it keeps well in the refrigerator and gets more delicious as it rests. I also like to eat this scooped into romaine heart leaves as an appetizer.

½ cup dry white wine or vegetable or chicken broth

1 teaspoon kosher salt, plus more as needed

1 cup white quinoa, rinsed and drained

3 Roma (plum) tomatoes, seeded and cut into small dice

1 cup small diced seedless English or Persian cucumber, unpeeled

½ medium red onion, cut into small dice

1 cup minced fresh flat-leaf parsley (about 2 large bunches)

¼ cup fresh lemon juice (from about 2 lemons)

¼ cup olive oil

1 In a medium pot, combine the wine, salt, and 1 cup of water and bring to a simmer over medium heat. Add the quinoa and bring back to a simmer. Cover, reduce the heat to very low, and simmer for 15 minutes. Remove from the heat and let sit for 15 to 20 minutes. Remove the lid, fluff the quinoa with a fork, and transfer to a large bowl to cool.

2 Add the tomatoes, cucumber, red onion, and parsley and gently toss everything together. Add the lemon juice and the oil and toss to combine. Season with salt and transfer to a serving bowl.

QUINOA is one of nature's perfect foods. It is super high in two important flavonoids, quercetin and kaempferol, along with many others that make it a strong tool against inflammation.

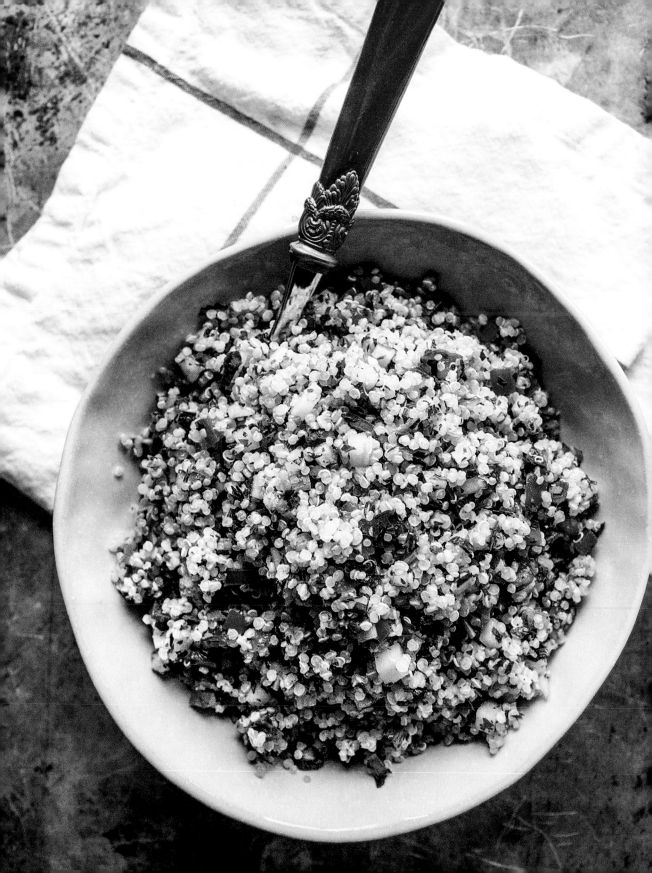

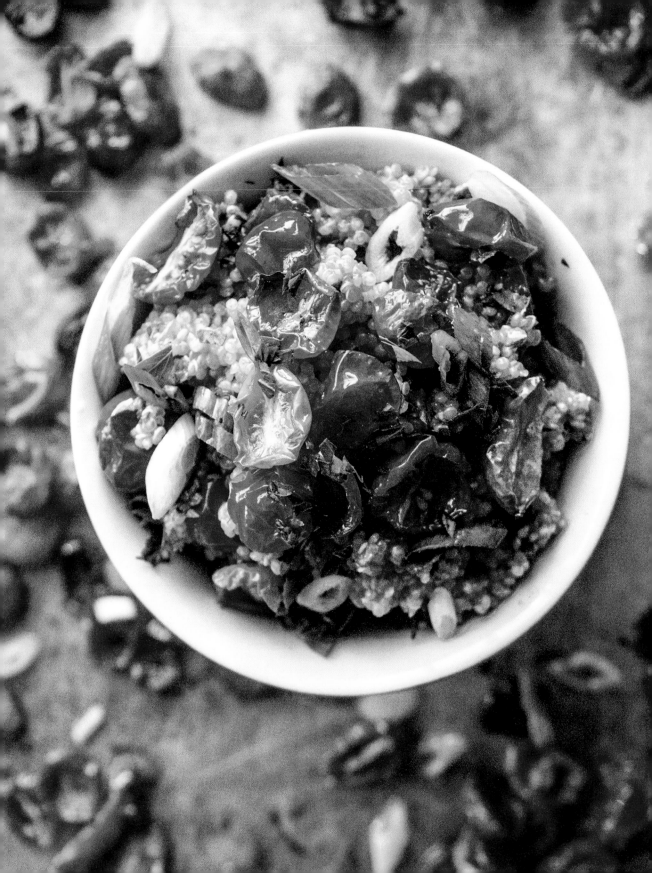

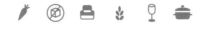

QUINOA WITH OVEN-DRIED TOMATOES AND SMOKY TOMATO VINAIGRETTE

PREPARATION 20 MINUTES   **COOK TIME** 1 HOUR 30 MINUTES   **SERVINGS** 6 TO 8

This is a dish that celebrates the flavor of fresh tomato and basil all year round. I often make this in the months when you can still get cherry tomatoes, but they are not at their peak. By oven drying the tomatoes, you get the concentrated flavor of the tomato, with a chewy and crispy texture that I adore. I serve this as a side dish, but it also makes for easy lunches and snacks throughout the week. It might even taste better after sitting for a day or two and is great cold.

OVEN-DRIED TOMATOES

1 pound cherry tomatoes, halved

3 tablespoons olive oil

1 teaspoon kosher salt, plus more as needed

• • •

2 cups white quinoa, rinsed and drained

½ cup dry white wine or vegetable or chicken broth

SMOKY ROASTED TOMATO SAUCE

1 garlic clove, coarsely chopped

¼ cup red wine vinegar

¼ cup olive oil

1 teaspoon smoked paprika

• • •

Kosher salt

2 green onions, thinly sliced

½ cup minced fresh flat-leaf parsley

1 To make the oven-dried tomatoes: Preheat the oven to 250°F.

2 Arrange the cherry tomato halves in a single layer on a rimmed baking sheet and drizzle them with the olive oil. Sprinkle with salt. Bake the tomatoes for 90 minutes, then set aside to cool.

3 Meanwhile, cook the quinoa: In a medium pot, combine the wine, the 1 teaspoon salt, and 1 cup water and bring to a simmer over medium heat. Add the quinoa and bring back to a simmer. Cover, reduce the heat to very low, and simmer for 15 minutes. Remove from the heat and let sit for

15 to 20 minutes. Remove the lid, fluff the quinoa with a fork, and transfer to a large bowl to cool.

4 To make the smoky roasted tomato sauce: In a blender, combine ¼ cup of the juiciest oven-dried tomatoes, the garlic, vinegar, olive oil, and paprika. Purée on high until smooth. Season with salt.

5 Add the tomato sauce to the quinoa and mix well. Add more salt if necessary. Gently fold in the remaining oven-dried tomatoes, green onions, and parsley and serve immediately or store in the refrigerator for up to 5 days.

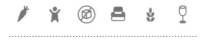

PUMPKIN POLENTA

PREPARATION 10 MINUTES   **COOK TIME** 25 MINUTES   **SERVINGS** 4 TO 6

I make this pumpkin polenta countless times in the cold months. It is a divine side dish for any type of braised meat, but it's also hearty enough to be a meatless main dish topped with a generous portion of Red Wine Mushrooms (page 152). The pumpkin keeps the polenta nice and creamy despite the fact that there is no dairy in this recipe.

4 cups vegetable or chicken broth

2 teaspoons kosher salt, plus more as needed

1 cup polenta

½ cup canned pumpkin purée

2 tablespoons soy-free vegan butter

1 In a large pot, bring the broth to a simmer over medium heat. Add the salt, then pour in the polenta, stirring as you add it to prevent lumps from forming. Cook for 15 minutes, stirring very frequently to ensure it doesn't scorch or stick.

2 Add the pumpkin purée and continue to stir and cook for 5 minutes more. The polenta should be cooked through and thick but somewhat fluid in consistency.

3 Turn off the heat and stir in the vegan butter until melted and well incorporated. Season with salt and serve hot.

NOTE: You can also pour the polenta onto a greased rimmed baking sheet and refrigerate until ready to use. The polenta will firm up as it chills. Cut the polenta into shapes and pan-fry them or warm them up in the oven for 10 minutes at 350°F.

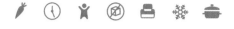

GINGER SUNFLOWER BUTTER BUCKWHEAT NOODLES

PREPARATION 10 MINUTES   **COOK TIME** 7 MINUTES   **SERVINGS** 4

This is the most fantastic, zesty, garlicky, gingery, creamy noodle dish. It is so full of bright, kicky flavors and makes such a delicious side. The noodles hold up really well to the sauce and are great for taking to potlucks or to work for lunch. I consider them a must with crispy salmon or alongside Asian Pulled Pork (page 245).

1 pound soba noodles

3 garlic cloves

1 (3-inch) piece fresh ginger, peeled and thinly sliced

⅓ cup sunflower butter

¼ cup unsweetened coconut milk

½ cup rice vinegar

2 tablespoons sambal oelek (Asian red chili garlic paste)

2 green onions, thinly sliced

1 Bring a large pot of water to a boil. Add the soba noodles and cook for 6 to 7 minutes. Drain and rinse with cold water until the noodles have cooled completely. Drain again and transfer to a large bowl.

2 In a food processor, pulse the garlic and ginger together until they are finely minced. Add the sunflower butter, coconut milk, vinegar, and sambal and pulse until the sauce is smooth.

3 Gently toss the noodles with the sauce until they are well coated and sprinkle with the green onions. Serve immediately or refrigerate and serve chilled.

BUCKWHEAT is not a grain; it is actually a fruit seed and related to rhubarb and sorrel! However, some people who have allergies to other fruit seeds may find that they have issues with buckwheat as well.

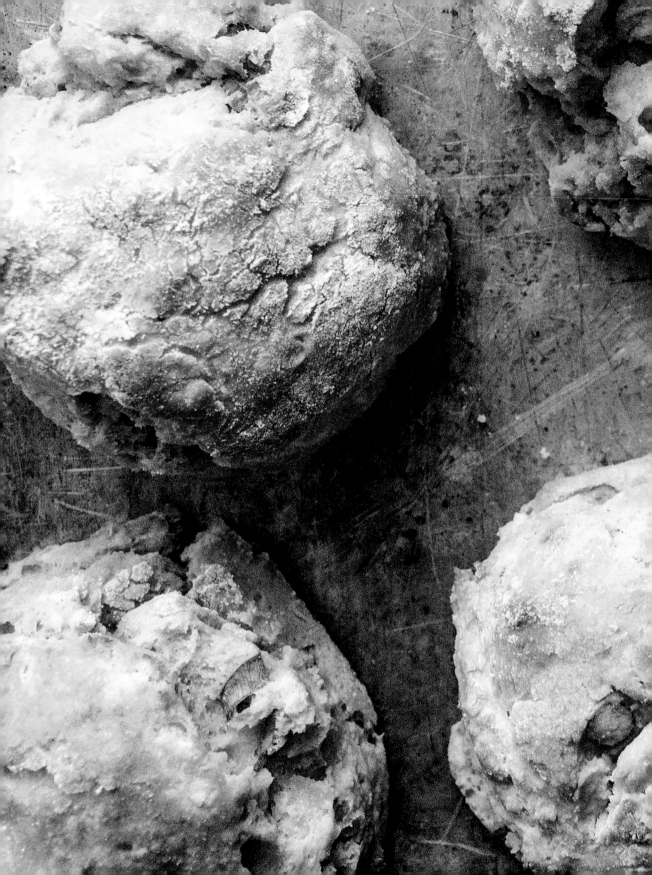

baked goods

Breads, crackers, rolls—these foods are the foundation of the average American diet, and we still want them even when it becomes necessary to modify our diets to eliminate allergens and inflammatory foods. We will always want bread for our sandwiches and our morning toast, buns for our burgers, and cornbread for our chili. Crackers for our hummus. You get the idea. We are a culture of bread eaters and carb lovers and that is consistently one of the hardest things for the average person to let go of when they make "the change." There are more and more products coming out that are gluten-free, but most still have dairy, eggs, and soy in them. But be deprived no longer! Breads, buns, and crackers are here to help. These recipes can transform your meals and fulfill your cravings, and are so good you won't know the difference. I hope these baked goods bring the same level of comfort and happiness to you as they have brought to my family!

◄ Green Onion Sweet Potato Biscuits (page 182)

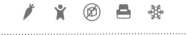

SANDWICH BREAD

PREPARATION 10 MINUTES   **COOK TIME** 60 MINUTES   **SERVINGS** 8 TO 10

Here's an incredibly easy alternative to yeast-leavened bread. The beer and baking soda react to give it all the lift it needs, producing a really fluffy rise as well as a natural sweetness without any added sugar. It's perfect for sandwiches and toasting. Store this bread in an airtight resealable bag. It will stay fresh for a day or two, and then is best eaten toasted. You can also slice and freeze the bread, thawing what you need when you would like a portion of bread or toast.

4 cups all-purpose gluten-free flour

1 tablespoon kosher salt

2 teaspoons baking soda

1½ teaspoons xanthan gum (see page 34)

2 tablespoons soy-free vegan butter, melted

1 (12-ounce) bottle gluten-free beer (I use pale ale)

1 Preheat the oven to 350°F. Grease an 8 × 5-inch loaf pan with oil or vegan butter.

2 In the bowl of a stand mixer fitted with the whisk attachment, combine the flour, salt, baking soda, and xanthan gum. With the mixer on low, add the melted vegan butter and the beer. Whip until you have a uniformly smooth, wet dough.

3 Transfer the dough to the prepared loaf pan and smooth the top with an offset spatula or butter knife dipped in water.

4 Bake for about 60 minutes, until the top is puffed up very high and nicely golden. Let cool in the pan for about 20 minutes before turning out onto a cutting board and slicing.

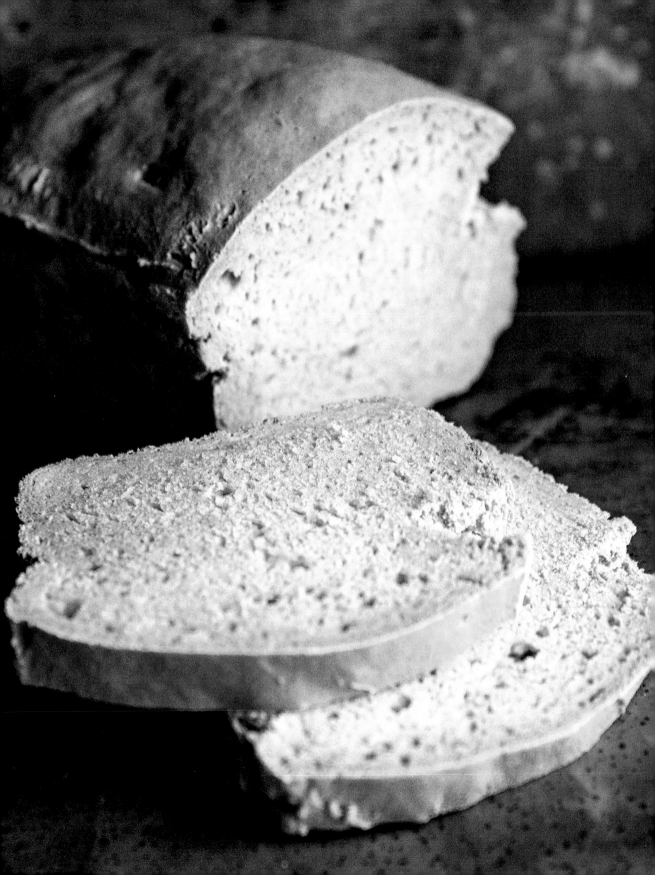

HAMBURGER BUNS

PREPARATION 30 MINUTES   **COOK TIME** 20 MINUTES   **SERVINGS** 8

It's fine to eat a burger between two pieces of regular bread, I guess . . . But wouldn't you rather eat a burger in a bun? That's shaped like a bun? Better still, one with a sweet glaze and sesame seeds sprinkled on top? While these are a little complicated to make, the result is a thick, toothsome bun that has a nice chew to it but is still soft. You can make and refrigerate the dough for up to several days before you bake it. You will want to bake them right before serving, as they get stale quickly, but reheating them in the oven can revive them a day later.

1 (¼-ounce) packet active dry yeast

1¼ cups hot water (110°F to 115°F)

8 tablespoons plus 1 teaspoon granulated beet sugar

1 cup tapioca starch

1 cup sorghum flour

1 cup potato starch

½ cup brown rice flour

½ cup gluten-free millet flour

1 tablespoon baking powder

2 teaspoons xanthan gum (see page 34)

1½ teaspoons kosher salt

¼ cup good olive oil

6 tablespoons canned garbanzo bean liquid

2 teaspoons apple cider vinegar

1 teaspoon toasted sesame seeds

1 Preheat the oven to 400°F. Grease two baking sheets with olive oil.

2 In a small bowl, combine the yeast, hot water, and 1 teaspoon of the sugar. Stir and set aside for 10 minutes to proof; it should become bubbly and frothy.

3 In the bowl of a stand mixer fitted with the whisk attachment, whisk together the tapioca starch, sorghum flour, potato starch, brown rice flour, millet flour, baking powder, xanthan gum, salt, and 5 tablespoons sugar. Beat in the olive oil, garbanzo bean fluid, and vinegar and then add the yeast mixture. Continue to beat until the dough

is creamy, smooth, and not too thick, similar to a soft cookie dough in consistency. At this point, you can bake the dough or store it in a tightly sealed container in the fridge to use within a few days.

4 Divide the dough into 8 portions and transfer the dough to the prepared baking sheets. With wet hands, smooth the dough into circles with rounded tops (think about the shape of a hamburger bun). The dough is *very* soft, so be sure to keep your hands damp; if you touch it with dry hands, it will tear away from the pan. Take your time and get the surfaces as smooth as possible.

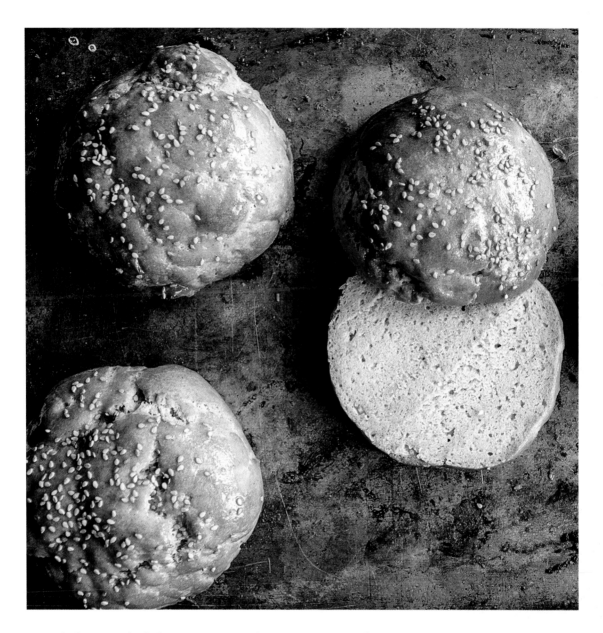

5 Set the buns in a draft-free spot to rest and rise for 15 minutes.

6 Meanwhile, in a small pan, combine the remaining 3 tablespoons sugar and 3 tablespoons water. Mix well and cook over medium heat, stirring, until the sugar has melted, about 2 minutes.

7 Brush the bun tops with the sugar syrup and sprinkle with the sesame seeds. Bake for 15 to 17 minutes, or until golden brown and then let them rest on the baking sheets until somewhat cooled but still warm. Slice in half horizontally and use immediately.

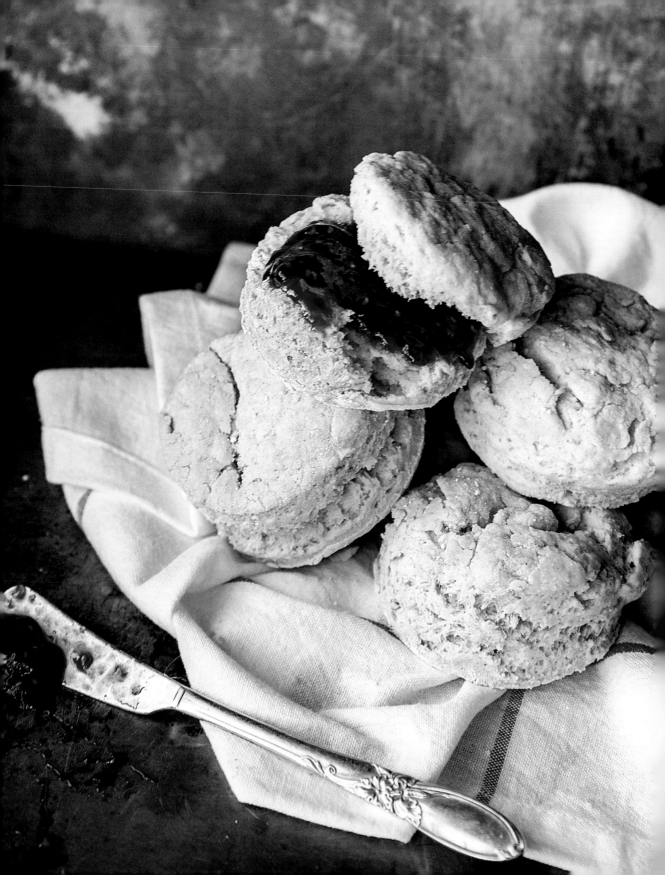

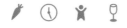

"BUTTERMILK" BISCUITS

PREPARATION 10 MINUTES **COOK TIME** 12 MINUTES **SERVINGS** 6 TO 8 BISCUITS

These are exactly what you want to make for your family on a weeknight. It's such a special treat to have fresh-baked *anything* on a weeknight, and when it is this easy to bake up fresh biscuits, it's hard to say no. When I make soup (which is all the time), these are practically a given. My children and husband eat at least two each, and then I can heat up the leftover biscuits in the morning to serve with jam.

1 cup unsweetened coconut milk

1 tablespoon apple cider vinegar

2½ cups all-purpose gluten-free flour, plus more for dusting

4 teaspoons baking powder

1½ teaspoons xanthan gum (see page 34)

1 teaspoon kosher salt

½ cup (1 stick) cold soy-free vegan butter, cut into chunks

1 Preheat the oven to 450°F. Line a baking sheet with a silicone baking mat or parchment paper.

2 In a small bowl, stir together the coconut milk and vinegar and set aside.

3 In a medium bowl, combine the flour, baking powder, xanthan gum, and salt. Add the cold vegan butter and using a pastry cutter or your fingers, cut the butter into the flour until you have a mixture with pea-size chunks of flour and butter.

4 Make a well in the center and add the coconut milk mixture. Using your hands, gently mix everything together to make a wet, sticky dough.

5 Turn the dough out onto a lightly floured surface and gently pat the dough into a disk about 1 inch thick. Use a biscuit cutter or a juice glass to cut the dough. You will get 6 to 8 biscuits depending on the size of the cutter.

6 Transfer the biscuits to the prepared baking sheet and bake for 12 minutes, until lightly golden on top. Serve hot or at room temperature. Store in an airtight container for an extra day or two; you can reheat the biscuits in the oven.

GREEN ONION SWEET POTATO BISCUITS

PREPARATION 15 MINUTES   COOK TIME 15 MINUTES   SERVINGS 8

Just as easy and delicious as my basic "Buttermilk" Biscuit recipe (page 181), these are amped up a little bit with sweet potato purée and a liberal dose of green onions, and made fluffy with beer. Serve them alongside a big pot of hot soup or bake up a batch around the holidays to accompany the Roast Turkey Breast and Cranberry Chutney (page 243) or to make ham or turkey sandwiches with.

½ cup unsweetened coconut milk

1 tablespoon apple cider vinegar

2½ cups all-purpose gluten-free flour, plus more for shaping the dough

½ teaspoon xanthan gum (see page 34)

4 teaspoons baking powder

1 tablespoon granulated beet sugar

1 teaspoon kosher salt

½ cup chopped green onions

½ cup cold soy-free vegan butter, cut into chunks

½ cup sweet potato purée, canned or homemade (page 34)

½ cup gluten-free beer

1 Preheat the oven to 400°F. Line a baking sheet with a silicone baking mat or parchment paper.

2 In a small bowl, combine the coconut milk and vinegar and set aside.

3 In a medium bowl, combine the flour, xanthan gum, baking powder, sugar, salt, and green onions. Add the vegan butter and using either a pastry cutter or your fingers, cut or pinch the butter into the dry ingredients until you have crumbly dough.

4 Make a well in the center and add the sweet potato purée and the coconut milk mixture. Using your hands, partially mix together, then add the beer and gently combine to make a thick, wet dough.

5 Use up to ¼ cup additional gluten-free flour to help transfer the dough to a countertop and shape it into an even disc. Using a knife or a biscuit cutter, divide the dough into 8 biscuits and place them on the prepared baking sheet.

6 Bake for 13 to 15 minutes, until golden and puffy. These are best when served immediately.

CORNBREAD

PREPARATION 15 MINUTES   **COOK TIME** 20 MINUTES   **SERVINGS** 6 TO 8

People tend to be passionate about cornbread, with some in the sweet camp and others who believe adding any sweetness to cornbread is sacrilege. I'm in the first camp, and to my palate this cornbread has just the right amount of sweet and is unbelievably moist. You can add green onions, jalapeños, fresh chives—there are a ton of options! Serve it hot with honey (unless you are vegan) or alongside a big bowl of spicy chili.

2 tablespoons chia seeds

1 cup plus 2 tablespoons unsweetened coconut milk

1 tablespoon apple cider vinegar

1 cup all-purpose gluten-free flour

1 cup fine cornmeal

⅓ cup granulated beet sugar

1 teaspoon xanthan gum (see page 34)

2 teaspoons baking powder

½ teaspoon baking soda

1 teaspoon kosher salt

¼ cup coconut oil, melted

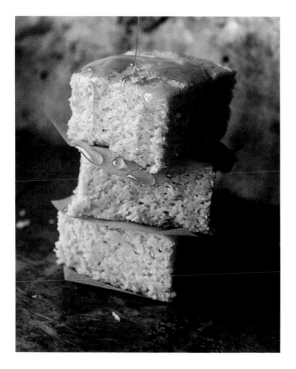

1 In a small bowl, combine the chia seeds with 6 tablespoons hot tap water. Let sit until the mixture becomes jellylike, at least 10 minutes.

2 In a separate small bowl, combine the coconut milk and vinegar and set aside.

3 Preheat the oven to 425°F and grease an 8 × 8-inch glass baking dish with coconut oil.

4 In a medium bowl, whisk together the flour, cornmeal, sugar, xanthan gum, baking powder, baking soda, and salt until well combined.

5 Add the melted coconut oil, the coconut milk mixture, and chia seed jelly and stir to make a uniform batter. Transfer the batter to the baking dish and bake for 20 minutes. Let cool in the pan for at least 20 minutes before slicing.

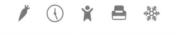

FLATBREAD

PREPARATION 20 MINUTES   **COOK TIME** 10 MINUTES   **SERVINGS** 6

Flatbreads are all kinds of useful. They are the best for scooping up hummus as well as for making wrap sandwiches. This one has a nice flavor and a great chewy texture. This basic recipe is also a great canvas for improvisation; you could add fresh garlic to the dough or even sprinkle the top with toasted sesame seeds or za'atar (a Middle Eastern spice) before baking for extra depth of flavor.

1 (¼-ounce) packet active dry yeast

2 teaspoons granulated beet sugar

5¼ cups all-purpose gluten-free flour

1½ teaspoons xanthan gum (see page 34)

2 teaspoons onion powder

1½ tablespoons kosher salt

⅓ cup plus 6 tablespoons olive oil

1 Preheat the oven to 400°F.

2 In a small bowl, combine the yeast, sugar, and 2 cups hot tap water. Set aside to proof for about 10 minutes. It will become frothy and bubbly.

3 In the bowl of a stand mixer fitted with the paddle attachment, combine the flour, xanthan gum, onion powder, and salt. Add the proofed yeast mixture and beat on medium speed until combined. With the mixer running on medium, pour in ⅓ cup of the olive oil in a thin stream. Mix until the dough is smooth and well combined.

4 Divide the dough into 6 equal balls. Gently roll each ball into a circle about ⅓ inch thick. Carefully transfer the dough to three baking sheets. (Two dough rounds will fit on each baking sheet.) Brush the dough rounds with 3 tablespoons of the olive oil.

5 Bake the flatbreads for 10 minutes. Remove from the oven and brush with the remaining 3 tablespoons olive oil. Serve hot or at room temperature. You can store these in an airtight resealable plastic bag for a few days; they reheat well.

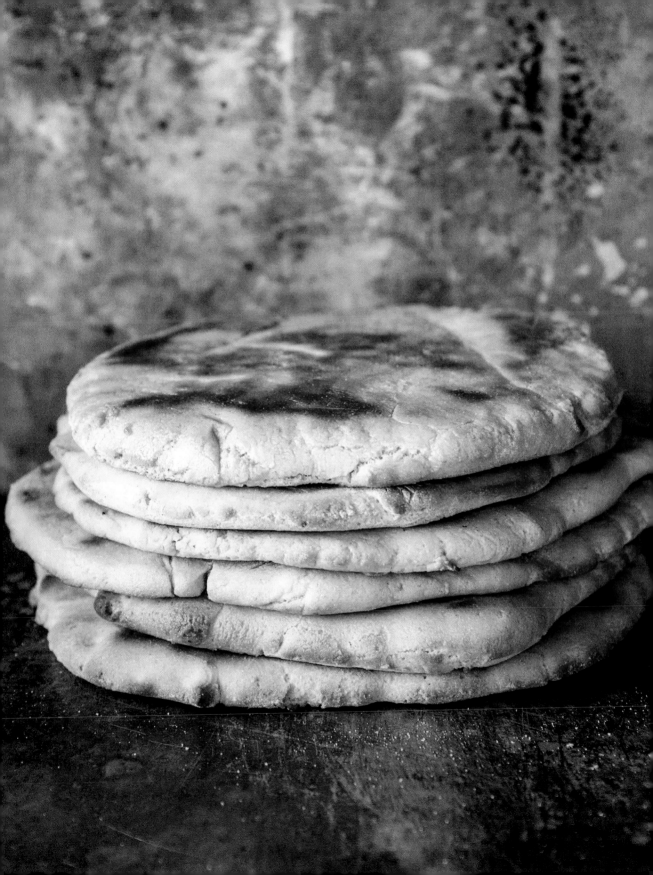

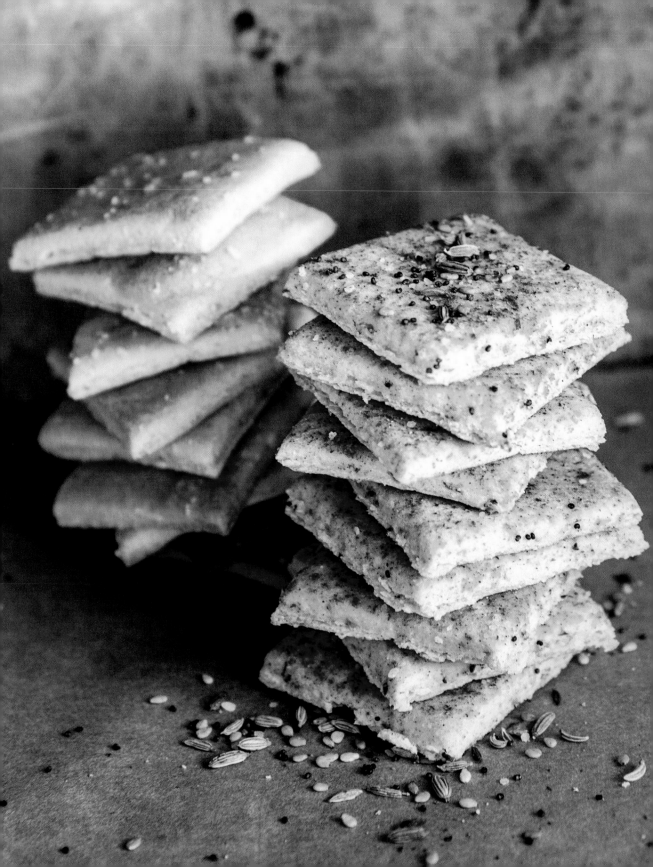

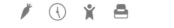

ROSEMARY CRACKERS
AND EVERYTHING CRACKERS

PREPARATION 15 MINUTES   **COOK TIME** 15 MINUTES   **SERVINGS** 6 TO 8

One cracker dough, two versions: The simple flavor of fresh rosemary and salt is a good choice to serve with cheeses, while the over-the-top blend inspired by everyone's favorite bagel is perfect for snacks all on its own.

CRACKERS

1 cup plus 3 tablespoons all-purpose gluten-free flour, plus more for dusting

½ teaspoon kosher salt

1 tablespoon minced fresh rosemary (for Rosemary Crackers) or 1 teaspoon onion powder (for Everything Crackers)

2 tablespoons soy-free vegan butter

1 teaspoon honey (or agave for vegans)

⅓ cup ice water

EVERYTHING TOPPING

½ teaspoon poppy seeds

½ teaspoon fennel seeds

½ teaspoon toasted sesame seeds

¼ teaspoon smoked paprika

¼ teaspoon onion powder

¼ teaspoon kosher salt

1 Preheat the oven to 350°F.

2 In the bowl of a food processor, combine the flour, salt, and rosemary or onion powder. Cut the vegan butter into chunks and add it to the bowl. Pulse to make a crumbly dough. Add the honey and the ice water and pulse until the dough is smooth and holds together.

3 Transfer the dough to a sheet of parchment paper and sprinkle with a little gluten-free flour. Place a second sheet of parchment paper on top. Gently roll the dough as thinly as you can without tearing it; the thinner the dough, the crispier the crackers will be. Gently peel off the top sheet of parchment paper. Transfer the dough along with its bottom sheet of parchment paper to a baking sheet. Use a pizza cutter or a sharp knife to score the dough into square or rectangular crackers of your desired size.

4 If making rosemary crackers, sprinkle the dough with a little salt. If making everything crackers, combine the topping ingredients in a small bowl and sprinkle over the dough.

5 Bake the crackers for 12 to 15 minutes, until pale golden. Let them cool completely to crisp up and then break them apart along the scored lines and store in an airtight container.

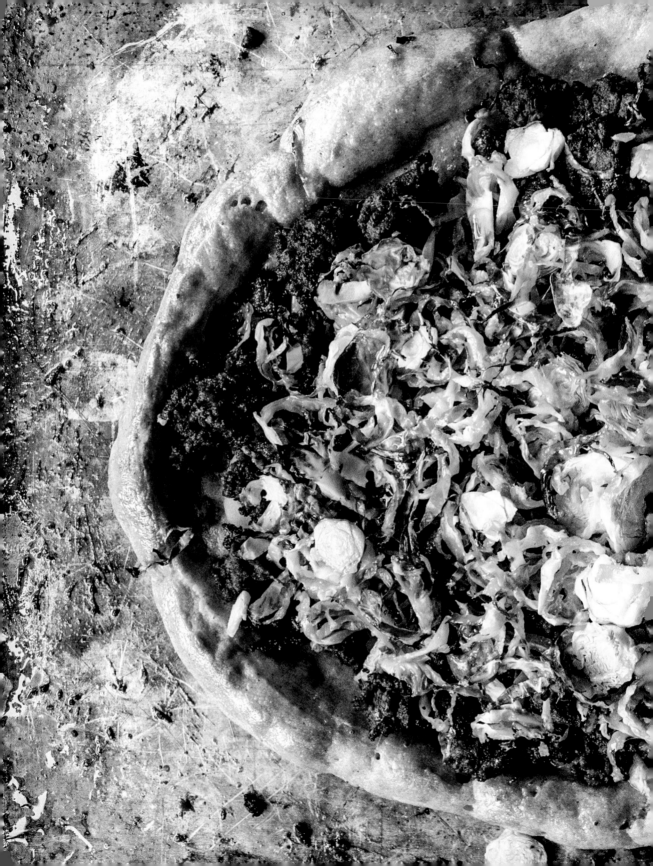

pizza and burgers

If there's one request I get more than any other, it's for an allergen-free pizza, and I understand why all too well: for years and years, Thursday nights meant calling our favorite takeout place to order up two large pizzas dripping with cheese and all our favorite toppings. Now we have new pizza traditions—and no stomachaches afterward. I worked overtime to create pizzas with a beautiful golden crust and a nice chewy tooth, one that is crisp enough to stand up to toppings without flopping over and, of course, tastes great.

With cheese out of the picture as far as toppings go, I tend to gravitate toward really flavorful ingredients and unusual combinations, like beet purée with baby arugula, or potatoes, spicy chorizo, and lemony Brussels sprouts. Get as creative as you want. The recipes in this chapter should give you a nudge in the right direction.

Most folks love a good burger now and then, and you'll find those here in spades. I am pretty sure you aren't thinking about the fact that they aren't draped in melted cheese when faced with a juicy lamb burger topped with in homemade ketchup and topped with spicy cucumbers, or a tender Asian Salmon Burger piled high with pickled onions.

◀ Potato, Chorizo, and Brussels Sprouts Pizza (page 196)

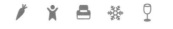

PIZZA CRUST

PREPARATION 30 MINUTES   **COOK TIME** 20 MINUTES
SERVINGS MAKES ONE LARGE PIZZA SERVING 4-6

Making this pizza is more about the technique than the ingredients, and you may need to try it a few times before you get it exactly right. Don't be afraid of the olive oil here—it helps ensure that you get a nice chewy crust with great flavor. Take the time to form the crust with wet hands; the smoother your dough, the better it will look and bake. If you make a crackly crust, then it will bake up that way, too. And make sure you leave ample space around the edge for a nice chewy, pillowy crust.

If you prefer, you can mix up the batter for the dough up to 3 days ahead of time and store it in the fridge. Note, however, that while it tastes the same, it is easiest to work with right after you make it. This dough makes one large pizza or you can divide the dough and make two small pizzas.

1 (¼-ounce) packet active dry yeast

1 teaspoon plus 3 tablespoons granulated beet sugar

1¼ cups hot water (110°F to 115°F)

1 cup tapioca starch

1 cup sorghum flour

½ cup gluten-free millet flour

½ cup potato starch

½ cup dehydrated potato flakes

1 tablespoon baking powder

2 teaspoons xanthan gum (see page 34)

1½ teaspoons kosher salt, plus more for sprinkling

2 tablespoons onion powder

⅓ cup canned garbanzo bean liquid (page 35)

¼ cup olive oil, plus more for drizzling

2 tablespoons apple cider vinegar

1 Preheat the oven to 425°F and arrange two racks in the center of the oven.

2 In a small bowl, stir together the yeast, 1 teaspoon of the sugar, and the warm water. Set aside in a draft-free place to proof for at least 10 minutes or until the yeast is puffed and bubbly.

3 In the bowl of a stand mixer fitted with the paddle attachment, combine the tapioca starch,

sorghum flour, millet flour, potato starch, potato flakes, baking powder, xanthan gum, salt, onion powder, and remaining 3 tablespoons sugar.

4 In a small bowl, whisk together the garbanzo bean liquid, olive oil, and vinegar.

5 With the mixer on low, pour the proofed yeast into the dry ingredients and combine. Add the garbanzo bean liquid mixture.

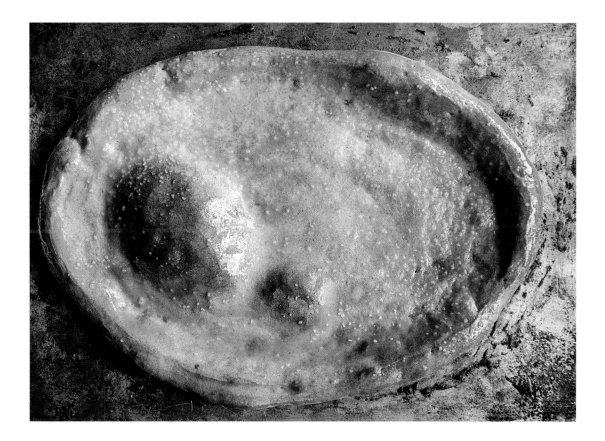

6 Turn the mixer to medium and beat the dough until the batter is smooth and sticky, with the consistency of a soft cookie dough. (At this point, you can use it immediately or store it in a sealed container in the fridge to use within a few days.)

7 Place the dough on the center of an ungreased baking sheet. Place a little bowl of warm water next to the pan. Wet your hands, then lightly press and flatten the dough to create a thin, even shell with slightly raised edges. Keep wetting your hands as you work the dough, as it is *very* soft and will stick and tear away from the pan if you use dry hands. Get the dough as thin and smooth as possible, making the outer 1½ inches a bit thicker.

8 Set the pizza crusts in a draft-free spot to rest for 15 minutes. Drizzle generously with olive oil and sprinkle with salt.

9 Bake the crusts for 15 minutes, until golden. Remove the crust from the oven and use a spatula to lift the dough from the pan (it will be sticking, so a hard flat spatula is helpful). Brush with a little olive oil, top as desired, then return to the oven and bake for 2 to 3 minutes more, or until your toppings are hot and the crust is a deep golden color. Slice and serve immediately.

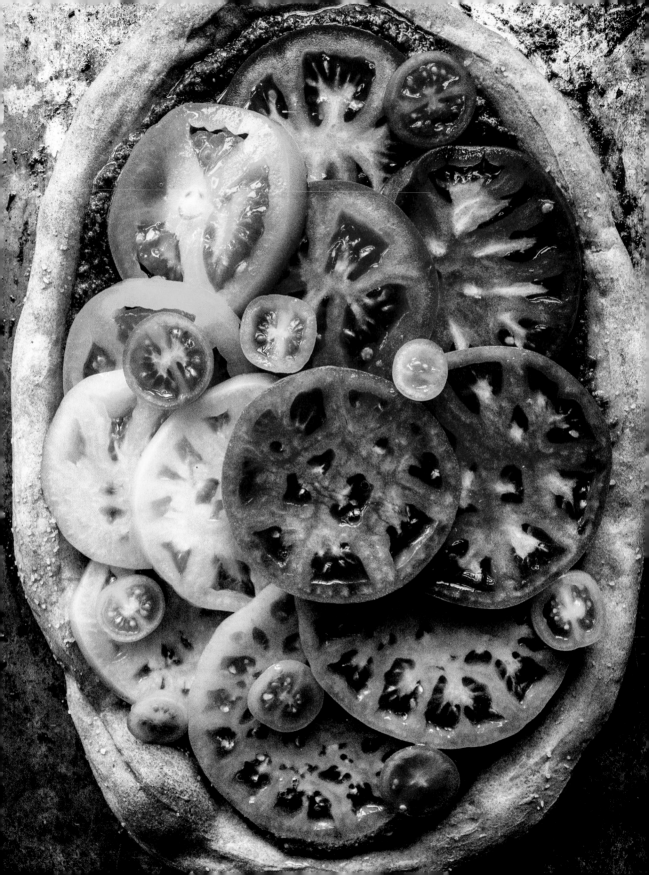

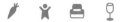

HEIRLOOM TOMATO AND PESTO PIZZA

PREPARATION 45 MINUTES   **COOK TIME** 25 MINUTES   **SERVINGS** 6

For the most beautiful presentation, take advantage of the colorful variety of heirloom tomatoes you can find these days. Of course, this recipe is most wonderful in the heat of summer when the tomatoes are sweet and plentiful and the basil is at its most fragrant, but thanks to greenhouse growers, it's possible to get heirloom tomatoes nearly all year long. This pizza will win you lots of praise, I promise.

1 recipe Pizza Crust dough (page 190)

3 garlic cloves

4 cups lightly packed basil leaves

¼ cup olive oil, plus more as needed

2 tablespoons fresh lemon juice

4 fresh heirloom tomatoes, thinly sliced

Kosher salt

1 Preheat the oven to 425°F and arrange a rack in the center of the oven.

2 Place a pizza crust dough ball on the center of an ungreased baking sheet. Place a little bowl of warm water next to the pan. Wet your hands, then lightly press and flatten the dough to create a thin, even shell with slightly raised edges. Keep wetting your hands as you work the dough, as it is *very* soft and will stick and tear away from the pan if you use dry hands. Get the dough as thin and smooth as possible, making the outer 1½ inches a bit thicker.

3 Set the pizza crust in a draft-free spot to rest for 15 minutes. Drizzle generously with some olive oil and sprinkle with salt.

4 Bake the crust for 15 minutes, until golden.

5 While the crust is baking, in a blender, combine the garlic, basil, olive oil, and lemon juice and purée until smooth.

6 Remove the crust from the oven and brush with a little olive oil. Spread the basil purée over the crust and bake for 2 to 3 minutes more, until hot. Remove from the oven and arrange the tomato slices evenly over the top. Sprinkle with salt and drizzle with more olive oil. Slice and serve immediately.

TOMATOES are packed with antioxidants like vitamin C and beta-carotene and great amounts of manganese and vitamin E. They're also full of phytonutrients that support the cardiovascular system and bone health and have incredible anticancer benefits.

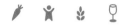

BEET PIZZA WITH BABY ARUGULA

PREPARATION 50 MINUTES **COOK TIME** 40 MINUTES **SERVINGS** 6 TO 8

Beets and pizza may not be the most likely of friends, but this flavor combination is extraordinary. And I'm pretty sure that magnificent shade of fuchsia hasn't been lost on you. Give this one a try and become a believer.

6 small beets, trimmed and scrubbed

Kosher salt

1 recipe Pizza Crust dough (page 190)

4 garlic cloves

1 tablespoon olive oil, plus more for drizzling

2 tablespoons balsamic vinegar

¼ cup baby arugula, for garnish

1 Preheat the oven to 425°F and arrange a rack in the center of the oven.

2 Put the beets in a medium pot and add water to cover. Salt the water and bring to a simmer over medium heat. Cook until the beets are tender, about 20 minutes.

3 Rinse the beets until cool enough to handle and rub the skins off. Cut them into quarters and transfer to the bowl of a food processor. Add the garlic, olive oil, and vinegar. Pulse until really well combined. Season with salt.

4 While the beets are cooking, place a pizza crust dough ball on the center of an ungreased baking sheet. Place a little bowl of warm water next to the pan. Wet your hands, then lightly press and flatten

the dough to create a thin, even shell with slightly raised edges. Keep wetting your hands as you work the dough, as it is *very* soft and will stick and tear away from the pan if you use dry hands. Get the dough as thin and smooth as possible, making the outer 1½ inches a bit thicker.

5 Set the pizza crust in a draft-free spot to rest for 15 minutes. Drizzle generously with olive oil and sprinkle with salt.

6 Bake the crust for 15 minutes, until golden. Remove the crust from the oven and brush with a little olive oil. Spread the beet purée evenly over the crust. Return the pizza to the oven and bake for 2 to 3 minutes more. Sprinkle with the arugula and drizzle with a bit more olive oil. Slice and serve hot!

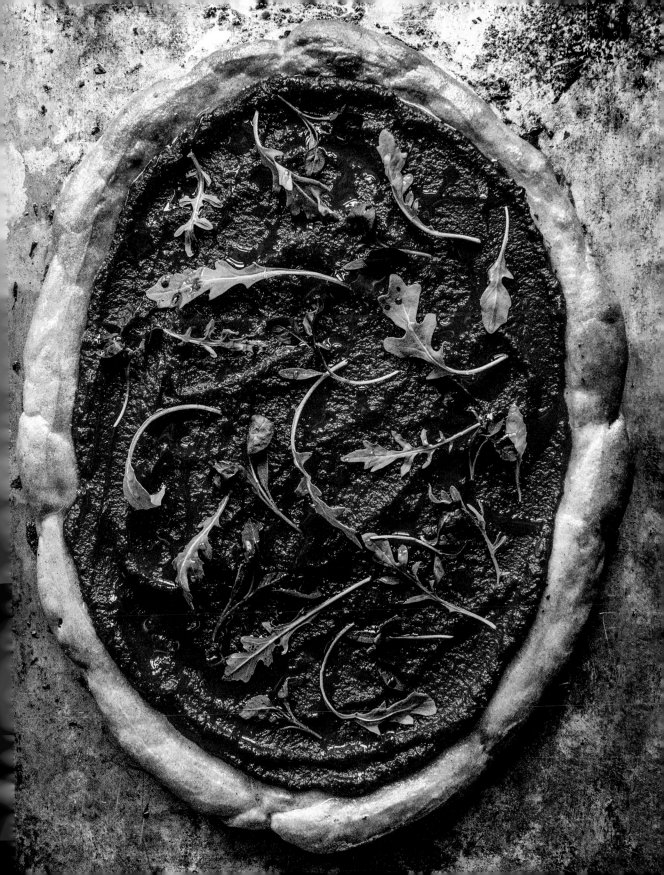

POTATO, CHORIZO, AND BRUSSELS SPROUTS PIZZA

PREPARATION 45 MINUTES   **COOK TIME** 17 MINUTES   **SERVINGS** 6 TO 8

My affinity for Brussels sprouts is no secret, and when they are shredded they have a crunchy texture that I find especially irresistible. This pizza may be as unconventional as they come, but it is a serious crowd-pleaser (photograph on page 188).

1 recipe Pizza Crust dough (page 190)

3 tablespoons olive oil

Kosher salt

1 large Yukon Gold potato, peeled and very thinly sliced

½ pound fresh Spanish chorizo

1 garlic clove, minced

½ pound Brussels sprouts, very thinly sliced

Juice of 1 lemon

1 Preheat the oven to 425°F and arrange a rack in the center of the oven.

2 Place a pizza crust dough ball on the center of an ungreased baking sheet. Place a little bowl of warm water next to the pan. Wet your hands, then lightly press and flatten the dough to create a thin, even shell with slightly raised edges. Keep wetting your hands as you work the dough, as it is *very* soft and will stick and tear away from the pan if you use dry hands. Get the dough as thin and smooth as possible, making the outer 1½ inches a bit thicker.

3 Set the pizza crust in a draft-free spot to rest for 15 minutes. Drizzle generously with olive oil and sprinkle with salt.

4 Bake the crust for 15 minutes until golden. Remove the crust from the oven and brush with a little olive oil.

5 Bring a small saucepan of salted water to a boil. Add the potato slices and boil for 5 minutes, or until just tender. Drain and pat dry, then arrange evenly over the pizza crust. Drizzle with 1 tablespoon of olive oil and sprinkle with salt. Bake for 5 to 7 minutes.

6 Meanwhile, in a medium pan, heat 1 teaspoon of olive oil over medium heat. Add the chorizo and cook, breaking it up with a wooden spoon.

7 In a separate large pan, heat the remaining 2 tablespoons olive oil over high heat. Add the garlic and cook for 1 minute. Add the Brussels sprouts and cook, stirring continuously, until softened, 2 to 3 minutes. Add the lemon juice and season with salt.

8 When the chorizo is completely cooked, spread it over the potatoes. Top with the hot Brussels sprouts. Slice and serve hot.

ROASTED RED PEPPER PIZZA WITH ARTICHOKE HEARTS, PEAS, AND PROSCIUTTO

PREPARATION 45 MINUTES   COOK TIME 5 MINUTES   SERVINGS 6 TO 8

Spanish flavors were the inspiration for this pizza; the red pepper sauce is similar to a romesco, and the artichokes, peas, and prosciutto are all ingredients you might encounter in a tapas bar. On a pizza, the combo is nothing short of showstopping. (Photograph on page 7.)

RED PEPPER SAUCE

1 (4-ounce) jar water-packed roasted red peppers

2 garlic cloves

2 teaspoons red wine vinegar

2 tablespoons olive oil

Kosher salt

PIZZA

1 recipe Pizza Crust dough (page 190)

Olive oil, for drizzling

Kosher salt

1 cup frozen artichoke hearts, thawed

⅓ cup shelled green peas (about ½ pound in the pod)

4 ounces prosciutto

2 tablespoons minced fresh curly parsley

1 Preheat the oven to 425°F and arrange a rack in the center of the oven.

2 To make the red pepper sauce: In a food processor or blender, combine all the sauce ingredients and purée until thick and well combined. Season with salt.

3 Place a pizza crust dough ball on the center of an ungreased baking sheet. Place a little bowl of warm water next to the pan. Wet your hands, then lightly press and flatten the dough to create a thin, even shell with slightly raised edges. Keep wetting your hands as you work the dough, as it is *very* soft and will stick and tear away from the pan

if you use dry hands. Get the dough as thin and smooth as possible, making the outer 1½ inches a bit thicker.

4 Set the pizza crust in a draft-free spot to rest for 15 minutes. Drizzle generously with olive oil and sprinkle with salt.

5 Bake the crust until golden, about 15 minutes. Remove the crusts from the oven and brush with a little olive oil. Spread the red pepper sauce liberally over the crust. Add the artichoke hearts, peas, and prosciutto and then drizzle liberally with olive oil. Bake the pizza for 5 minutes more. Sprinkle the parsley over top, slice, and serve hot.

MEDITERRANEAN PIZZA

PREPARATION 45 MINUTES   COOK TIME 25 MINUTES   SERVINGS 6 TO 8

The bold, intense flavors of this Mediterranean-inspired pizza are quite addictive—I know I have personally eaten the bulk of one of these myself!

ROASTED GARLIC

1 head of garlic

1 tablespoon olive oil, plus more as needed

Kosher salt, plus more as needed

BASIL PESTO

2 garlic cloves

4 ounces fresh basil leaves and stems (about 4 cups lightly packed)

¼ cup olive oil

2 teaspoons red wine vinegar

Kosher salt

PIZZA

1 recipe Pizza Crust dough (page 190)

Olive oil, for drizzling

1 cup shredded cooked chicken breast

2 roasted red peppers, thinly sliced

⅓ cup pitted kalamata olives

1 Preheat the oven to 425°F and arrange a rack in the center of the oven.

2 Slice the top quarter off the head of garlic to expose the cloves and place on a small sheet of aluminum foil. Drizzle with the olive oil and add a generous pinch of salt. Bring the edges of the foil together and twist closed. Roast the garlic for 20 minutes and then set aside.

3 Meanwhile, make the basil pesto: Combine all the pesto ingredients in a food processor and pulse until thick and well combined. Season with salt.

4 Place a pizza crust dough ball on the center of an ungreased baking sheet. Place a little bowl of warm water next to the pan. Wet your hands, then lightly press and flatten the dough to create a thin, even shell with slightly raised edges. Keep wetting your hands as you work the dough, as it is *very* soft and will stick and tear away from the pan if you use dry hands. Get the dough as thin and smooth as possible, making the outer 1½ inches a bit thicker.

5 Set the pizza crust in a draft-free spot to rest for 15 minutes. Drizzle generously with olive oil and sprinkle with salt.

6 Bake the crust for 15 minutes, until golden. Remove the crust from the oven and brush with a little olive oil.

7 Spread the crust with the pesto, then squeeze the garlic cloves on top. Top with the chicken, peppers, and olives.

8 Bake for 2 to 3 minutes until hot. Drizzle with a bit more olive oil, slice, and serve.

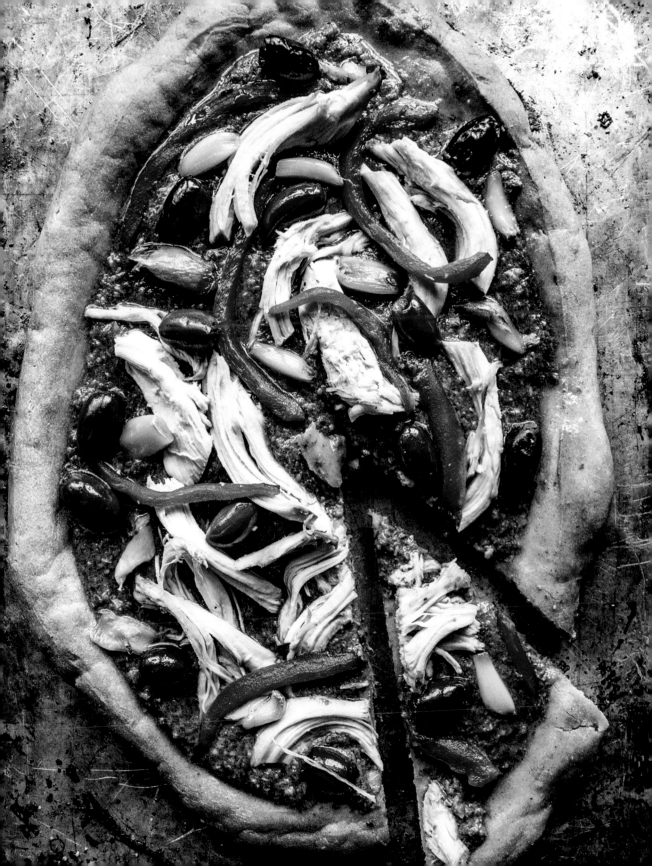

TUNA TARTARE PIZZA

PREPARATION 45 MINUTES   **COOK TIME** 15 MINUTES   **SERVINGS** 6

This may be one of the coolest twists on pizza I've ever come up with, essentially a mash-up of pizza and a spicy tuna sushi roll, and the result is really quite wonderful. The unusual combination is always a hit with cocktails.

1 recipe Pizza Crust dough (page 190)

Olive oil

Kosher salt

WASABI COCONUT CREAM

1 cup unsweetened coconut cream, chilled

2 teaspoons prepared wasabi paste

3 garlic cloves, minced

Zest of 1 lime, minced

1 tablespoon fresh lime juice

2 tablespoons minced fresh cilantro

Kosher salt

TOPPINGS

1 avocado, pitted, peeled, and thinly sliced

6 ounces sashimi-grade tuna, thinly sliced

⅔ cup thinly sliced seedless cucumber

Sweet and Spicy Pickled Onions (page 94)

2 tablespoons fresh cilantro leaves

1 red Fresno chile, thinly sliced

1 jalapeño, thinly sliced

1 Preheat the oven to 425°F and arrange a rack in the center of the oven.

2 Place a pizza crust dough ball on the center of an ungreased baking sheet. Place a little bowl of warm water next to the pan. Wet your hands, then lightly press and flatten the dough to create a thin, even shell with slightly raised edges. Keep wetting your hands as you work the dough, as it is *very* soft and will stick and tear away from the pan if you use dry hands. Get the dough as thin and smooth as possible, making the outer 1½ inches a bit thicker.

3 Set the pizza crust in a draft-free spot to rest for 15 minutes. Drizzle generously with olive oil and sprinkle with salt.

4 Bake the crust for 15 minutes, until golden. Remove the crust from the oven and brush with a little olive oil.

5 To make the wasabi coconut cream: In a small bowl, whisk together the coconut cream, wasabi, garlic cloves, lime zest, lime juice, and cilantro. Season with salt. Refrigerate until ready to use.

6 Spread the wasabi coconut cream evenly over the cooled pizza crust. Top with the avocado slices and then the tuna. Add the cucumbers slices and pickled onions, then sprinkle with the cilantro and chiles. Slice and serve.

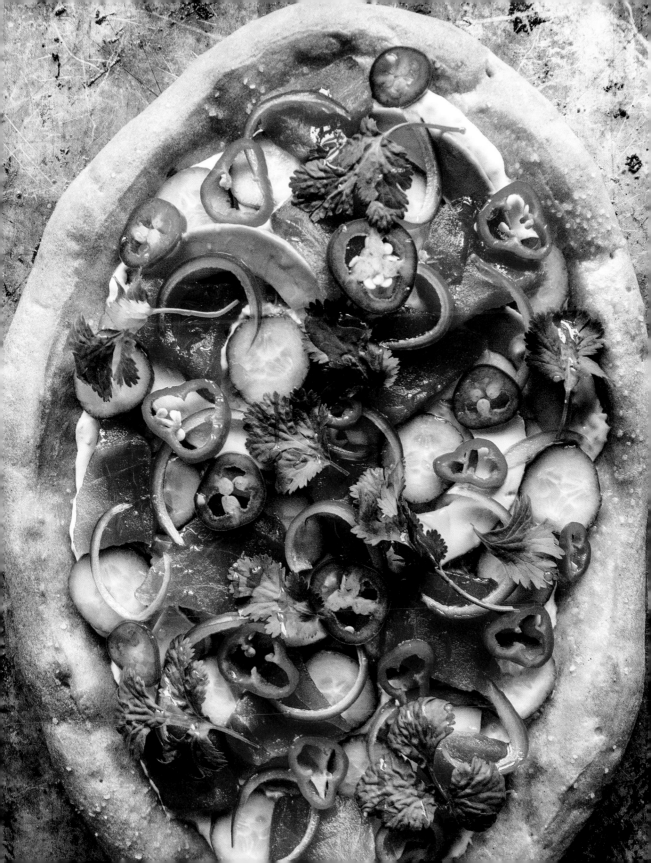

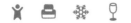

ASIAN SALMON BURGERS

PREPARATION 30 MINUTES, PLUS AT LEAST 1 HOUR OF REFRIGERATION TIME
COOK TIME 8 MINUTES **SERVINGS** 6

Elevate your backyard BBQ with these herbaceous and tender salmon patties. Topped with creamy smashed avocado, spicy pickled cucumbers, and pickled onions, they pack more flavor per bite than you could imagine. If you like, you can form the burgers and refrigerate them until you are ready to grill—I will often make these in the morning for an evening grill.

SPICY PICKLED CUCUMBERS

1 cup rice vinegar

¼ cup granulated beet sugar

2 teaspoons kosher salt

¼ teaspoon crushed red pepper flakes

1 large English cucumber, thinly sliced

BURGERS

2 pounds boneless, skinless salmon fillet

1 cup thinly sliced green onions

½ cup minced fresh cilantro

¼ cup minced fresh flat-leaf parsley

1 jalapeño, seeded and minced

¼ cup plus 2 tablespoons dehydrated potato flakes

2 tablespoons toasted sesame oil

1 teaspoon kosher salt

1 large avocado, pitted, peeled, and thinly sliced

6 Hamburger Buns (page 178)

Kosher salt

Sweet and Spicy Pickled Onions (page 94)

1 To make the spicy pickled cucumbers: In a small saucepan, combine the vinegar, sugar, salt, and red pepper flakes. When you have brought the mixture to a simmer, whisk well to make sure the sugar and salt have dissolved. Transfer the pickling liquid to a nonreactive bowl and let it cool completely.

2 When the liquid is cool, add the cucumber slices. Refrigerate until ready to serve.

3 To make the burgers: Using a large sharp knife, finely dice the salmon. Place in a large bowl.

4 Add the green onions, cilantro, parsley, jalapeño, ¼ cup of the potato flakes, the sesame oil, and the salt.

5 Mix really well and refrigerate for about an hour or up to 3 hours ahead of time.

6 Preheat a BBQ grill to medium heat. Line a rimmed baking sheet with parchment paper.

7 When the burger mixture is nice and cold, mix in the remaining 2 tablespoons potato flakes with clean hands. Form the mixture into 6 equal patties and set them on the prepared baking sheet. Place the patties directly onto the grill and cook them for about 4 minutes on each side, until golden.

8 Arrange the avocado slices on the bottom half of the buns and sprinkle with salt. Use a fork to gently smash the avocado. Top each with a grilled salmon patty and top with pickled cucumbers, pickled onions, and the bun tops.

NOTE: You could also serve these burgers sans bun on a bed of greens, like the Kale Power Salad with Garlic Honey Sesame Dressing (page 108).

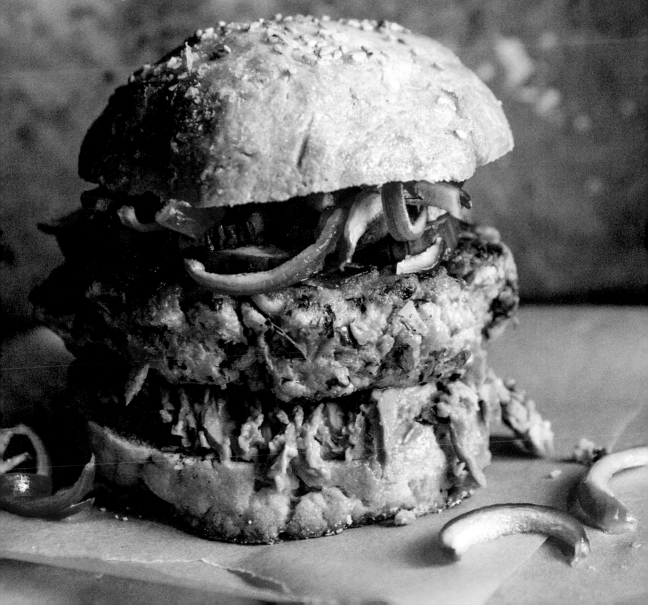

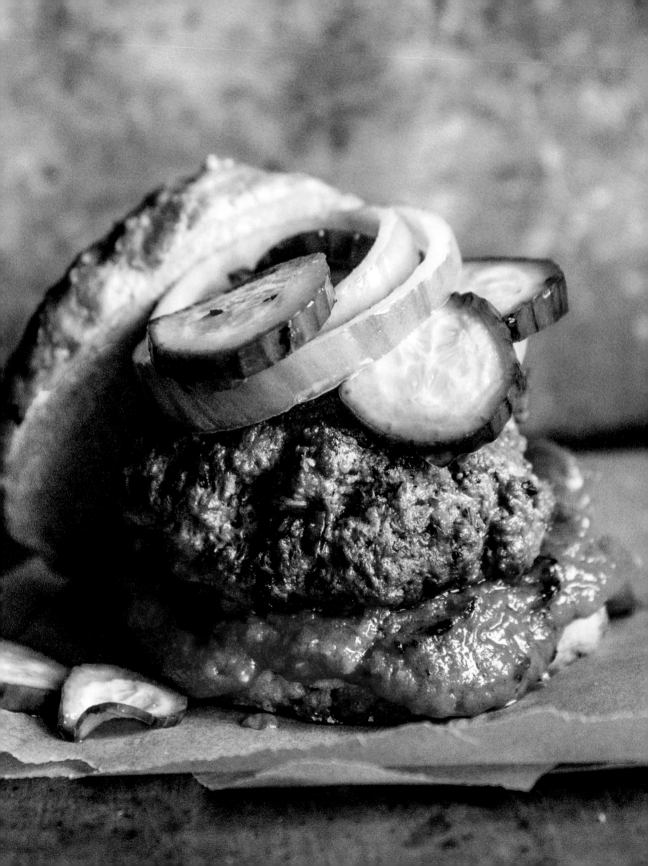

GREEK LAMB BURGERS WITH CHILE-RED ONION KETCHUP

PREPARATION 15 MINUTES COOK TIME 20 MINUTES SERVINGS 6

Nothing pairs better with ground lamb than garlic, fresh herbs, and red wine. With a slathering of semi-homemade ketchup, red onions, and spicy pickled cucumbers, you will have people lining up for this rather gourmet burger. Pair with Quinoa Tabbouleh (page 168) and Fresh Tomato Salad (page 114) or Broccoli Chopped Salad (page 111).

CHILE-RED ONION KETCHUP

1 tablespoon olive oil

1/2 red onion, chopped

1 red Fresno chile, seeded and minced

11/2 cups ketchup

Kosher salt

BURGERS

1½ pounds ground lamb

2 garlic cloves, minced

⅓ cup minced green onions

2 tablespoons minced fresh mint

2 tablespoons minced fresh oregano

¼ cup dehydrated potato flakes

2 tablespoons dry red wine

1½ teaspoons kosher salt

Spicy Pickled Cucumbers (page 202)

4 Hamburger Buns (page 178)

Sliced red onion, for garnish

1 To make the chile–red onion ketchup: In a medium sauté pan, heat the oil over medium heat. Add the onion and the chile and fry until they are golden, about 5 minutes. Transfer to a blender with the ketchup and purée until smooth and creamy. Season with salt. Refrigerate until ready to use.

2 To make the burgers: In a large bowl, use your clean hands to break up the ground lamb.

3 Add the garlic, green onions, mint, and oregano, then add the potato flakes and the wine and mix everything together really well. Add the salt and mix well.

4 Form the lamb mixture into 6 patties and set them on a baking sheet pan lined with parchment paper. Cover the pan with plastic wrap and refrigerate the burgers until you are ready to cook. I like to make them early in the day so that the flavors marry really well.

5 Preheat your grill to medium and oil the grill grates so the burgers won't stick.

6 Grill the burgers for 5 to 6 minutes on each side, or until medium and still a little pink in the center. Place a burger on a bun and top with with the chile–red onion ketchup, spicy pickled cucumbers, sliced red onion, and the bun tops.

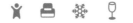

TURKEY BURGERS WITH CRANBERRY MUSTARD

PREPARATION 20 MINUTES   **COOK TIME** 12 MINUTES   **SERVINGS** 4

These burgers lie in a very happy place somewhere between Thanksgiving dinner and a really good breakfast sausage. The turkey patties are so savory and juicy, and then the gorgeous cranberry mustard, with all its sweet, sour, and spicy flavors, really give these burgers a kick. I like a handful of arugula and crunchy red onions for extra flavor.

CRANBERRY MUSTARD

⅓ cup fresh cranberries

2 tablespoons honey

3 tablespoons rice vinegar

¼ cup whole-grain mustard

Kosher salt

BURGERS

1½ pounds ground turkey

¼ cup minced fresh sage

½ cup finely diced yellow onion

1 garlic clove, minced

1½ teaspoons kosher salt

⅓ cup dehydrated potato flakes

6 Hamburger Buns (page 178)

Red onion slices

2 cups fresh arugula

1 To make the cranberry mustard: In the bowl of a food processor, combine the cranberries, honey, and vinegar. Pulse on high until you have a pulp. Add the mustard and pulse until well combined. Season with salt.

2 To make the burgers: In a large bowl, use your clean hands to mix together the turkey, sage, onion, garlic, salt, and potato flakes until completely combined. Form the mixture into 4 equal patties and set them on a baking sheet lined with parchment paper. (At this point, you could refrigerate them until you need to grill them, up to a day.)

3 When you are ready to cook, preheat your grill to medium and oil the grill grates so that the burgers don't stick.

4 Grill the burgers for 5 to 6 minutes on each side, or until cooked through.

5 Slather the bottom of the buns with the cranberry mustard and place a turkey burger on each. Top with red onion slices and arugula. Top with the other half of the bun and serve hot.

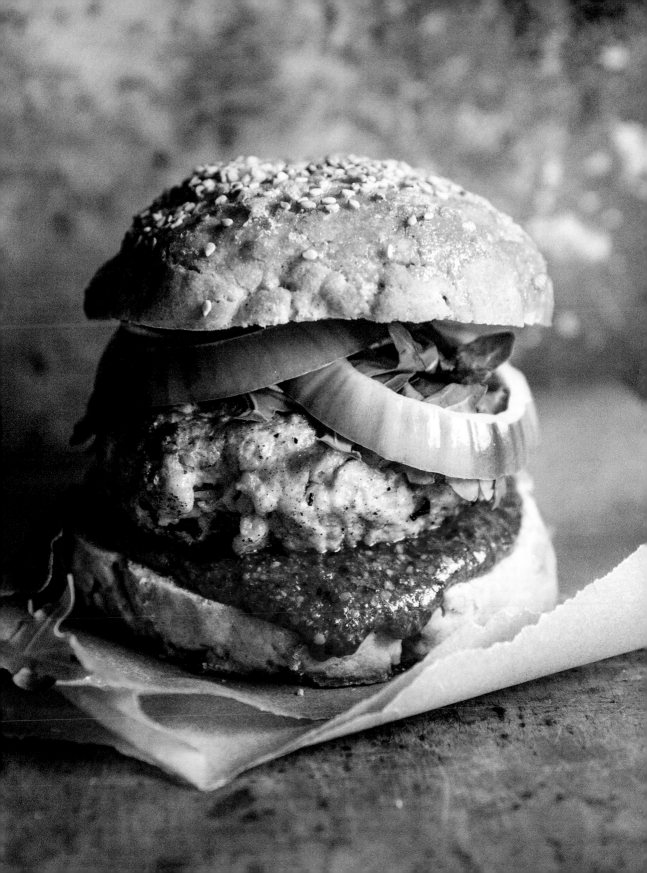

PORTOBELLO MUSHROOM BURGERS WITH CREAMY RED PEPPER SPREAD AND ROASTED SHALLOTS AND CHERRY TOMATOES

PREPARATION 30 MINUTES, PLUS 30 MINUTES MARINATING TIME
COOK TIME 10 TO 12 MINUTES   **SERVINGS** 4

I don't think I voluntarily ate a mushroom until I was in college, but when our friend Kirby included them in a barbecue spread, I realized what I had been missing all those years. He had marinated these huge meaty portobellos for hours and then grilled them, giving them a very similar flavor to the flank steak they were next to—I was completely shocked and totally hooked. I have been cooking a variety of mushrooms ever since, but still really have a thing for marinated and grilled portobellos, so I am sharing them here. They make an excellent replacement for meat in a burger and are perfect for entertaining, since you can make the sauce and marinate the mushrooms the day before.

RED PEPPER BASIL SAUCE

2 garlic cloves, chopped

1 whole roasted red pepper

½ cup fresh basil leaves

¼ cup olive oil

3 tablespoons red wine vinegar

Kosher salt

½ cup chilled unsweetened coconut cream

MARINATED MUSHROOMS

4 large portobello mushrooms

3 garlic cloves, minced

¼ cup balsamic vinegar

½ teaspoon kosher salt

1 tablespoon olive oil

ROASTED SHALLOTS AND CHERRY TOMATOES

2 large shallots, thinly sliced

1 cup cherry tomatoes

2 tablespoons olive oil

Kosher salt

• • •

4 Hamburger Buns (page 178)

1 cup arugula

1 Preheat the oven to 450°F.

2 To make the red pepper basil sauce: In a food processor, combine the garlic, red pepper, basil, olive oil, and vinegar. Pulse until smooth and season with salt.

3 Transfer ¼ cup of the sauce to a large resealable bag and put the rest in a bowl. Gently mix the chilled coconut cream into the sauce in the bowl until thoroughly combined. Season with salt and refrigerate. As the sauce chills, it will firm up. (You can make the sauce the day before.)

4 To make the marinated mushrooms: Trim the stems from the portobello mushrooms and set aside. To the plastic bag with the ¼ cup red pepper basil sauce, add the garlic, vinegar, and salt. Add the mushrooms and seal the bag. Really shake and move the mushrooms around to coat them. Marinate them in the refrigerator for at least 30 minutes or up to overnight.

5 In a large heavy grill pan or skillet, heat the olive oil over medium heat. Add the mushrooms, top down. Cook the mushrooms for 4 to 5 minutes, then flip and cook for 4 to 5 minutes more.

6 Meanwhile, to make the roasted shallots and cherry tomoatoes: Place the shallots and cherry tomatoes on a sheet of aluminum foil. Add the olive oil and a sprinkle of salt and wrap the foil up tightly. Roast directly on the oven rack for 10 minutes. Remove and set aside, without opening.

7 Cut the buns in half and spread the bottom half with a generous amount of the creamy red pepper spread. Top each with a mushroom and a handful of fresh arugula leaves. Open the foil with the roasted shallots and cherry tomatoes and spoon some on top of each burger. Serve hot or at room temperature.

MUSHROOMS, and specifically cremini or portobello mushrooms, provide unique support to the immune system and fight inflammation, and, in particular, battle the onset of arthritis.

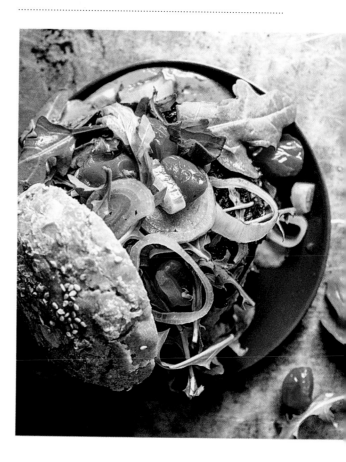

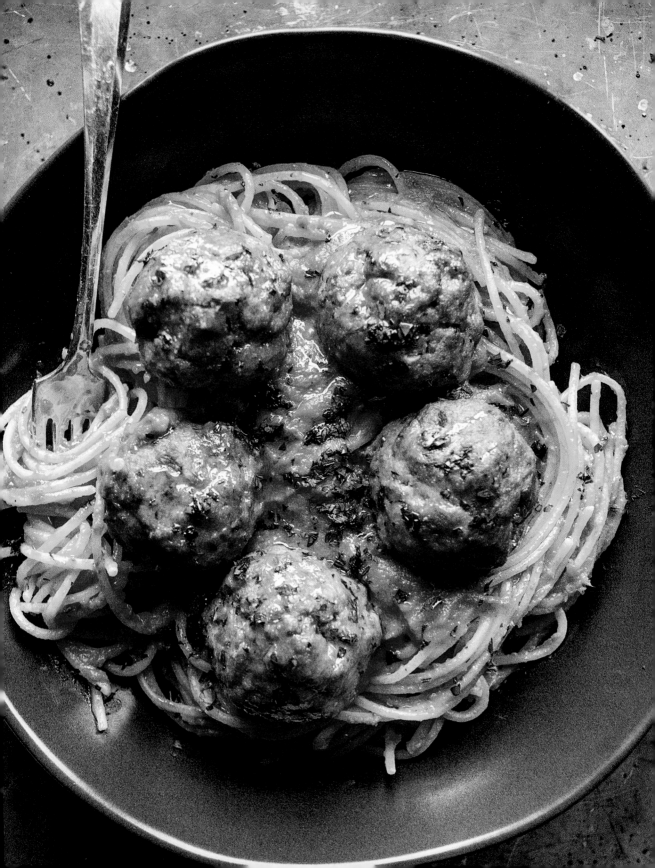

pasta

If I designate soup as my soul food, then my husband would lay claim to pasta. And for busy weeknights, it's a family go-to, especially when I'm reduced to raiding the fridge and pantry for a quickly thrown-together entrée. Thanks to the incredible selection of gluten-free varieties available now, having allergies hasn't thrown my pasta game off too much. The easiest varieties to find are brown rice, quinoa, and corn pastas. In my experience, brown rice pasta is the most finicky and tends to go mushy quickly, so I always undercook it by a few minutes to keep an al dente texture. I have found that I like corn pasta the best, because it most closely mimics traditional semolina pasta and has a nice tooth to it. Then I just substitute a lot of fresh produce, olive oil, and bright flavors for the traditional cheese and cream. Thank goodness for coconut cream, which gives many of the sauces here—like the Creamy Mushroom Pasta and Creamy Tomato-Vodka Sauce—richness and a smooth texture. Every dish in this section takes thirty minutes or less to make and pleases a wide range of appetites, and I've added plenty of ideas for adjusting the flavor profiles and ingredients to suit your tastes, so you can truly make these dishes your own.

◄ Old-Fashioned Spaghetti and Meatballs (page 212)

OLD-FASHIONED SPAGHETTI AND MEATBALLS

PREPARATION 15 MINUTES **COOK TIME** 15 MINUTES **SERVINGS** 4 TO 6

For years my sister made me spaghetti and meatballs on my birthday and it has always been at the very top of my desert island–meal list—I love it that much. So when all this allergy stuff happened, I literally wept at the thought that I would never again feast on her silky spaghetti and melt-in-your-mouth meatballs. And then a friend shared the magical solution to binding the meatball mixture and keeping them tender without eggs, cheese, or bread crumbs: dehydrated potato flakes. Laugh if you will, but then go pick up a box at the store and see if you don't agree. Because everything cooks simultaneously, it takes me only a half hour to get this onto the table. (Photograph on page 210.)

MEATBALLS

½ cup chopped red onion

3 garlic cloves, minced

3 tablespoons pepitas

1 tablespoon plus 1 teaspoon Worcestershire sauce

1 tablespoon olive oil

2½ teaspoons kosher salt

1 teaspoon crushed red pepper flakes

1 pound ground beef (80% lean)

1 pound ground pork

½ cup dehydrated potato flakes

⅓ cup minced fresh flat-leaf parsley

1 tablespoon minced fresh oregano

TOMATO SAUCE

3 tablespoons olive oil

1 yellow onion, coarsely chopped

½ red onion, coarsely chopped

2 garlic cloves, coarsely chopped

1 (28-ounce) can crushed tomatoes

2 teaspoons dried oregano

Kosher salt

• • •

1 pound gluten-free spaghetti

1 To make the meatballs: Preheat the oven to 375°F. Line a rimmed baking sheet with parchment paper.

2 In a food processor, combine the red onion, garlic, pepitas, Worcestershire sauce, olive oil, salt, and red pepper flakes and pulse until well combined.

3 In a large bowl, use your clean hands to break up the ground beef and pork. Add the contents of the food processor, the potato flakes, parsley, and oregano, and mix well until everything is completely combined.

4 Form the mixture into 24 medium meatballs and line them up on the prepared baking sheet. Bake until the meatballs are lightly golden and cooked through, about 15 minutes.

5 Meanwhile, to make the tomato sauce: In a large saucepan, heat the olive oil over medium heat. Add the onions and sauté until soft and tender, 5 to 7 minutes. Add the garlic and cook for 2 minutes more. Stir in the tomatoes.

6 Transfer the mixture to a blender and purée on high until smooth. Return the purée to the pan and add the oregano. Season to taste with salt. Cover the pan and reduce the heat to low.

7 Meanwhile, bring a large pot of salted water to a boil. Add the spaghetti and cook until al dente according to the package directions.

8 Add the meatballs to the sauce and simmer while the pasta cooks.

9 Drain the pasta and return it to the pot. Pour the sauce and meatballs over the pasta and toss to coat. Serve hot.

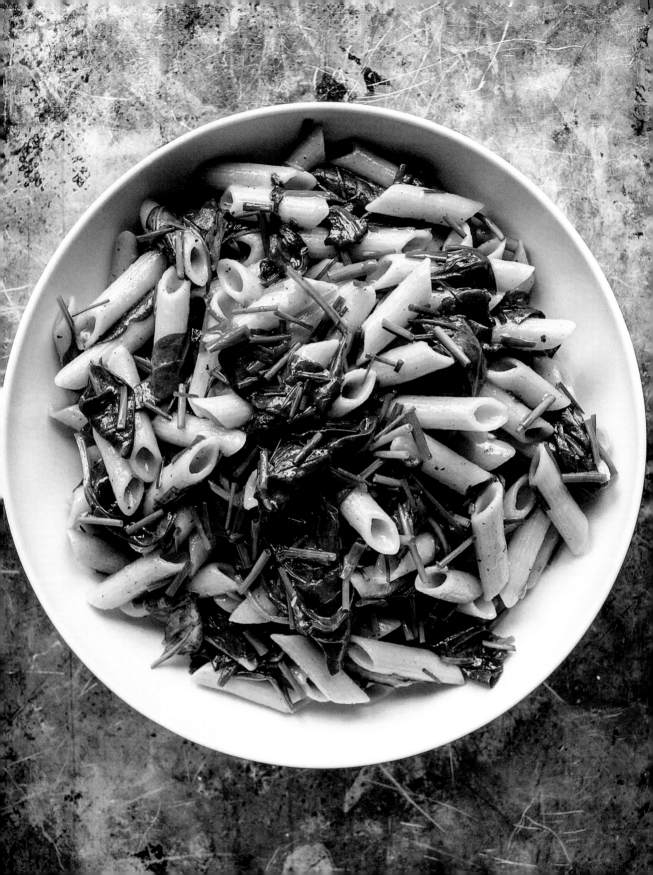

PASTA WITH BACON, SPINACH, AND CHIVES

PREPARATION 5 MINUTES   **COOK TIME** 10 MINUTES   **SERVINGS 4**

You can't argue with the brilliance of a dish as lovely as this one, which can be made in just one pot in about fifteen minutes. I make it often during the summer, when I can pick chives and spinach in my garden, but truthfully, it is wonderful any time of year. I prefer tender small baby spinach leaves in this recipe, as they are really just wilted by the heat of the pasta, not cooked through. If you like, add a generous pinch of red pepper flakes along with the garlic. It gives some nice heat to the dish.

Kosher salt

1 pound gluten-free penne

4 thick-cut uncured bacon slices, chopped into ½-inch pieces

1 garlic clove, minced

2 tablespoons olive oil

2 tablespoons red wine vinegar

4 cups fresh baby spinach

½ cup minced fresh chives

1 Bring a large pot of salted water to a boil. Add the pasta and cook, stirring often, just until al dente, according to package directions. Reserve ½ cup of the pasta cooking water and drain the pasta.

2 While the pasta cooks, in a large heavy skillet, cook the bacon over medium heat until the fat has rendered and the bacon is crisp, about 5 minutes. Add the garlic and cook until fragrant and lightly browned, 2 minutes more.

3 Add the drained pasta and the reserved pasta water to the skillet and mix well. In a small bowl, mix together the olive oil and vinegar, then drizzle the mixture over the pasta. Add the spinach, toss to combine, and season with salt. Sprinkle with the chives, toss, and serve immediately.

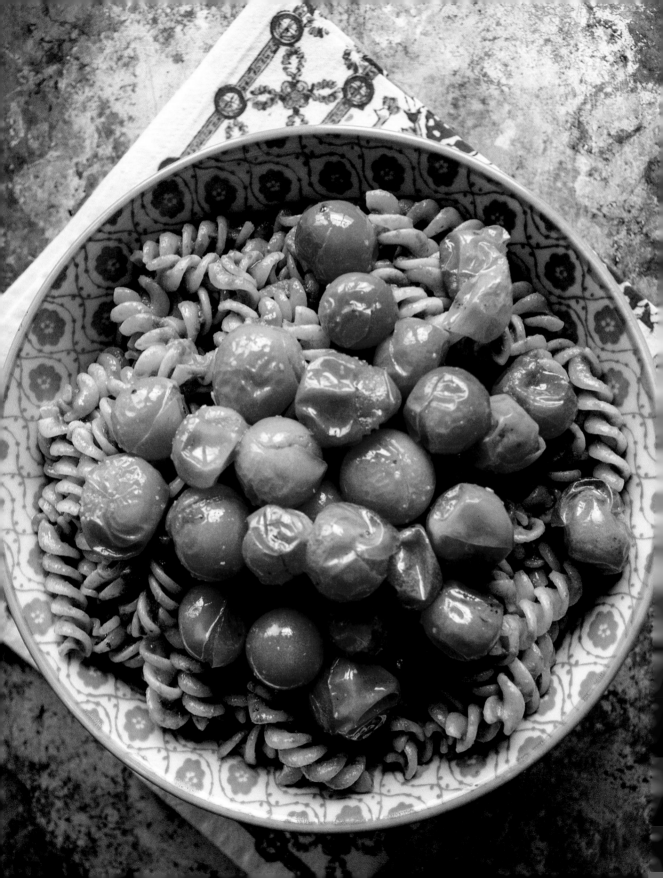

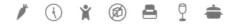

PASTA WITH ROASTED TOMATOES AND HOT BASIL VINAIGRETTE

PREPARATION 5 MINUTES   **COOK TIME** 15 MINUTES   **SERVINGS** 4

The vibrant flavor and bright colors of this warm vinaigrette are completely addictive. Heating the vinaigrette enhances the basil's aroma while mellowing the bite of the garlic. All of that is beautifully balanced by the sweet, juicy, roasted cherry tomatoes, which burst in your mouth when you happen to catch one on your fork. By the way, this is also delicious served as a cold pasta salad.

PASTA

Kosher salt

1 pint cherry tomatoes

¼ cup olive oil

1 pound gluten-free short pasta, such as rotini

BASIL VINAIGRETTE

3 garlic cloves, coarsely chopped

4 ounces fresh basil leaves (about 4 cups, loosely packed)

¼ cup olive oil

3 tablespoons red wine vinegar

Kosher salt

1 Preheat the oven to 400°F. Bring a large pot of salted water to a boil.

2 Arrange the cherry tomatoes on a rimmed baking sheet add and drizzle with the olive oil. Sprinkle with a little salt. Roast for 10 minutes.

3 Add the pasta to the boiling water and cook to al dente, according to the package directions, stirring often to keep the pasta from sticking.

4 Meanwhile, make the basil vinaigrette: In a blender, combine the garlic, basil, olive oil, and vinegar. Purée until you have a smooth dressing. Season with salt.

5 Drain the pasta and return it to the pot. Add the basil vinaigrette and toss with the hot pasta, adding salt to taste if needed. Transfer the pasta to a serving platter and top with the roasted tomatoes. Drizzle any juices from the pan over the pasta. Serve immediately.

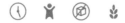

PASTA WITH SAUSAGE, WHITE BEANS, AND MUSTARD GREENS

PREPARATION 10 MINUTES   **COOK TIME** 15 MINUTES   **SERVINGS** 4

The combination of a less-used green with spicy sausage and creamy white beans may seem unusual, but trust me on this one. The peppery greens boldly flavor the pasta, and the sausage and beans contribute tons of protein. This is exactly the kind of dish you want to cozy up to in the middle of fall or winter.

Kosher salt

1 pound gluten-free penne

12 ounces spicy pork or chicken sausage, casings removed

2 tablespoons olive oil, plus more for drizzling

1 red onion, thinly sliced

5 cups coarsely chopped mustard greens

1 (15-ounce) can cannellini beans, drained and rinsed

1 Bring a large pot of salted water to a boil. Add the pasta and cook to al dente, according to package directions, stirring often to prevent the pasta from sticking. Reserve ½ cup of the pasta cooking water, then drain the pasta and set aside.

2 While the pasta is cooking, in a large heavy pan or skillet, cook the sausage over medium heat, breaking it up with a wooden spoon as you cook until lightly browned, about 5 minutes.

3 Add the olive oil and the red onion to the skillet and cook until the onion is softened, about 3 minutes more. Add the mustard greens and sauté just until the greens are wilted, 1 minute.

4 Add the white beans and the drained pasta to the pan along with the reserved pasta water, tossing everything together and cooking for 1 to 2 minutes until the water has been absorbed. Add Kosher salt, drizzle with a bit of olive oil and serve immediately.

MUSTARD GREENS. 1 cup of mustard greens has almost 1,000 percent of your recommended daily vitamin K, 100 percent of your vitamin A, and 50 percent of your vitamin C!

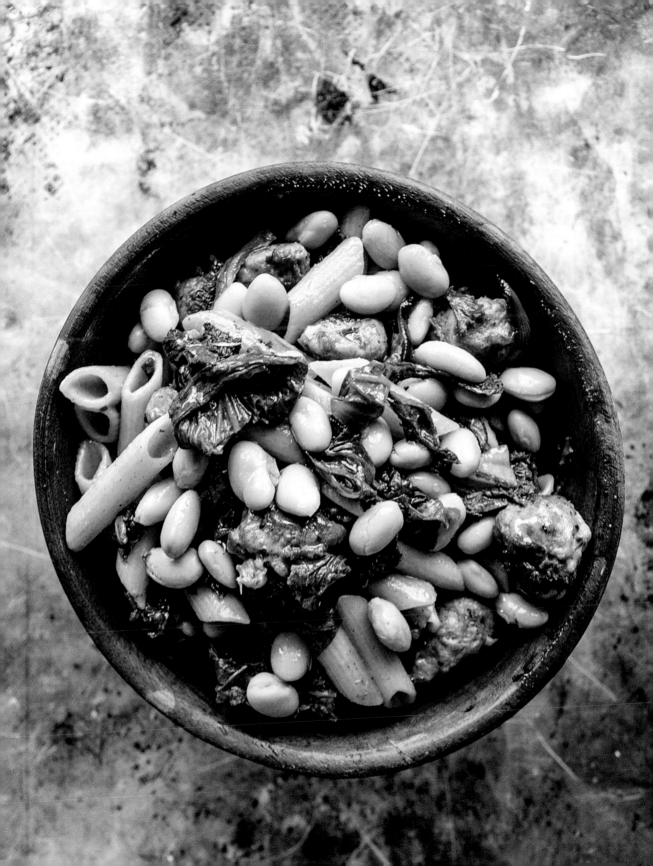

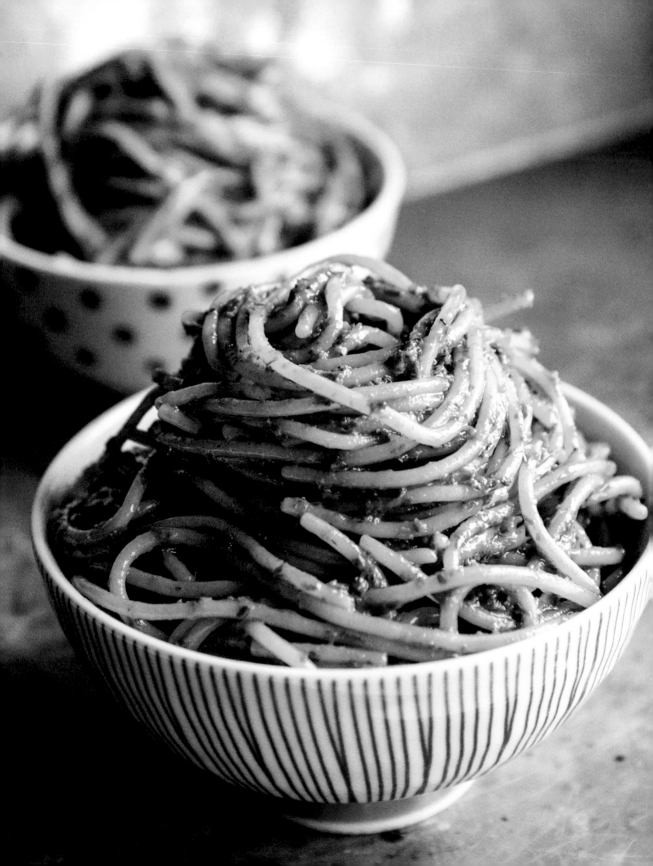

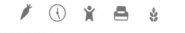

KALE PESTO PASTA

PREPARATION 10 MINUTES   **COOK TIME** 10 MINUTES   **SERVINGS** 4

I came late to the kale party; sautéed kale was just so tough, so healthy, so *green*! Where I found acceptance and later love was with raw kale, first in salads and then in this sauce. It is still *sooooo* green, but it also has complex herbal notes as well. It's a most delicious way to get a major dose of your daily greens! Serve topped with a pinch of red pepper flakes if you like.

KALE PESTO

4 cups kale leaves, stems removed and coarsely chopped

2 garlic cloves, coarsely chopped

2 tablespoons fresh lemon juice

¼ teaspoon crushed red pepper flakes

¼ cup olive oil

Kosher salt

PASTA

Kosher salt

1 pound gluten-free spaghetti

Olive oil, for drizzling

1 Make the kale pesto: In a food processor, combine all the pesto ingredients and pulse until smooth. Season with salt. Set aside.

2 Bring a large pot of salted water to a boil. Cook the pasta just until al dente, according to package directions; drain and transfer to a serving bowl.

3 Toss the pasta with the pesto until well coated; add more salt to taste. Drizzle with olive oil and serve immediately.

KALE. 1 cup of kale has 1,180 percent of your daily recommended vitamin K! It also has 98 percent of your vitamin A and 71 percent of your vitamin C. Amazing! Kale has more than forty-five different varieties of flavonoids. All those kale flavonoids combine with the antioxidant and anti-inflammatory benefits in a unique way to help fight chronic inflammation. Kale is known to be a specific soldier in the fight against bladder, breast, colon, ovarian, and prostate cancers.

CARROT PESTO PASTA

PREPARATION 15 MINUTES   COOK TIME 10 MINUTES   SERVINGS 4 TO 6

One of the great things about this light and flavorful pasta is that carrots are in season any time of the year. With only six simple ingredients in the whole dish, you really get to taste the freshness of the carrots. You can vary the color of this sauce depending on what variety of carrots you use, getting hues from deep orange to yellow.

Kosher salt

4 cups carrots, peeled and chopped into 1-inch pieces

3 garlic cloves

2 tablespoons rice vinegar

1 cup olive oil

1 pound gluten-free pasta

Chives and edible flowers for garnish (optional)

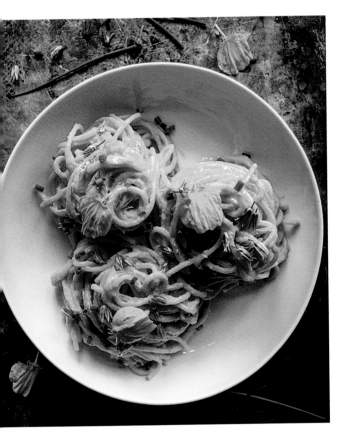

1 Bring a large pot of salted water to a boil. Add the carrots to the pot and boil them for 10 minutes. Using a slotted spoon, remove the carrots from the water, shaking off the extra water; don't discard the cooking water.

2 Place the drained carrots in a blender and add the garlic, vinegar, and oil. Purée until very smooth. Season generously with salt.

3 Bring the pot of water back to a boil and add the pasta. Cook just to al dente (a few minutes short of the manufacturer's directions). When the pasta is cooked, drain and return it to the empty pot. Add the carrot pesto and toss to coat.

4 Transfer the pasta to a serving platter, garnish with edible flowers and chives, if desired, and serve hot.

PASTA WITH SPICY GARLIC CHICKEN AND TOMATOES

PREPARATION 5 MINUTES   **COOK TIME** 15 MINUTES   **SERVINGS** 4

I ate something like this just about every week growing up—it's my mom in a bowl. I loved it then and still do today, and luckily, my kids do, too (although I usually leave out the red pepper flakes for them). It's a fast-and-easy dish at its finest, with pasta, veggies, and chicken all in one—perfect for uncomplicated weekday cooking. (Photograph on page 7.)

2 tablespoons olive oil

3 garlic cloves, minced

½ teaspoon crushed red pepper flakes

½ pound boneless, skinless chicken breasts

½ cup dry white wine

1 pound cherry tomatoes

Kosher salt

1 pound gluten-free pasta

1 cup finely chopped fresh flat-leaf parsley

Juice of 1 lemon

1 In a large sauté pan, heat the olive oil over medium heat. Add the garlic and red pepper flakes and cook for about 1 minute. Add the chicken breast and cook for 2 minutes, until golden brown on the bottom. Turn the chicken, add the wine, and stir to scrape up any browned bits from the bottom of the pan. Add the cherry tomatoes and cover the pan. Cook for about 5 minutes, or until the chicken is cooked through.

2 Transfer the chicken to a plate and in the same pan, cook the tomatoes for about 2 minutes.

3 Chop the chicken into bite-size pieces and return it to the pan. Cook the tomatoes and chicken for 2 to 3 minutes more, until some of the tomatoes are just beginning to burst. Cover and keep warm on low heat.

4 Bring a large pot of salted water to a boil. Add the pasta and cook to al dente, according to package directions, stirring often to prevent the pasta from sticking.

5 Drain the pasta and add it to the skillet. Gently fold the pasta into the chicken and tomatoes.

6 Add the parsley, lemon juice, and salt to taste. Serve immediately.

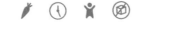

CREAMY MUSHROOM PASTA

PREPARATION 5 MINUTES   **COOK TIME** 20 MINUTES   **SERVINGS** 4

There is something so comforting and nostalgic about this creamy mushroom pasta. I still have fond memories of the many things my grammy used to make with good old cream-of-mushroom soup. This is about a million times fresher and more delicious, but it still pulls off that rich, creamy, comfort food feeling.

Kosher salt

2 tablespoons soy-free vegan butter

1 yellow onion, finely chopped

6 cups sliced cremini or button mushrooms

1 pound gluten-free pasta

½ cup dry sherry

½ cup mushroom or chicken broth

½ cup unsweetened coconut cream

2 teaspoons fresh thyme leaves

1 Bring a large pot of salted water to a boil.

2 In a large heavy pan or skillet, melt the vegan butter over medium-high heat. Add the onion and cook until soft and tender, about 5 minutes. Add the mushrooms and cook until they have released their juices, their liquid cooks off, and the pan is dry, about 5 minutes more.

3 At this point, add the pasta to the boiling water and cook to al dente, according to the package directions, stirring often to prevent it from sticking. Reserve ½ cup of the pasta cooking water, then drain the pasta.

4 Add sherry to the pan with the mushrooms and scrape up any browned bits from the bottom of the pan. Add the broth and cook until the mushrooms are tender and the broth has reduced, 5 to 7 minutes more.

5 Stir in the coconut cream to make a creamy sauce. Stir in the thyme, then add the pasta, tossing to coat well. If the pasta seems dry, add the reserved pasta water a little at a time and stir until desired consistency is achieved. Season with salt and serve immediately.

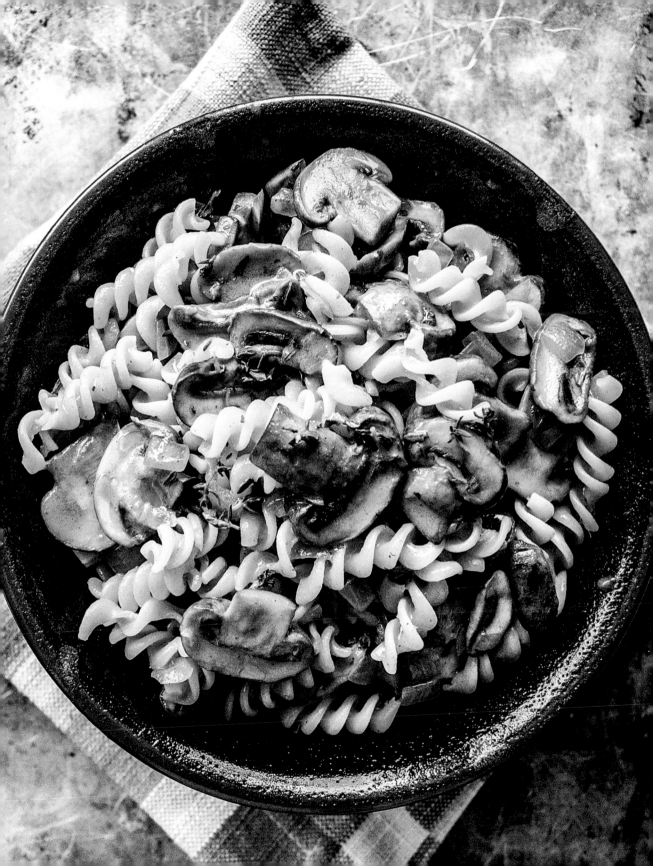

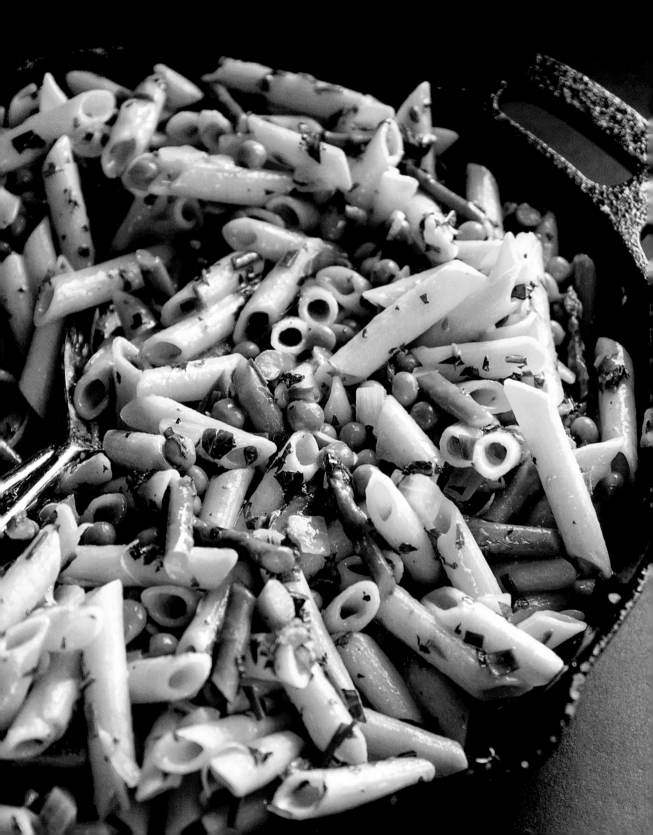

PASTA VERDE

PREPARATION 5 MINUTES **COOK TIME** 15 MINUTES **SERVINGS** 4

Bright, fresh, and springlike are good ways to describe this beautiful pasta dish. It makes a perfect vegan entrée and would also be lovely accompanied by a fillet of crispy salmon. Either way, it is even better with a glass of white wine (as so many things are . . .).

Kosher salt

1 pound gluten-free pasta

¼ cup olive oil

½ yellow onion, finely chopped

¾ cup dry white wine

2 cups shelled green peas (about 2 pounds in the pod)

1 pound asparagus, trimmed and cut into thirds

Grated zest of 1 lemon

2 tablespoons fresh lemon juice

¼ cup minced fresh chives

⅓ cup finely chopped fresh mint

1 Bring a large pot of salted water to a boil. Add the pasta and cook to al dente, according to the package directions, stirring often to keep the pasta from sticking.

2 While the pasta is cooking, in a large skillet or heavy pan, heat the oil over medium heat. Add the onion and sprinkle with salt, then cook until the onion is soft and tender but not browned, about 5 minutes. Add the wine, stir well, and cook until the wine has reduced, 1 to 2 minutes more.

3 Add the peas and asparagus and simmer until they are just cooked through and bright green, about 2 minutes.

4 Drain the pasta then add it directly to the pan with the vegetables. Add the lemon zest, lemon juice, chives, mint, and salt to taste and toss to combine. Serve hot.

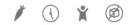

PENNE WITH
CREAMY TOMATO-VODKA SAUCE

PREPARATION 5 MINUTES **COOK TIME** 25 MINUTES **SERVINGS** 4

I think the reason so many people are fans of penne with vodka sauce is the way the sauce fills up the pasta tubes, so you get a ton of it in each bite. This version satisfies that requirement and more.

3 tablespoons soy-free vegan butter

1 yellow onion, finely chopped

3 garlic cloves

½ cup vodka

¼ teaspoon crushed red pepper flakes

1 (28-ounce) can crushed tomatoes

Kosher salt

1 pound gluten-free penne

⅔ cup unsweetened coconut cream

1 In a heavy pan or skillet, melt the butter over medium heat. Add the onion and cook for 5 minutes, until tender. Add the garlic and cook until it is golden, 2 minutes more. Add the vodka slowly to the center of the pan and stir carefully to prevent lighting the pan on fire! (Alcohol is flammable.) Cook for about 1 minute.

2 Add the red pepper flakes and the tomatoes and cook for 2 minutes. Transfer the contents of the pan to a blender and purée until smooth. Season with salt. Return the sauce to the pan and simmer over low heat for 15 minutes to thicken.

3 Meanwhile, bring a large pot of salted water to a boil. Add the penne and cook until just shy of al dente, according to the package directions.

4 Stir the coconut cream into the sauce and adjust the seasoning. Add the drained pasta to the pan and cook with the sauce for 2 minutes. Add salt as needed and serve hot.

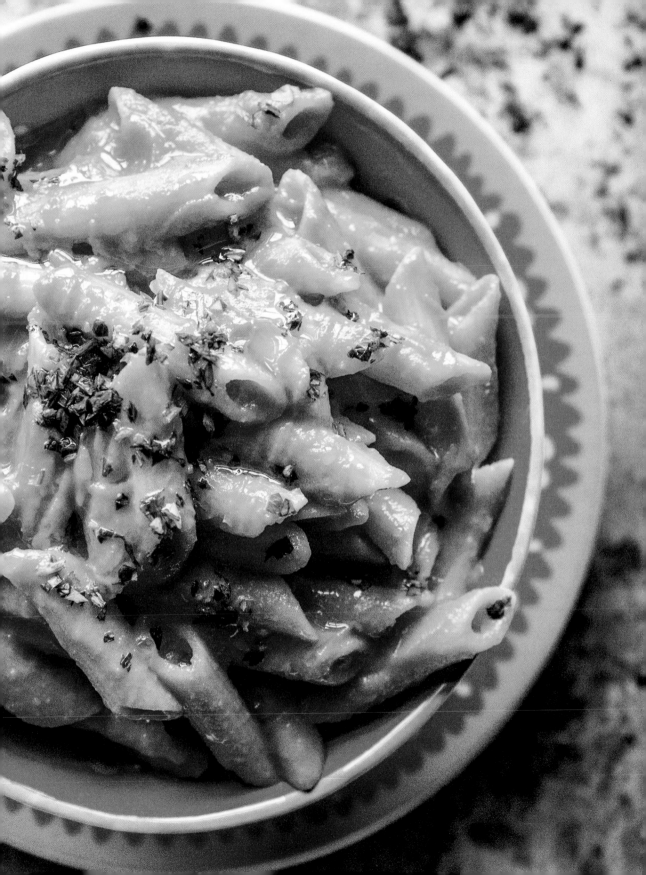

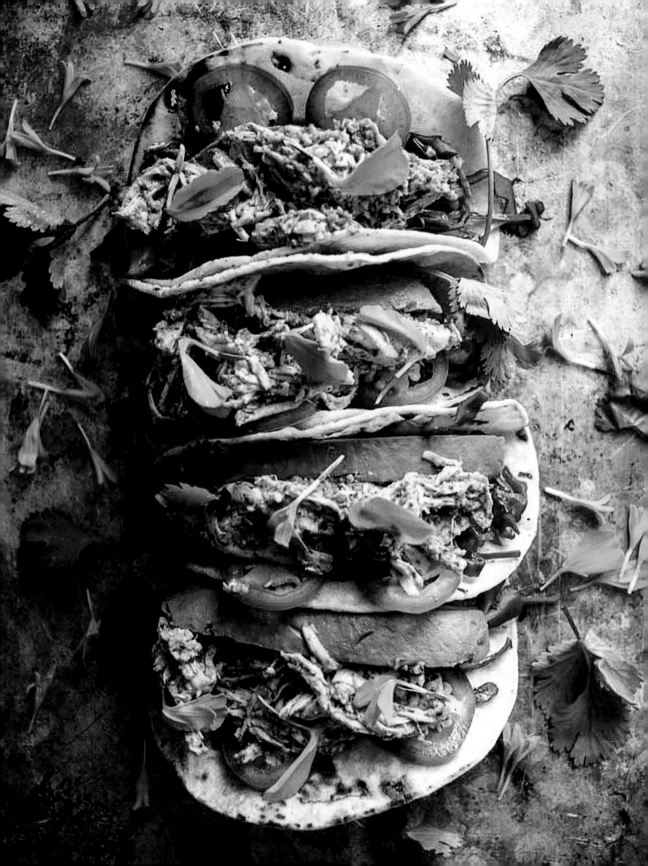

mains

Adjusting ingredients to make savory recipes allergen-free is much less complicated than adapting recipes for baking. It's about letting go of your butter (remember, you've still got olive oil!) and cream (you'll come to love coconut cream!) and cheese (can't help you there, I'm afraid, but I promise you're not even going to notice its absence). In every instance, though, the basic promise should be the same: a savory, fresh, full-of-flavor dish that nourishes and satisfies.

In this chapter you'll find everything from ultimate comfort food like classic Meat Loaf and Greek Stuffed Peppers to slow-cooked meats like Pork Ragù and Beer-Braised Brisket, Spicy Shredded Beef Tostadas, and Asian Pulled Pork. Get to know light and fresh dishes like Roasted Halibut with Strawberry-Basil Salsa, and explore one of the beautiful salmon dishes I've provided. Feeling exotic? Try the Red Vegetable Curry or the Spicy Tuna Sushi Bowl. Looking for a happy substitute for drive-through fare? Chicken nuggets or fish and chips should satisfy that craving for young *and* old. In fact, there is something (and more) for everyone here, including lots of tips on how you can make subtle changes to create other flavor profiles, and make a dish stretch over two meals or more. Get cooking!

◀ Chicken Tacos with Cilantro Pesto (page 244)

CHICKEN TERIYAKI

PREPARATION 5 MINUTES   **COOK TIME** 20 MINUTES   **SERVINGS** 4

I discovered this classic combo in high school when my friends and I would head to a local spot and scrape our change together to buy chicken teriyaki. I basically repeated the same situation in college, when I discovered a great spot around the corner from where I lived. As an adult, I would sometimes venture back to that same college haunt with Pete and bring takeout home to eat with disposable chopsticks in front of the TV. When Pia and Coco became fans, too, I figured out how to make that same great sauce allergen-free. Sometimes we make teriyaki chicken breasts, but here I wanted to honor chicken thighs, which are traditional.

TERIYAKI SAUCE

¼ cup coconut amino acids

¼ cup honey

2 garlic cloves, grated

2 tablespoons grated fresh ginger

2 tablespoons rice vinegar

2 teaspoons sesame oil

1 tablespoon cornstarch

CHICKEN

2 tablespoons vegetable oil

1½ pounds boneless, skin-on chicken thighs

Steamed white rice and broccoli, for serving

Thinly sliced green onions and sesame seeds, for garnish

1 Make the teriyaki sauce: In a sauté pan, combine the amino acids, honey, garlic, ginger, vinegar, sesame oil, and ½ cup hot water. Whisk and simmer over low heat until smooth.

2 In a small jar, combine the cornstarch and ¼ cup cold water and shake until smooth. Add the cornstarch slurry to the saucepan and whisk while cooking over medium heat until the teriyaki sauce thickens, about 2 minutes. Set aside.

3 Heat the oil in a heavy pan over medium-high heat. Add the chicken, skin-side down, and cook for about 6 minutes, until the fat has rendered and the chicken skin is golden and crisp.

4 Turn the chicken pieces over and add ¼ cup water to the pan and cover with a lid so that the chicken steams and cooks through, about 5 minutes more. Add any liquid that has accumulated in the pan to the teriyaki sauce. (If the sauce has gotten too thick, just add ¼ cup water and whisk over low heat until smooth.)

5 Cook the chicken in the sauce for 1 to 2 minutes more, turning the chicken to coat it in the sauce. Serve hot with steamed white rice and broccoli and garnished with green onions and sesame seeds.

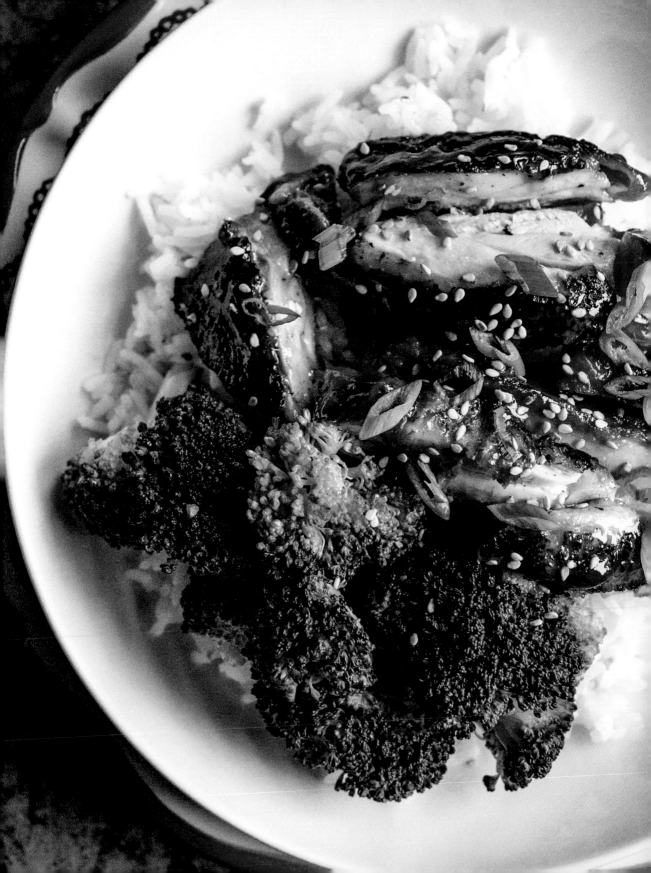

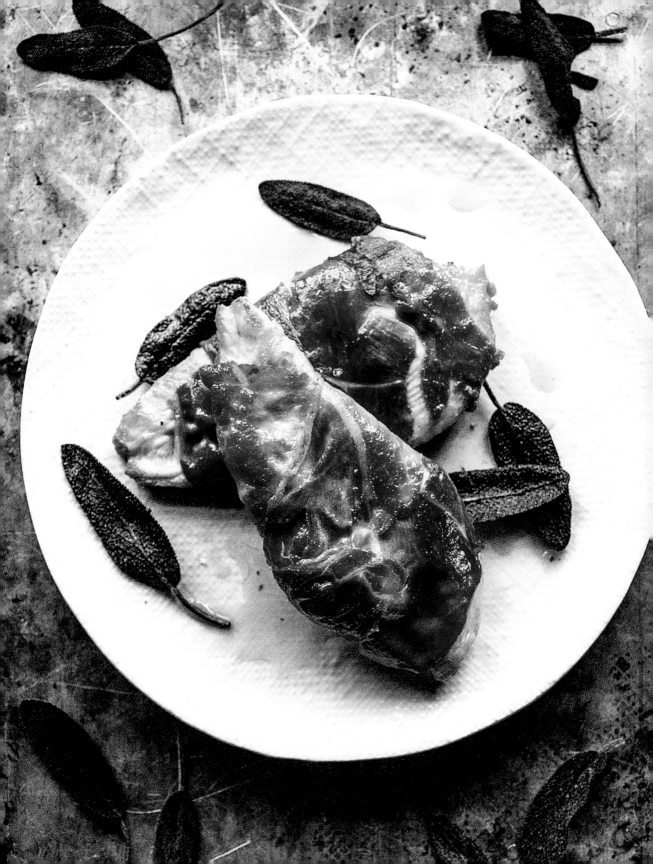

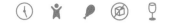

PROSCIUTTO-WRAPPED CHICKEN BREASTS
WITH CRISPY SAGE

PREPARATION 10 MINUTES **COOK TIME** 12 MINUTES **SERVINGS** 4

Prosciutto gives a simple chicken breast a nice golden exterior and lots of extra flavor. The crispy sage leaves and squeeze of fresh lemon bring the whole plate to life. As my mom says, this recipe makes it so easy to turn plain old chicken breasts into something really special!

4 thin boneless, skinless chicken breasts

4 large slices prosciutto

¼ cup olive oil

8 fresh sage leaves

4 lemon wedges

1 Wrap each chicken breast tightly with a piece of prosciutto. Set aside.

2 In a heavy pan, heat the olive oil over medium-high heat. Add the sage leaves and fry until crisp, 3 to 5 minutes. Drain on a paper towel.

3 Add the chicken breasts to the same pan and cook until the prosciutto is crispy and the chicken is cooked partially through, about 3 minutes.

Carefully turn the chicken and cook until just cooked through. (With a thin breast, it will be about 2 minutes more, or cook to done according to the thickness of the chicken.)

4 Transfer to a serving plate and top with a drizzle of the oil from the pan. Garnish with a couple of crispy sage leaves and a lemon wedge to squeeze over the chicken.

CRISPY CHICKEN NUGGETS WITH POPPY SEED-HONEY-MUSTARD DIPPING SAUCE

PREPARATION 45 MINUTES   **COOK TIME** 15 MINUTES   **SERVINGS** 2 TO 4

McDonald's Chicken McNuggets will forever be a guilty pleasure, at least in my memories. My brothers and I pined for them as children, and if we were lucky, my dad would sneak us down for a "fast-food hit" when my mom wasn't looking. I think it would be fair to say I am not alone in my fondness for deep-fried chunks of chicken. And if you're among that crew, you're welcome.

DIPPING SAUCE

¼ cup Dijon mustard

¼ cup honey

2 tablespoons unsweetened coconut cream

Kosher salt

½ teaspoon poppy seeds

CHICKEN NUGGETS

1½ cups rice flour

2 teaspoons onion powder

¼ teaspoon cayenne

2 teaspoons kosher salt

1 (12-ounce) bottle gluten-free beer or pale ale

Vegetable oil, for frying

1 pound boneless, skinless chicken breasts, cut into 2-inch chunks

1 To make the dipping sauce: In a small saucepan, whisk together the mustard and honey over medium heat until smooth and hot. Remove from the heat and whisk in the coconut cream. Season to taste with salt, then whisk in the poppy seeds. Set aside.

2 In a medium bowl, whisk together the rice flour, onion powder, cayenne, and salt. Pour in the beer and mix to make a smooth, pasty batter. Refrigerate for at least 30 minutes.

3 Pour the vegetable oil into a large heavy pot and clip a deep-fry or candy thermometer to the side. Bring the oil up to 375°F.

4 Dip the chicken chunks into the batter one at a time, coating them thickly. Quickly and gently lower the chicken chunks into the hot oil. Fry about 5 chunks of chicken at a time, adjusting the heat so that the oil does not dip below 350°F.

5 Cook the chicken nuggets, stirring and turning them often, until they are a deep golden brown, about 5 minutes. Use a spider strainer or slotted spoon to transfer them to a paper towel to drain. Sprinkle lightly with salt.

6 Repeat the process with the remaining chicken. You can keep the nuggets hot in a 250°F oven. Serve hot, with the dipping sauce.

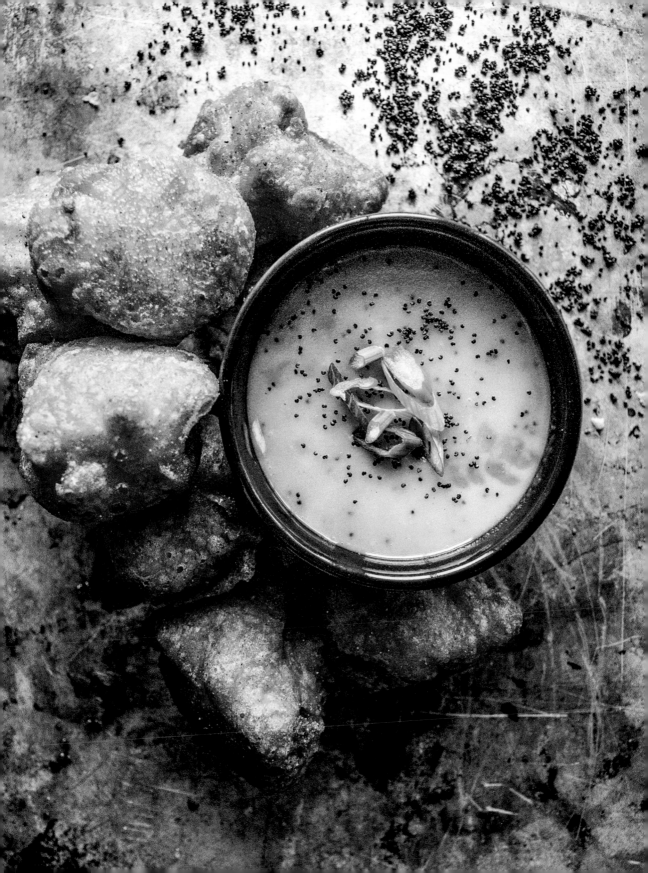

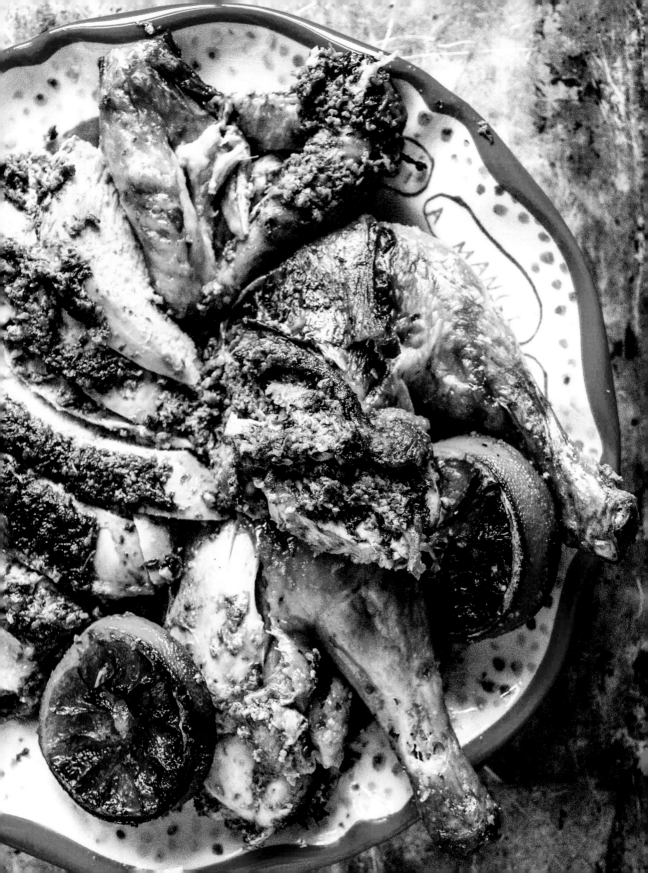

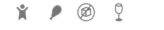

PESTO ROASTED CHICKEN

PREPARATION 20 MINUTES   **COOK TIME** 90 MINUTES   **SERVINGS** 4

Roasting up a chicken at least once each week is a big part of how I keep my family on track with healthy eating. It's dinner one night, then the leftovers go into a salad or soup. This particular version is made especially vibrant with a basil pesto thickened with pepitas.

PEPITA PESTO

6 garlic cloves

4 ounces fresh basil leaves (about 4 cups loosely packed)

¼ cup toasted pepitas

¼ cup olive oil

¼ cup fresh lemon juice

Kosher salt

CHICKEN

1 (3½- to 4-pound) whole chicken, rinsed and patted dry

Kosher salt

1 lemon, halved

1 Preheat the oven to 350°F.

2 To make the pesto: In a food processor, combine the garlic, basil, pepitas, olive oil, and lemon juice. Pulse to make a smooth pesto. Season with salt.

3 Set the chicken in a roasting pan. Separate the skin over the chicken breasts by gently working your fingers underneath. Spoon or rub the pesto all over the breasts under the skin. Rub the rest of the pesto over the skin of the chicken. Sprinkle the chicken with salt.

4 Stuff the halved lemon into the chicken's cavity. Roast the chicken for 90 minutes, or until the skin is golden and crispy and the meat is juicy and falling from the bone.

5 Let the chicken rest for 5 to 10 minutes and then cut it up and transfer to a serving platter. Garnish with the roasted lemon halves from inside the chicken.

CHICKEN PAILLARD WITH FRISÉE AND ARTICHOKE SALAD AND RED PEPPER SAUCE

PREPARATION 20 MINUTES   **COOK TIME** 6 MINUTES   **SERVINGS** 4

I love the way the hot chicken contrasts with the cool salad, and enjoy it the most with a fresh squeeze of lemon juice. At home, I serve this with a bowl of Spring Minestrone (page 74).

RED PEPPER SAUCE

½ cup water-packed roasted red peppers, drained

2 garlic cloves, chopped

2 tablespoons chopped fresh flat-leaf parsley

¼ cup olive oil

2 tablespoons fresh lemon juice

Kosher salt

FRISÉE AND ARTICHOKE SALAD

1 head frisée (curly endive), leaves torn into bite-size pieces

12 ounces frozen artichoke hearts, thawed and drained

1 cup halved cherry tomatoes

2 teaspoons olive oil

Kosher salt

CHICKEN PAILLARD

4 thinly sliced, boneless, skinless chicken cutlets

1 cup unsweetened coconut milk

1 tablespoon cider vinegar

½ cup fine cornmeal

½ cup corn flour

1 teaspoon kosher salt

½ teaspoon cayenne

Lemon wedges, for serving

1 To make the red pepper sauce: In a blender, combine the roasted red peppers, garlic, parsley, olive oil, and lemon juice. Purée until smooth and season with salt. Set aside.

2 To make the frisée and artichoke salad: In a medium bowl, gently combine the frisée, artichoke hearts, cherry tomatoes, and olive oil. Sprinkle with salt and set aside.

3 To make the chicken paillard: In a medium bowl, submerge the chicken in the coconut milk and the vinegar. Soak for 10 minutes.

4 Heat a skillet or griddle over very high heat. Combine the cornmeal, corn flour, salt, and cayenne in a shallow bowl or plate.

5 Remove a chicken breast from the soaking liquid and gently dredge the breast in the cornmeal mixture. Pat the coating onto the chicken and set aside. Repeat with the remaining chicken breasts.

6 Coat the bottom of the skillet with a layer of vegetable oil. When the oil is very hot, add the chicken breasts to the pan. Cook for 2 to 3 minutes

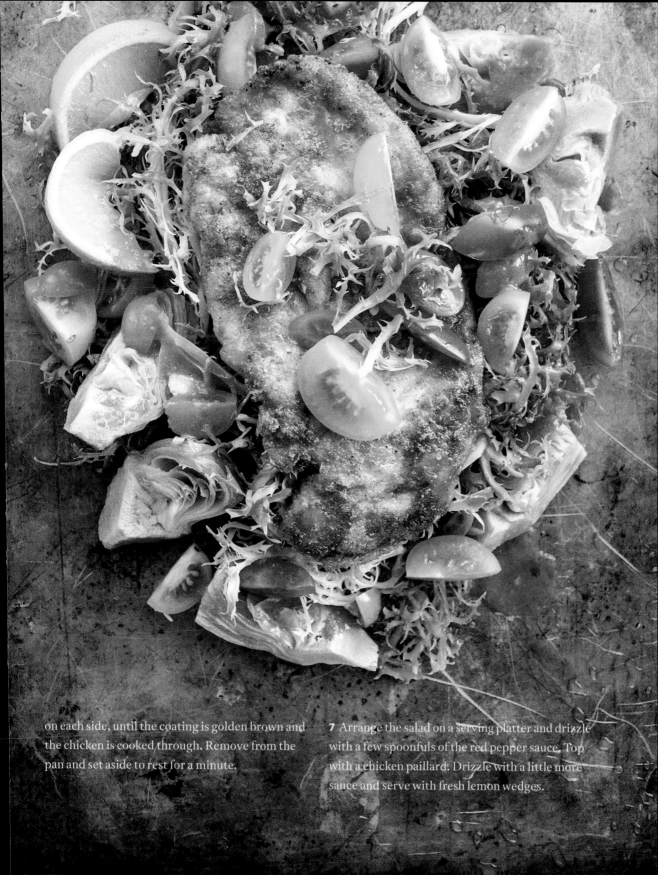

on each side, until the coating is golden brown and the chicken is cooked through. Remove from the pan and set aside to rest for a minute.

7 Arrange the salad on a serving platter and drizzle with a few spoonfuls of the red pepper sauce. Top with a chicken paillard. Drizzle with a little more sauce and serve with fresh lemon wedges.

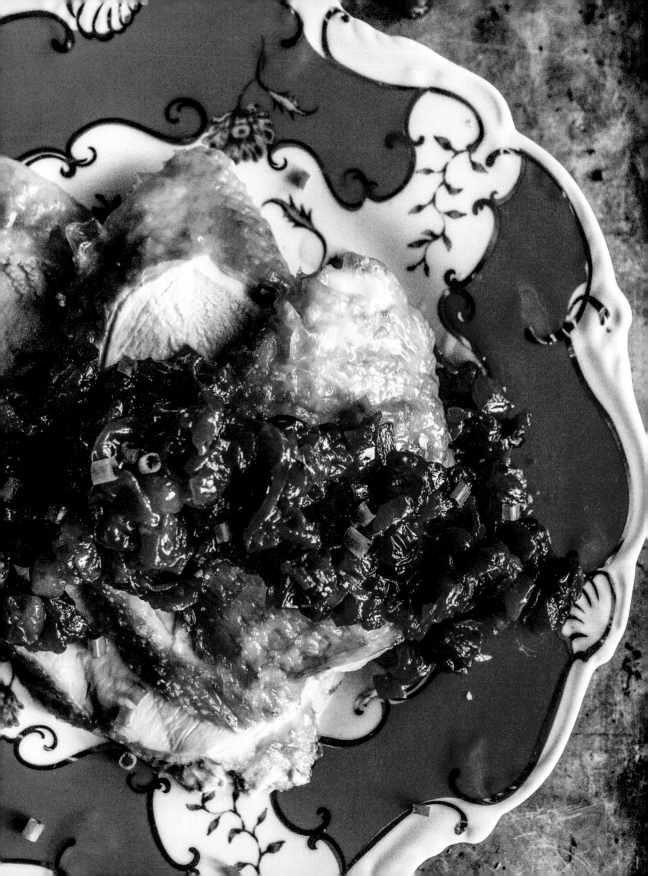

ROAST TURKEY BREAST
WITH CRANBERRY CHUTNEY

PREPARATION 20 MINUTES   **COOK TIME** 60 MINUTES   **SERVINGS** 4

It's such a shame that the spectacular combination of roast turkey and cranberry only gets proper credit at Thanksgiving, and is basically ignored the rest of the year. When turkey is piled high with this sweet, sour, and savory cranberry chutney, you'll want to serve it all year long. A turkey breast can vary in weight from 3 to 6 pounds, so you will need to adjust the cooking time accordingly.

TURKEY

1 bone-in, skin-on turkey breast

1 large yellow onion, cut into thick rounds

2 tablespoons olive oil

Kosher salt

CRANBERRY CHUTNEY

1 red onion, finely diced

1 tablespoon olive oil

2 cups fresh or frozen cranberries

Zest of 1 orange

2 tablespoons red wine vinegar

½ cup beet or coconut sugar

¼ teaspoon ground cinnamon

1 Rinse the turkey breast and pat dry.

2 Arrange the onion rounds in a single layer in a baking dish or on a rimmed baking sheet and place the breast on top. Rub the breast with the coconut oil and sprinkle generously with salt.

3 Preheat the oven to 450°F, letting the turkey come up to room temperature while the oven heats.

4 Put the turkey in the oven, then immediately reduce the heat to 350°F. Roast for 1 hour before checking the internal temp with an instant-read thermometer. When it reaches 165°F, it is done. If you don't have a thermometer, make sure the juices run clear, and feel free to cut into the center to make sure that the turkey breast is cooked through.

5 Let the turkey rest for at least 10 to 15 minutes, then slice it against the grain.

6 While the turkey is roasting, make the cranberry chutney: In a medium saucepan, cook the onion in the olive oil over medium heat until soft and tender, 5 to 7 minutes. Add the cranberries, orange zest, vinegar, sugar, and cinnamon. Cook for 2 minutes, stirring often, then reduce the heat to low and simmer, stirring occasionally, for 10 minutes. The cranberries should have burst and the sugar should have melted into the sauce. Season with salt to taste.

7 Serve the turkey topped with the cranberry chutney.

CHICKEN TACOS WITH CILANTRO PESTO

PREPARATION 10 MINUTES   **COOK TIME** 15 MINUTES   **SERVINGS** 4

Pork, steak, and fish tacos may seem more exciting than your average chicken taco, but the cilantro pesto on these makes them a strong contender for best taco on the block. The addition of the pepita-thickened garlicky cilantro pesto is what makes it so interesting to me. I like to serve them with charred corn tortillas and fresh slaw. (Photograph on page 230.)

SLAW

3 cups thinly sliced purple cabbage

1 cup coarsely chopped cilantro

4 green onions, thinly sliced

Juice of 1 lime

2 tablespoons vegetable oil

Kosher salt

CHICKEN

1 tablespoon vegetable oil

1¼ pounds boneless, skinless chicken breasts

CILANTRO PESTO

1 large bunch cilantro

4 garlic cloves, chopped

½ to 1 jalapeño coarsely chopped (seeded or not, depending on how spicy you like it)

⅓ cup pepitas

⅓ cup vegetable oil

Juice of 1 lime

Kosher salt

TO SERVE

8 corn tortillas

1 tablespoon vegetable oil

1 large avocado, thinly sliced

1 jalapeño, thinly sliced

1 To make the slaw: In a large bowl, combine the cabbage, cilantro, green onions, lime juice, and vegetable oil. Toss, then season with salt. Set aside.

2 In a heavy pan or skillet, heat the vegetable oil over medium heat. Add the chicken breasts and cook for 3 to 4 minutes per side (depending on thickness), until they are just cooked through in the center. Transfer to a plate and set aside.

3 To make the cilantro pesto: In a food processor, combine the cilantro, garlic, jalapeño, pepitas, vegetable oil, and lime juice. Pulse until well combined and season with salt.

4 Using two forks, shred the chicken. Combine the chicken with the cilantro pesto in a mixing bowl and toss to coat. Add salt if needed.

5 Rub the tortillas with the vegetable oil and set them directly over a gas burner until they are slightly charred and hot, about 10 seconds, turning them with tongs. You can also heat them directly in the bottom of a very hot dry skillet or heavy pan, using tongs to turn them. Stuff each tortilla with some of the chicken mixture and a scoop of the slaw, and garnish with a few slices of avocado and jalapeño. Serve immediately.

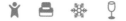

ASIAN PULLED PORK WITH COCONUT RICE

PREPARATION 15 MINUTES   **COOK TIME** 4 HOURS   **SERVINGS** 8

This pork dish is full of fantastic flavors: savory, spicy, and slightly sweet. It's equally good served in a sandwich like traditional pulled pork or over steamed rice. Have it for dinner one night and then make a delicious Bánh Mì Salad (page 94) later in the week.

PORK

2 tablespoons vegetable oil

1 (4-pound) pork shoulder

Kosher salt

2 yellow onions, quartered

4 garlic cloves, thinly sliced

2 jalapeños, thinly sliced, with seeds

¼ cup coconut amino acids

½ cup rice vinegar

¼ cup beet or coconut sugar

4 cups chicken broth

SWEET AND SPICY SAUCE

1 tablespoon coconut amino acids

2 tablespoons Sriracha

2 tablespoons honey

1 tablespoon rice vinegar

TO SERVE

Coconut-Cilantro Rice (page 166), for serving

Sweet and Spicy Pickled Onions (page 94), for serving

Lime wedges, fresh cilantro, and sliced red chiles, for garnish

1 In a large heavy pot, heat the vegetable oil over high heat. Sprinkle the pork shoulder generously with salt, then add it to the pot and sear on all sides until browned, 8 to 10 minutes total. Add the onions, garlic, jalapeños, amino acids, vinegar, sugar, and broth. The liquid will not completely cover the meat. Bring the liquid to a simmer, then cover the pot and reduce the heat to low. Simmer the pork for 3½ to 4 hours, turning the meat halfway through. Cook until the pork is completely tender and falling apart.

2 To make the sweet and spicy sauce: In a small bowl stir, together the sauce ingredients until well combined. Set aside.

3 Transfer the meat to a platter with tongs and let cool slightly. Use a fork to pull the meat into shreds, discarding the fat, gristle, and bone. Return the shredded meat to the pot with the cooked-down broth, onions, and jalapeños left from the braising. Cook over medium heat until some of the liquid has further reduced and the meat is very moist. Season with salt.

4 Serve hot with the sauce over coconut-cilantro rice, garnished with lime wedges, pickled onions, fresh cilantro, and red chiles.

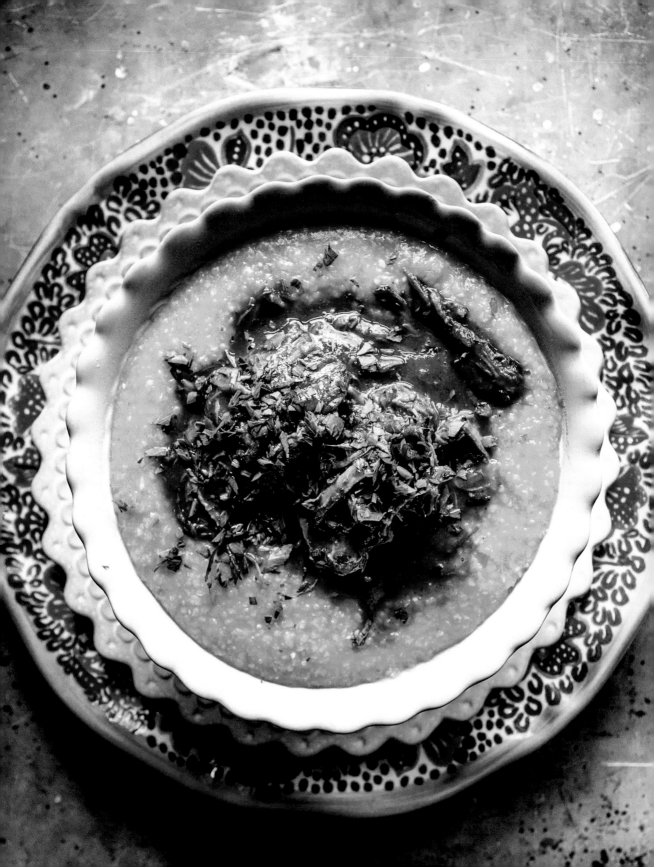

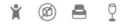

SLOW-BRAISED PORK RAGÙ

PREPARATION 20 MINUTES   **COOK TIME** 4 HOURS   **SERVINGS** 6 TO 8

This pork ragù is cooked low and slow until it is falling-off-the-bone tender, and the broth becomes a silky red wine sauce. Because the prep time is brief, I make this on weekdays when I am working from home, but it's also a wonderful dish for entertaining. You can completely prepare the pork the day before, then refrigerate it in the pot in its sauce. I serve it over Pumpkin Polenta, but it's just as good with Creamy Mashed Potatoes (page 154) or rice, or even tossed with pasta.

1 (3- to 4-pound) boneless pork shoulder

2 teaspoons kosher salt

7 tablespoons olive oil

1 yellow onion, chopped

3 carrots, cut into large chunks

3 celery stalks, cut in half

2 garlic cloves, minced

2 tablespoons tomato paste

2 bay leaves

1 (750 ml) bottle red wine (I use a Cabernet or Cab blend)

4 cups beef broth

Creamy Pumpkin Polenta (page 172)

1 Generously rub the pork shoulder on all sides with salt.

2 In a large heavy pot, heat 4 tablespoons of the olive oil over high heat. Add the pork shoulder and sear on all sides until it is golden brown; this should take 10 to 15 minutes total. Transfer the meat to a rimmed baking sheet.

3 Add the remaining 3 tablespoons olive oil to the pot along with the onion, carrots, celery, and garlic. Cook over high heat, stirring often, for 2 to 3 minutes.

4 Add the tomato paste and cook, stirring, for 1 minute. Add the bay leaves and return the pork to the pot, along with any juices that have gathered on the baking sheet. Add the wine and

the broth. Bring to a boil, then reduce the heat to low, cover, and simmer for 4 hours, turning the meat after it has cooked for about 2 hours. It will be very tender and falling apart. Transfer the pork to a rimmed baking sheet and let it rest.

5 Discard the bay leaves and celery, then transfer the rest of the cooking liquid to a blender (you may have to do this in batches) and purée on high until smooth. Pour the sauce back into the pot and simmer over low heat for about 10 minutes.

6 Remove the strings from the pork shoulder and break the meat into large chunks, disposing of any fat or gristle. Add the chunks to the simmering sauce and cook until the sauce thickens, about 10 minutes. Add salt to taste. Serve the pork and sauce hot, over Pumpkin Polenta.

GINGER-MAPLE ROASTED PORK TENDERLOIN WITH MANGO CHUTNEY

PREPARATION 20 MINUTES, PLUS AT LEAST 1 HOUR REFRIGERATION TIME
COOK TIME 25 MINUTES   SERVINGS 4

I had a version of this dish on my catering menu for years, and it is not only delicious but really pretty. To serve a group, roast several tenderloins and double or triple the chutney recipe (which can be made a day ahead of time), then arrange it all artfully on a big platter, transforming something quite simple into something rather elegant for a dinner party or holiday gathering.

PORK TENDERLOIN

1 pork tenderloin (about 1¼ pounds)

2 teaspoons kosher salt

¼ cup pure maple syrup

3 tablespoons Dijon mustard

2 garlic cloves, minced

2 tablespoons minced fresh ginger

1 tablespoon olive oil

MANGO CHUTNEY

2 tablespoons olive oil

½ large yellow onion, finely diced

1 red Fresno chile, minced

1 large mango, peeled, pitted, and finely diced

2 whole star anise

2 tablespoons granulated beet sugar

2 tablespoons red wine vinegar

Kosher salt

1 To make the pork tenderloin: Preheat the oven to 400°F.

2 In a resealable plastic bag, combine the pork, salt, syrup, mustard, garlic, and ginger. Refrigerate for at least 1 hour and up to 12 hours.

3 Set a heavy ovenproof pan or skillet over high heat. When it is smoking hot, add the olive oil and then the pork. Sear the tenderloin for about 1 minute on each side. Transfer the pan to the oven and cook the tenderloin for 12 minutes. Place the pan on a wire rack, tent with aluminum foil, and let rest for 10 minutes.

4 To make the mango chutney: In a large pan, heat the olive oil over medium heat. Add the onion and cook, stirring often, until softened but not browned, 5 to 7 minutes. Add the chile, mango, and star anise and cook for 5 minutes, stirring frequently. Stir in the sugar, vinegar, and ½ cup water. Simmer the chutney over medium heat for 5 minutes, or until the liquid has cooked off and the onion and mango are tender. Season with salt.

5 Slice the pork tenderloin and serve hot with the mango chutney.

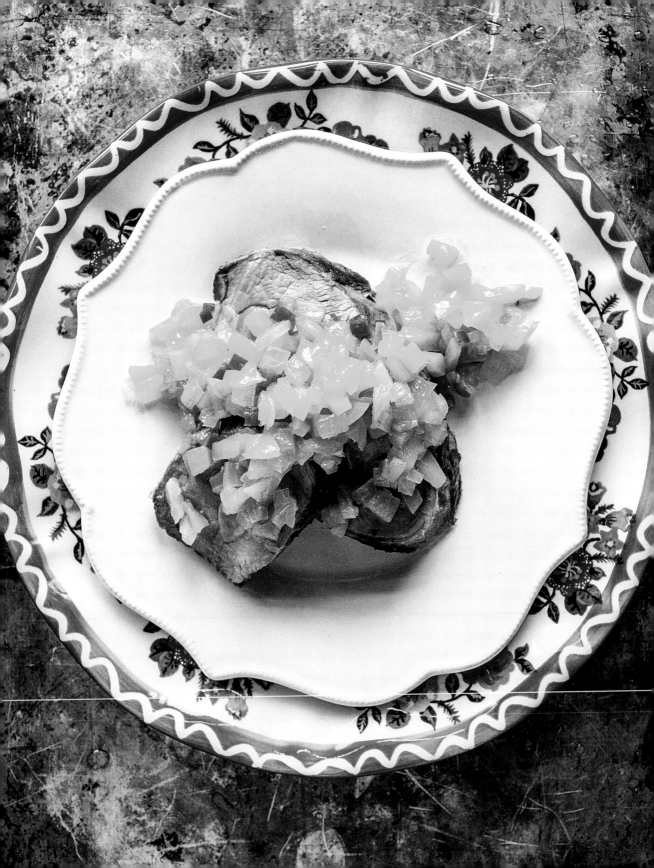

GRILLED SKIRT STEAK WITH CHIMICHURRI

PREPARATION 20 MINUTES, PLUS 4 HOURS MARINATING TIME

COOK TIME 6 MINUTES   **SERVINGS** 4 TO 6

In my opinion, very few things wouldn't be improved by a big old spoonful of chimichurri sauce, an herbaceous, intensely garlicky sauce spiced with red pepper and lightened up with lemon and vinegar. It's the traditional Argentinean accompaniment for grilled meat, but I also love it on roasted or grilled white-fleshed fish and tossed with quinoa or pasta for a side dish.

STEAK

2 skirt steaks (about 2 pounds)

6 garlic cloves, chopped

1 tablespoon kosher salt

2 tablespoons fresh oregano leaves

½ cup red wine vinegar

⅔ cup olive oil

CHIMICHURRI SAUCE

1 cup fresh flat-leaf parsley leaves

¼ cup fresh oregano leaves

3 green onions

3 garlic cloves

½ teaspoon crushed red pepper flakes

½ cup olive oil

¼ cup red wine vinegar

3 tablespoons fresh lemon juice

Kosher salt

• • •

4 cups sliced ripe tomatoes

½ red onion, thinly sliced

1 Place the meat in a resealable plastic bag and add the garlic, salt, oregano, vinegar, and olive oil. Seal the bag and mix the ingredients really well. Marinate in the refrigerator for at least 4 hours and up to 8 hours.

2 To make the chimichurri sauce: Finely mince the parsley, oregano, green onions, and garlic. Combine them in a medium bowl with the red pepper flakes, olive oil, vinegar, and lemon juice. Mix thoroughly and season with salt. This can be made up to a day ahead of time.

3 Preheat a grill to high. Pull the steaks from the marinade and place them on the grill. Dump the remaining marinade over the steaks (a little flare-up is okay!). Grill the steaks for 3 minutes on each side for medium rare. Transfer the steaks to a cutting board and let them rest for 10 minutes.

4 While the meat is resting, place the tomatoes and red onion in a medium bowl and add two generous spoonfuls of the chimichurri sauce. Gently toss the tomatoes and onions with the sauce and transfer them to a serving platter.

5 Slice the steak across the grain and pile it on top of the tomato salad. Serve with a generous amount of chimichurri sauce, which you can spoon on top before serving or pass in a bowl.

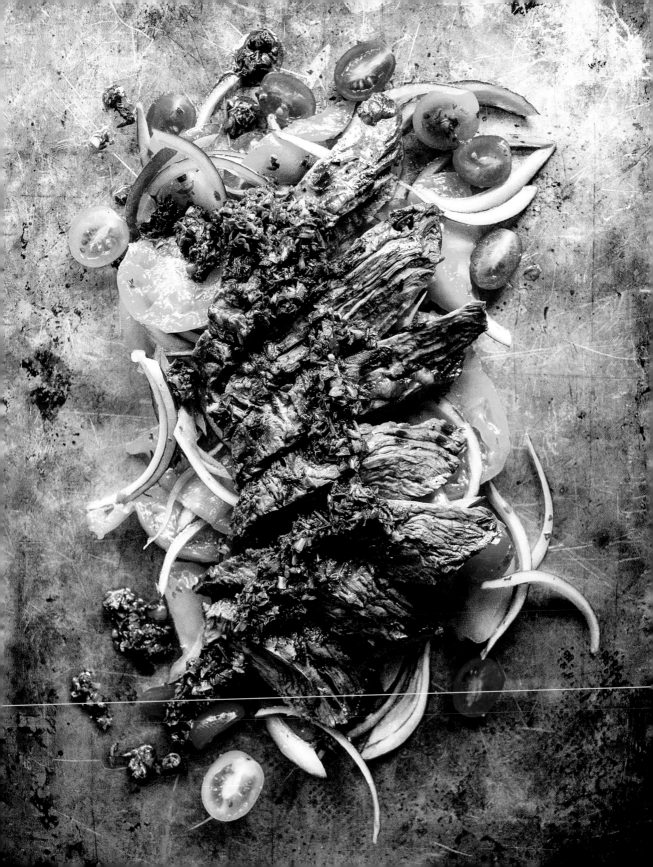

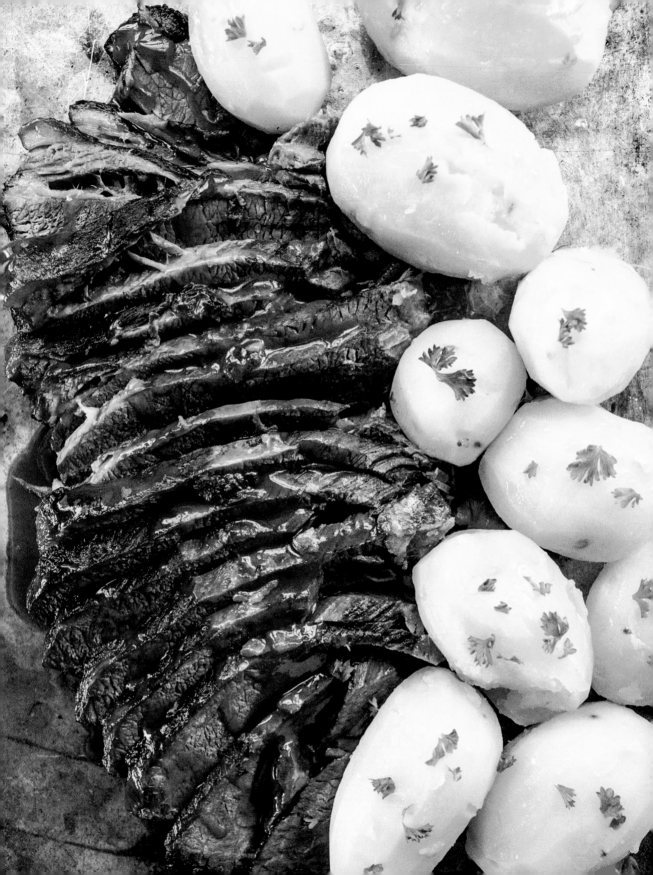

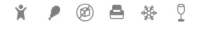

BEER-BRAISED BRISKET

PREPARATION 20 MINUTES   **COOK TIME** 4 HOURS 30 MINUTES   **SERVINGS** 8

This is the kind of dinner you want to put in the oven late on a Sunday morning when you have a whole day of stuff to get done. I will salt my brisket and then go do laundry, get the kids ready for the day, whatever, then come back and sear it, add the veggies and beer, and pop the lid on. At that point I can run errands, hit the garden or even the couch (I mean, it is a Sunday, after all!), and I just have to come back a few hours later, flip the meat, and go back to whatever I was doing. It takes about fifteen minutes to finish the dish and make the sauce when the meat is done cooking, and then you have a mouthwateringly rich, tender brisket that tastes as though you must have been slaving away on it all day. Serve with simple boiled potatoes, Creamy Mashed Potatoes (page 154), or Mustard-Crusted Potatoes (page 159).

1 (3- to 4-pound) beef brisket

Kosher salt

2 tablespoons olive oil

5 large carrots, cut into large chunks

2 yellow onions, cut into large chunks

2 bay leaves

4 cups beef broth

2 (12-ounce) gluten-free beers or pale ales

1 Generously salt the brisket at least an hour ahead of time and let sit at room temperature for 1 hour.

2 Heat a large Dutch oven or heavy pot over high heat until it's smoking. Cut the brisket in half so that both pieces will fit in the pot. Add the oil to the pot and then one piece of the brisket at a time. You want a nice deep golden sear on all sides of the brisket pieces; this should take about 10 minutes for each piece of brisket. Set aside on a plate.

3 Add the carrots, onions, and bay leaves and cook until the vegetables have some nice dark golden brown color to them, about 5 minutes. Add the broth, deglazing the pan and scraping up any browned bits.

4 Return the meat to the pot and pour in the beer. Cover and reduce the heat to low. Simmer the brisket for 2 hours, then flip the brisket over and simmer for 2 hours more.

5 Transfer the brisket (which should be very tender) to a cutting board and strain the sauce through a fine-mesh sieve. Return the sauce back to the pot and simmer over medium-low heat until the sauce reduces and thickens, 5 to 7 minutes. Season with salt.

6 While the sauce is simmering, thinly slice the brisket against the grain. Serve hot with the sauce over the top, or return the brisket to the sauce in the pot and keep it there until ready to serve.

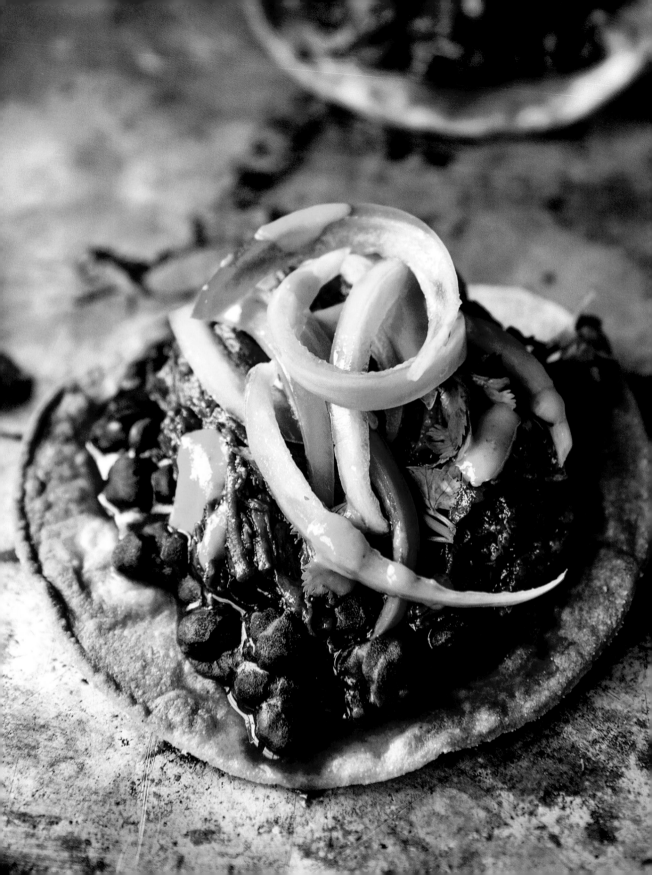

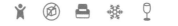

SHREDDED BEEF TOSTADAS

PREPARATION 20 MINUTES   **COOK TIME** 4 HOURS 30 MINUTES   **SERVINGS** 6

If there is one thing we all just go crazy for in my house, it's Mexican food. Coco always tells me how she "dreams" about delicious tacos. I don't feel differently. These shredded spicy beef tostadas are dream-worthy. The beef itself is incredible, but when paired with layers of delicious extras like homemade black beans, sweet pickled onions, and a homemade chile de árbol hot sauce, these are out-of-this-world amazing.

SLOW-COOKED BEEF

2 tablespoons ancho chile powder

2 tablespoons ground cumin

½ teaspoon cayenne

1 teaspoon kosher salt, plus more to taste

3 pounds beef shoulder

¼ cup vegetable oil, plus more for frying

1 yellow onion, thinly sliced

1 (28-ounce) can crushed tomatoes

4 cups beef broth

CHILE DE ÁRBOL HOT SAUCE (VERY SPICY!)

½ cup dried chiles de árbol

½ cup boiling water

2 garlic cloves

½ yellow onion, coarsely chopped

½ cup white vinegar

½ cup vegetable oil

¼ cup agave

Kosher salt

TO SERVE

12 corn tortillas

Restaurant-Style Black Beans (page 164)

Fresh cilantro

Sweet and Spicy Pickled Onions (page 94)

1 To make the slow-cooked beef: In a small bowl, combine the ancho chile powder, cumin, cayenne, and salt.

2 Rub the entire beef shoulder generously with salt and set aside.

3 In a large heavy pot, heat the vegetable oil over high heat. Add the beef shoulder and sear on all sides until the meat is golden and crisp on the outside, about 10 minutes total.

4 Add the onion, crushed tomatoes, and spice mixture to the pot and cook for 2 minutes more, then stir in the broth. Cover the pot and reduce the heat to low. Simmer the beef for 4 hours,

(recipe continues)

turning the meat over after it has cooked for 2 hours. When the meat is done, it should be very tender and falling apart.

5 To make the chile de árbol hot sauce: Place the whole, dried chiles in a medium bowl. Pour the boiling water over the chiles and cover the bowl with plastic wrap. Soak the chiles for about 30 minutes.

6 Drain the chiles, remove the stems, and place them in a blender along with the garlic, onion, vinegar, vegetable oil, and agave. Purée on high until you have a smooth orange sauce. Season with salt.

7 Transfer the beef to a cutting board. Turn the heat under the cooking liquid to medium and simmer, uncovered. Shred the beef, discarding any globs of fat or gristle. Return the shredded beef to the pot and cook until the sauce has reduced and become thick, about 20 minutes. Season with salt.

8 While the sauce is reducing, fry the tortillas. In a medium saucepan, heat ½ inch of vegetable oil until it registers 350°F to 375°F on a candy or deep-fry thermometer, or until a piece of tortilla immediately starts to bubble and floats to the top when dropped into the oil. Fry the tortillas one at a time, for about 30 seconds on each side until golden. Drain on a paper towel.

9 Top each tortilla with a spoonful of black beans and some shredded beef, fresh cilantro, and pickled onions. Top with a drizzle of the árbol hot sauce and serve immediately.

....

ANCHO CHILES are dried poblanos, and these peppers are high in iron and a good source of fiber. They also have high levels of vitamin A (25 percent of the recommended daily amount), a valuable antioxidant.

....

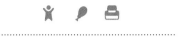

MEAT LOAF

PREPARATION 20 MINUTES   **COOK TIME** 45 MINUTES   **SERVINGS** 6 TO 8

In an ironic twist on the usual, I tried meat loaf for the very first time when I went to culinary school. I had always thought it was something to be feared, some type of mystery meat mash with a hard-boiled egg lurking inside. But after being force-fed a mouthful by a fellow student, I became a convert. Meat loaf is like a blank canvas for flavor, and almost anyone you ask will have their own ideas about what meats and seasonings should be included—and I'm no exception. My version is a mix of pork and beef, and includes a glaze that is the perfect sweet-and-savory crown for this awesome homage to American comfort food.

1 pound ground pork

1 pound 85% lean ground beef

1 pound 90% to 93% lean ground sirloin

1 small yellow onion, minced

2 garlic cloves, minced

½ cup dehydrated potato flakes

½ cup ketchup

2 tablespoons Worcestershire sauce

½ cup chopped fresh flat-leaf parsley

2 teaspoons kosher salt

GLAZE

¼ cup ketchup

2 tablespoons granulated beet sugar

2 tablespoons grainy Dijon mustard

1 teaspoon rice vinegar

1 Preheat the oven to 400°F.

2 Place the ground meats in a bowl, add the onion and garlic, and use your clean hands to combine just until incorporated. Add the potato flakes, ketchup, Worcestershire sauce, parsley, and salt. Form the mixture into an oval and place it in a 9 × 5-inch loaf pan.

3 To make the glaze: In a small bowl, stir together all the glaze ingredients until smooth.

4 Brush the glaze onto the top of the meat loaf and place the loaf pan on a rimmed baking sheet. Bake for 45 minutes. Let the meat loaf rest for 10 minutes before removing from the pan and slicing.

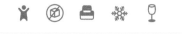

BEEF STEW

PREPARATION 10 MINUTES   **COOK TIME** 4 HOURS   **SERVINGS** 4 TO 6

I love to make this on days when I am working from home or on lazy Sundays when we stick close to the couch. Use cuts like chuck roast, round roast, rump roast, top round, etc., which will hold up well to the long slow braise getting extra tender in the process. The best thing about this is that you can let it cook all day while you get other things done.

4 pounds beef stew meat

Kosher salt

¼ cup vegetable oil

1 large yellow onion, diced

3 tablespoons tomato paste

1 cup dry red wine

2 bay leaves

8 cups beef broth

2 tablespoons balsamic vinegar

4 cups quartered white button mushrooms or cremini mushrooms

4 large carrots, cut into bite-size chunks

4 cups russet or Yukon Gold potatoes, peeled and cut into bite-size chunks

¼ cup cornstarch mixed with ¼ cup water

1½ cups frozen peas

1 cup unsweetened coconut cream

1 Generously sprinkle the beef chunks with salt.

2 In a large heavy pot or Dutch oven, heat 2 tablespoons of the vegetable oil over high heat. Add half the meat and cook until browned on all sides, about 8 minutes. Transfer the browned meat to a bowl. Add the remaining meat to the pot and cook until browned on all sides, then transfer the meat to the bowl.

3 In the same pot, heat the remaining 2 tablespoons oil. Add the onion and cook, stirring until the onion is very soft and tender, 5 to 7 minutes. Add the tomato paste and cook, stirring, for about 1 minute. Add the wine and scrape up any browned bits from the bottom of the pot.

4 Return the meat to the pot and add the bay leaves, broth, vinegar, and 2 cups water. Cover and reduce the heat to low. Simmer the stew for 3 hours.

5 Give the stew a good stir and add the mushrooms, carrots, and potatoes. Cover and simmer over low heat for 45 to 60 minutes more, until the carrots and potatoes are tender.

6 Stir in the cornstarch mixture and the peas and cook, uncovered, for 10 to 15 minutes, until the liquid has thickened.

7 Turn off the heat and stir in the coconut cream. Season with salt and serve hot.

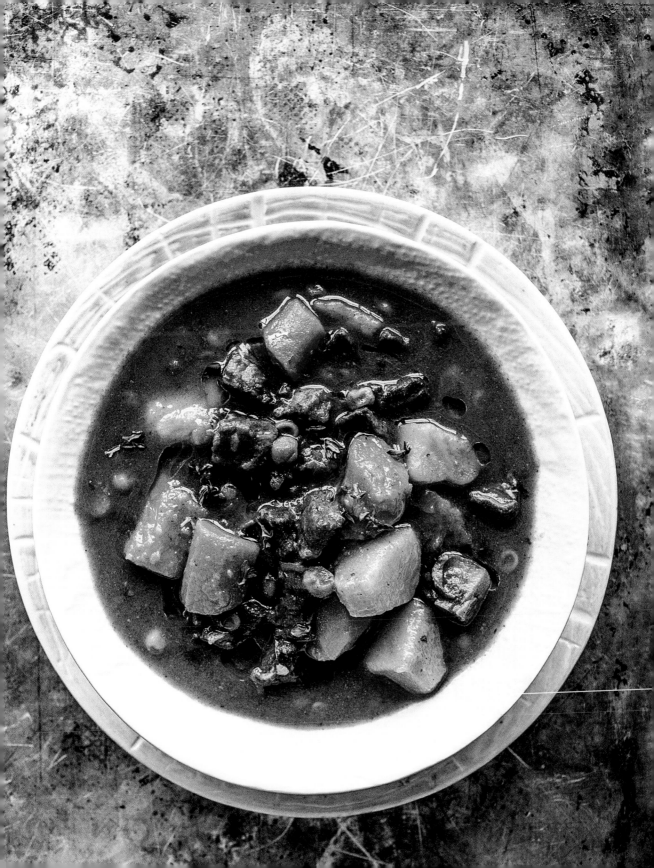

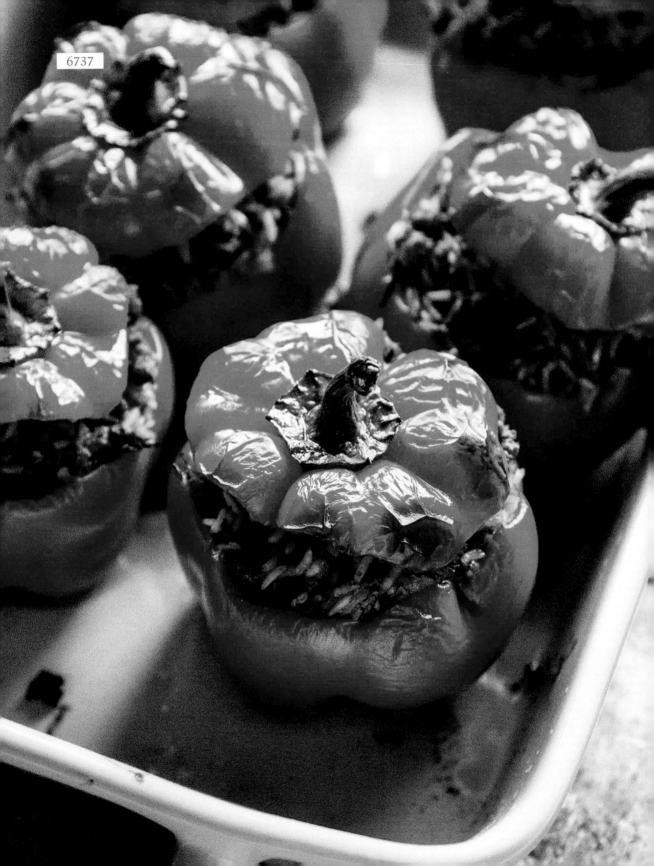

GREEK STUFFED PEPPERS
WITH RICE AND LAMB

PREPARATION 15 MINUTES   **COOK TIME** 60 MINUTES   **SERVINGS** 6

I have been lucky enough to pick up many of my mother-in-law's cooking techniques over the years, and this was one I was really determined to master. Good thing, too, because when I appeared on Food Network's *Cutthroat Kitchen* and they announced, "You will be making . . . stuffed peppers!" I just knew the competition was mine. Since the episode aired, I have been asked for this recipe thousands of times, and I'm betting you will be, too!

6 red, yellow, or orange bell peppers

1 pound ground lamb

3 tablespoons olive oil, plus more for brushing

1 yellow onion, finely diced

3 garlic cloves, minced

1 cup long-grain white rice

⅓ cup crushed tomatoes

½ cup white wine

1½ cups chicken or beef broth

⅔ cup minced fresh flat-leaf parsley

⅓ cup minced fresh mint

Kosher salt

1 Preheat the oven to 375°F.

2 Cut the tops off of the peppers. Remove the seeds and set the peppers and their tops aside.

3 In a large heavy pan, sauté the ground lamb over medium-high heat, sprinkling it with salt and breaking it up with a wooden spoon as it cooks. Cook until the meat is mostly cooked through, 3 to 4 minutes, then add the olive oil, onion, and garlic. Cook until the onion has softened and the garlic is fragrant, about 3 minutes.

4 Add the rice to the pan and stir to combine. Cook the rice for 3 to 4 minutes, then add the tomatoes and wine, making sure to scrape up any browned bits from the bottom of the pan.

5 Add 1 cup of the broth and reduce the heat to medium. Cook, stirring often, until most of the liquid has been absorbed, about 6 minutes.

6 Remove the pan from the heat and stir in the remaining ½ cup broth and the herbs. Season with salt.

7 Fill each bell pepper with a generous amount of stuffing and replace its cap. Place the filled peppers in a 9 × 13-inch baking dish and brush them with oil.

8 Bake for 45 minutes, until the rice is completely cooked through and the peppers are very soft. Serve hot.

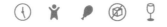

ROASTED HALIBUT WITH STRAWBERRY-BASIL SALSA

PREPARATION 10 MINUTES   COOK TIME 6 MINUTES   SERVINGS 2

The idea of pairing sweet, juicy berries with fish may seem odd at first, but trust me, it really works. The acid in the strawberries has an effect similar to that of the acid in a lemon. Serve this all summer long; it's easy to scale up to feed a crowd.

STRAWBERRY-BASIL SALSA

2 cups strawberries, cut into small dice

¼ cup small-diced red onion

½ cup loosely packed fresh basil leaves, very finely sliced into ribbons

¼ cup loosely packed fresh mint leaves, very finely sliced into ribbons

1 tablespoon red wine vinegar

1 tablespoon olive oil

Kosher salt

HALIBUT

2 (6-ounce) skin-on halibut fillets

Kosher salt

2 tablespoons vegetable oil

1 To make the strawberry-basil salsa: In a medium bowl, gently combine the salsa ingredients except the salt and add salt to taste. Set aside. (If you need to make this ahead, do so by only a few hours and then add the fresh herbs at the last minute, or they will discolor and the salsa will become soggy.)

2 Score the skin of the halibut fillets twice with a sharp knife to keep them from curling as they cook. Sprinkle both sides with salt.

3 In a heavy pan or skillet, heat the vegetable oil over medium-high heat. Place the halibut fillets in the pan skin-side down. Cook without moving for about 3 minutes, and then turn the fish skin-side up. Cook until the fish is crisp on the outside and just cooked through in the center, about 6 minutes total.

4 Spoon the salsa over the fish and serve immediately.

STRAWBERRIES. 1 cup of strawberries will give you more than 100 percent of your recommended daily amount of vitamin C, and they rank exceptionally high in terms of antioxidants packed into a small serving. When you eat strawberries at least three times a week, their anti-inflammation properties really kick in.

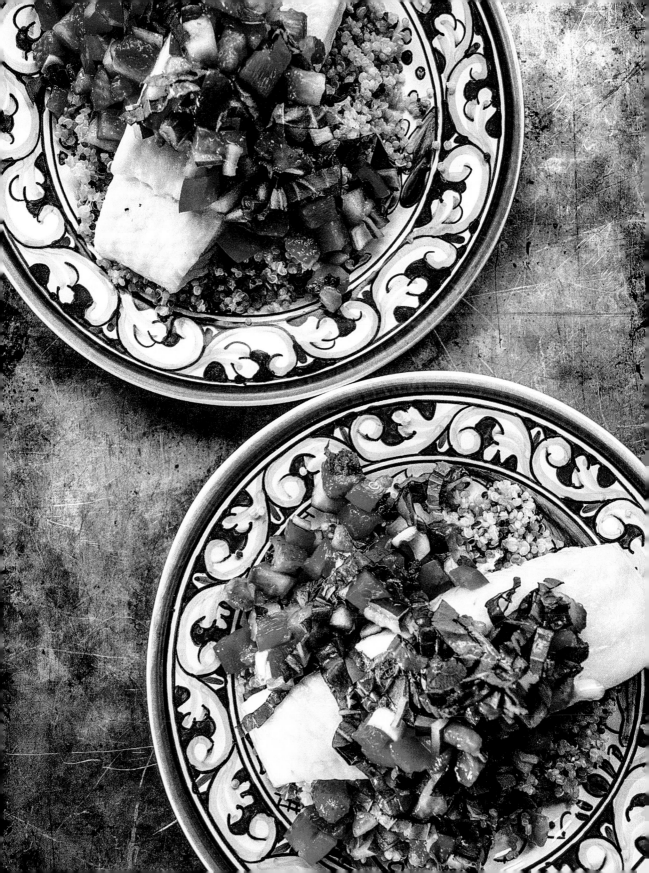

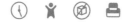

BROILED SALMON STEAKS WITH TOMATILLO-AVOCADO SAUCE

PREPARATION 10 MINUTES   **COOK TIME** 5 MINUTES   **SERVINGS** 4 (MAKES 3 CUPS SAUCE)

You're not going to believe you can make a dish that looks and tastes as incredible as this one in just fifteen minutes, but cooking is believing. The sauce can be made ahead and stored in the refrigerator, then used to top any kind of meat or fish. I guarantee this recipe will be dog-eared.

TOMATILLO-AVOCADO SAUCE

2 cups quartered tomatillos

⅓ cup fresh lime juice (from about 2 limes)

½ cup fresh cilantro stems and leaves

1 jalapeño, seeded and coarsely chopped

1 avocado, pitted and peeled

¼ yellow onion

2 garlic cloves

Kosher salt

SALMON

Zest and juice of 1 lime

2 tablespoons olive oil

4 (8-ounce) salmon steaks

Kosher salt

1 To make the tomatillo-avocado sauce: In a food processor, combine all the sauce ingredients except the salt and process until well combined. Season with salt and set aside.

2 Preheat the broiler.

3 In a small bowl, combine the lime zest, lime juice, and olive oil. Place the salmon steaks on a rimmed baking sheet and pour the lime juice mixture over them. Season generously with salt.

4 Broil the steaks for 5 minutes without turning; they will be golden around the edges and there may be a little white fat on the surface. Transfer the fish to serving plates and serve hot, topped with a generous scoop of the tomatillo-avocado sauce.

SALMON is a fantastic source of omega-3 fatty acids, which promote heart health and reduce the risk of stroke. Omega-3s also help to improve inflammation and immune disorders, like rheumatoid arthritis and Crohn's disease. It is also known to help alleviate mental issues, such as depression, and even help reduce the damage of Alzheimer's disease.

CRISPY SALMON SALAD
WITH HONEY-CHIPOTLE VINAIGRETTE

PREPARATION 10 MINUTES **COOK TIME** 3 TO 4 MINUTES **SERVINGS** 2

The extra-crispy salmon skin is the star of this salad and it also keeps the salmon fillet moist and flaky. When the spicy smoky chipotle chile and sweet honey combine with that rich crispy salmon and fresh romaine hearts, you have one memorable salad.

VINAIGRETTE

1 tablespoon ground chipotle pepper

3 tablespoons honey

¼ cup vegetable oil

3 tablespoons red wine vinegar

Kosher salt

SALMON SALAD

2 (3- to 4-ounce) skin-on salmon fillets, at room temperature

Kosher salt

3 tablespoons vegetable oil

2 hearts of romaine

1 large avocado, pitted, peeled, and cut into chunks

½ red onion, thinly sliced

¼ cup pepitas, toasted

1 To make the vinaigrette: In a blender, combine the chipotle, honey, vegetable oil, and vinegar. Purée until smooth. Season with salt.

2 Sprinkle the salmon fillets with kosher salt. In a heavy pan or skillet, heat the vegetable oil over high heat. When the pan is smoking hot, add the fish, skin-side down. Cook until the skin is crispy and browned, 2 minutes. Flip the fish and cook for 1 minute more. It will easily release from the pan when ready. Transfer the salmon to a plate and brush with a little of the chipotle vinaigrette. Set aside.

3 Arrange the romaine hearts, avocado, red onion, and pepitas on a serving platter or in a bowl. Drizzle with the vinaigrette and top with the salmon. Serve immediately.

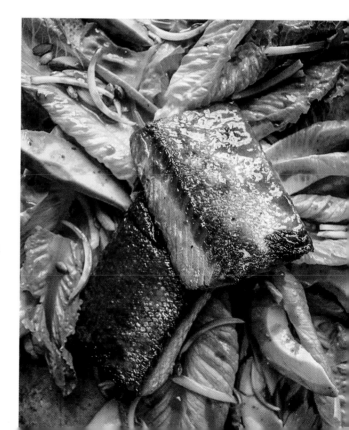

SPICY TUNA SUSHI BOWLS

PREPARATION 30 MINUTES   COOK TIME 20 MINUTES   SERVINGS 2

For those with allergies, Japanese cuisine is one of the easiest and most reliable to dine out on. But one can't go out every night! So I was thinking about how to bring sushi into the home kitchen. Fortunately my favorite combo, spicy tuna, cucumber, and avocado, works really well as a sushi bowl! If you are nervous about "raw" fish, don't be. The marinade partially cooks it, and as long as you get some good-quality fresh fish, you have nothing to worry about. The fish, crunchy cucumber, cilantro, and avocado makes a perfect bite.

RICE

1 teaspoon kosher salt

1½ cups short-grain white rice

1 tablespoon rice vinegar

SPICY TUNA

8 ounces sashimi-grade raw tuna

1 teaspoon sambal oelek (Asian red chili garlic sauce)

1½ teaspoons minced fresh ginger

1 tablespoon minced red Fresno chile

1 tablespoon minced green onion

1 tablespoon sesame oil

2 tablespoons coconut amino acids

2 tablespoons rice vinegar

GARNISHES

½ avocado, pitted, peeled, and sliced

⅓ cup thinly sliced seedless cucumber

Fresh cilantro and sesame seeds, for garnish

1 To make the rice: Pour 1¾ cups cold water into a small pot. Add the salt and rice and bring to a boil. Boil for 1 minute and then cover the pot tightly and reduce the heat to low. Cook for 15 to 17 minutes, until all the liquid has been absorbed. Turn off the heat, add the vinegar, and fluff the rice with a fork, then cover the rice and steam for 3 minutes. Set aside.

2 On a cutting board, cut the tuna into small dice. Use a large sharp knife or cleaver to mince the tuna.

3 In a medium bowl, combine the sambal, ginger, chile, green onion, sesame oil, amino acids, and vinegar. Reserve 1 tablespoon of the sauce. Add the tuna to the remaining sauce and gently combine. Set aside to marinate for up to 15 minutes.

4 Divide the rice between two bowls. Top each bowl of rice with half the avocado slices. Gently combine the cucumbers with the reserved 1 tablespoon sauce and add those to each bowl.

5 Top each of the bowls with the spicy tuna, cilantro, and sesame seeds, and serve immediately.

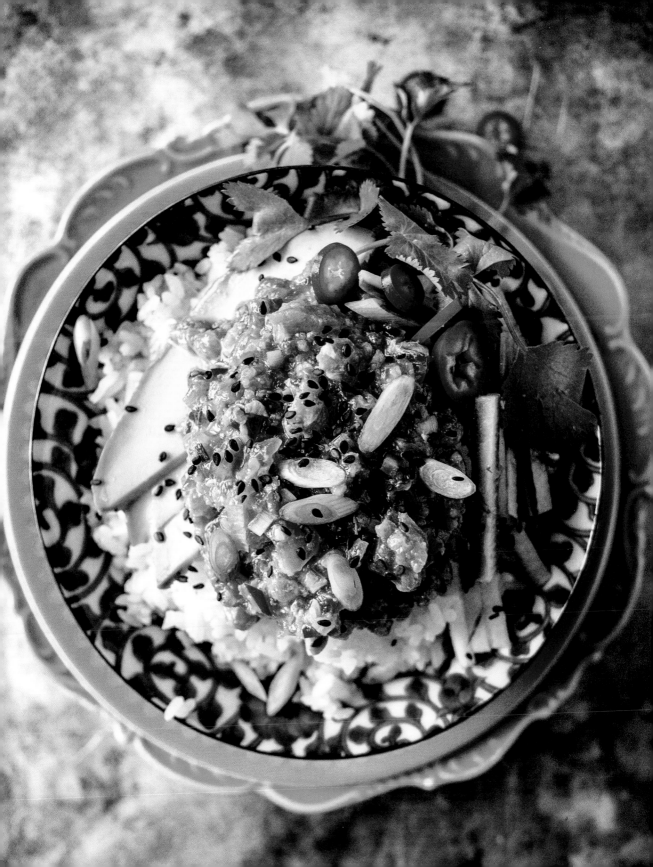

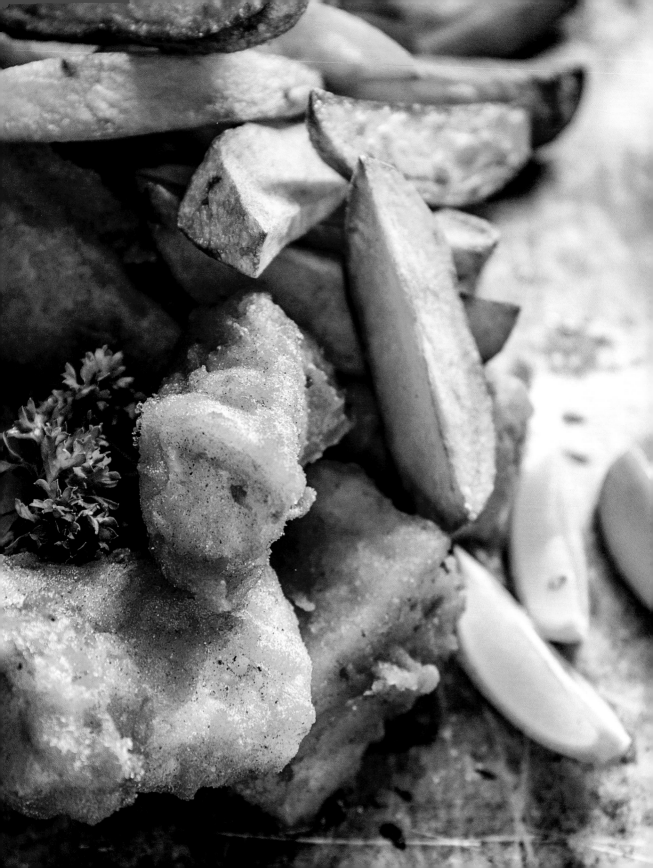

BEER-BATTERED FISH AND CHIPS

PREPARATION 45 MINUTES   **COOK TIME** 10 TO 15 MINUTES   **SERVINGS** 4 TO 6

When we were younger, my grampy and dad used to take my brothers and me to the fish-and-chips stand that popped up near Lake Washington each summer, and we absolutely loved those outings. The fish wasn't breaded, but had that even, fluffy, fried coating that you get from beer batter, with tender, juicy white fish inside. Just a squeeze of lemon and a sprinkle of salt made for a perfect bite. When I serve them, I make "chips" instead by cutting the potatoes into wedges instead of sticks and just adding a minute or two to the frying time.

2 pounds cod fillet	¼ teaspoon cayenne	Vegetable oil, for frying
1½ to 1¾ cups sweet rice flour	2 teaspoons kosher salt, plus more as needed	Kosher salt
2 teaspoons onion powder	1 (12-ounce) bottle gluten-free beer or pale ale	French Fries (page 157)
		Lemon wedges, for serving

1 Slice the fish into thick chunks, about 2 × 4 inches.

2 In a medium bowl, whisk together 1½ cups of the rice flour, the onion powder, cayenne, and salt. Pour in the beer and mix to make a smooth, pasty batter. Refrigerate for at least 30 minutes.

3 Pour the oil into a large heavy pot and clip a deep-frying or candy thermometer to the side. Bring the oil up to 375°F.

4 Dip each chunk of cod into the batter, coating it thickly, and then quickly and gently add the fish to the oil. Fry about 4 chunks of cod at a time, making sure to adjust the heat so that the oil does not dip below 350°F.

5 Cook the fish, stirring and turning the pieces often, until they are golden brown, about 5 minutes. Remove from the oil with a spider strainer or slotted spoon and transfer to a paper towel to drain. Sprinkle lightly with salt.

6 Repeat the process with the remaining fish. You can keep the fish hot in a 250°F oven. Serve hot, with french fries and lemon wedges.

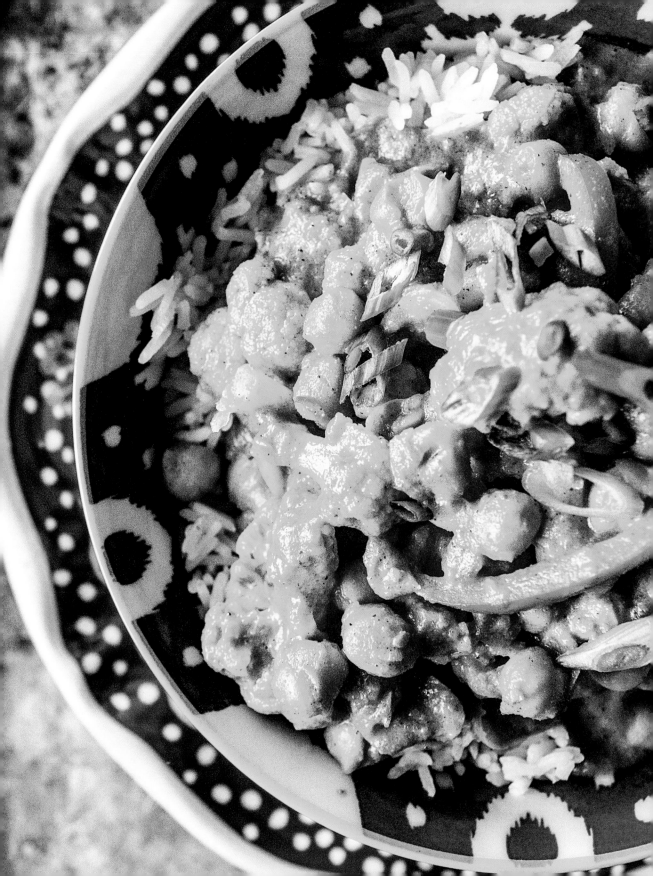

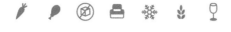

RED VEGETABLE CURRY

PREPARATION 15 MINUTES **COOK TIME** 1 HOUR **SERVINGS** 6

This dish has the earthy flavors of curry, ginger, and cumin typical of Indian cuisine. I tested it on some of my vegetarian and vegan friends, who gave it a thumbs-up not only for its exotic flavors but also for its balance of fiber, protein (from the beans), and carbs. It's a complete meal that's so hearty and filling that you'll never miss the meat.

¼ cup vegetable oil

1 yellow onion, coarsely chopped

4 garlic cloves, thinly sliced

1 (2-inch) piece fresh ginger, peeled and thinly sliced

2 jalapeños, thinly sliced, with seeds

2 tablespoons red curry paste

2 tablespoons curry powder

1 tablespoon ground cumin

1 (14-ounce) can garbanzo beans, drained and rinsed

1 head cauliflower, cut into bite-size pieces

1 red bell pepper, seeded and thinly sliced

3 cups vegetable broth

1 cup tomato sauce

1 (14-ounce) can unsweetened coconut milk

Kosher salt

Steamed jasmine or basmati rice, for serving

Thinly sliced green onions and chopped fresh cilantro, for garnish

1 In a large heavy pot, heat 2 tablespoons of the oil over medium heat. Add the onion and sauté until soft, 5 to 7 minutes. Add the garlic, ginger, and jalapeño and cook until fragrant and soft, 5 minutes more.

2 Add the curry paste, curry powder, and cumin and cook for a few minutes, stirring occasionally. Stir in ¼ cup water. Transfer the curry mixture to a food processor and purée until smooth.

3 Add the remaining 2 tablespoons oil to the same pot and heat over medium heat. Add the curry mixture and cook for 1 minute.

4 Add the beans, cauliflower, and bell pepper to the pot and stir to coat with the curry mixture. Add the broth, tomato sauce, and coconut milk. Stir and bring to a simmer. Reduce the heat to low, cover, and simmer for 30 minutes. Uncover the pot and cook for 15 minutes more to thicken. Season with salt and serve hot, over rice, garnished with green onions and cilantro.

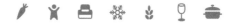

SPICY ROASTED VEGETABLE ENCHILADAS

PREPARATION 20 MINUTES   COOK TIME 45 MINUTES   SERVINGS 6

Our neighborhood taco joint sometimes sneaks smashed potatoes into their taco filling to make the meat go further. I stole that trick for these enchiladas. They may not have cheese, but they are every bit as delicious as the original.

ROASTED VEGETABLES

2 medium zucchini, thinly sliced lengthwise

1 red bell pepper, seeded and thinly sliced lengthwise

1 green bell pepper, seeded and thinly sliced lengthwise

2 small poblano chiles, thinly sliced lengthwise

1 red onion, thinly sliced lengthwise

2 cups thinly sliced button or cremini mushrooms

2 tablespoons vegetable oil

Kosher salt

SPICY RED ENCHILADA SAUCE

¼ cup vegetable oil

1 yellow onion, coarsely chopped

3 garlic cloves, coarsely chopped

1 large jalapeño, coarsely chopped

1 (28-ounce) can crushed tomatoes

2 teaspoons agave

Kosher salt

TO SERVE

3 cups Creamy Mashed Potatoes (page 154)

12 corn tortillas

Tomatillo-Avocado Sauce (page 264)

Fresh cilantro, for garnish

1 Preheat the oven to 400°F. Grease a 9 × 13-inch baking dish with a little vegetable oil.

2 Arrange the vegetables on a rimmed baking sheet and toss with the 2 tablespoons vegetable oil to coat. Sprinkle with salt and roast for 25 minutes. Set aside.

3 To make the spicy red enchilada sauce: In a large saucepan, heat the vegetable oil over medium heat. Add the onion, garlic, and jalapeño and cook until the vegetables begin to brown, about 5 minutes. Stir in the crushed tomatoes, cover, and cook over low heat for about 20 minutes.

4 Transfer the tomato mixture to a blender and add the agave. Purée on high until smooth. Season with salt, then set aside.

5 Smooth a few spoonfuls of mashed potatoes onto each tortilla and top with some of the roasted vegetables. Roll the tortillas and gently place in the prepared baking dish, seam-side down. Pour the red sauce over the enchiladas.

6 Bake for 20 minutes, until lightly golden. Top with the tomatillo-avocado sauce and cilantro and serve hot.

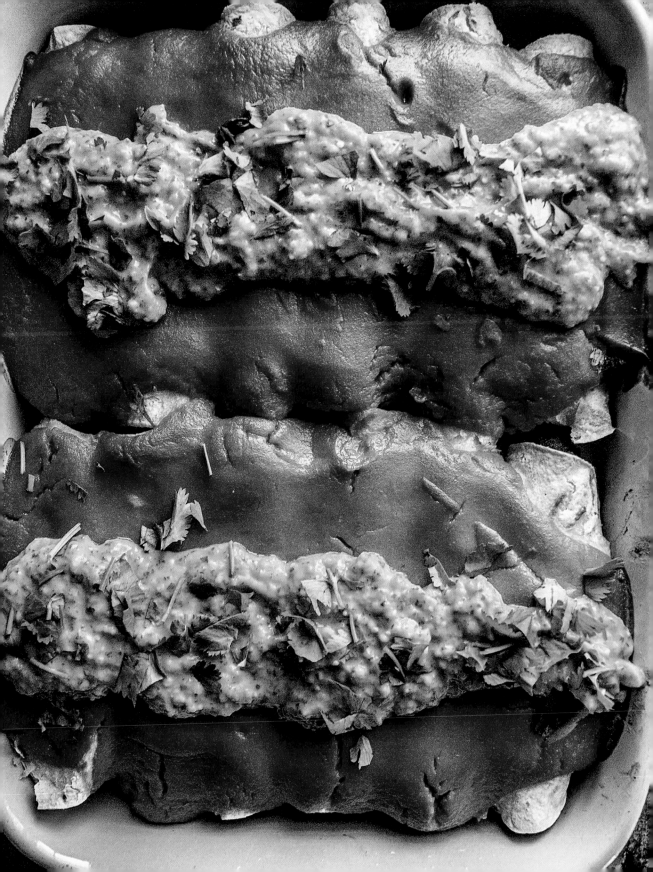

ROASTED TOMATO AND CORN RISOTTO WITH ARUGULA BASIL PESTO

PREPARATION 20 MINUTES   **COOK TIME** 30 MINUTES   **SERVINGS** 6 TO 8

Risotto is one of the most versatile recipes out there; you can add virtually any ingredients you like—from beets or red wine and bacon to zucchini or butternut squash—and create a beautiful, tasty, seasonal dish. Since this version omits the Parmesan cheese and butter typically added to risottos, it is a lighter dish, and the flavors of whatever ingredients you add really get a chance to shine. If you stir diligently, the final result will still be quite creamy. This pesto sauce features blanched garlic, arugula, and basil, which mellow the garlic flavor and gives the sauce a bright green color that doesn't turn brown like most other pestos.

ROASTED VEGETABLES

¼ cup raw corn kernels

2 cups cherry tomatoes

2 tablespoons olive oil

ARUGULA BASIL PESTO

3 garlic cloves

2 cups packed fresh basil leaves

4 cups packed arugula leaves

¼ cup olive oil

¼ cup rice vinegar

Kosher salt

RISOTTO

6 cups chicken stock

¼ cup olive oil

1 yellow onion, finely diced

1½ cups Arborio rice

1 cup raw corn kernels

Kosher salt

2 cups fresh arugula

1 avocado, peeled and diced

1 teaspoon olive oil

Kosher salt

Small fresh basil leaves, for garnish (optional)

1 To prepare the roasted vegetables: Preheat the oven to 450°F. Line a baking sheet with parchment paper. Arrange the corn kernels and the cherry tomatoes on the baking sheet and drizzle the oil over the top.

2 To make the arugula basil pesto: Bring a small pot of water to a boil. Fill a bowl with ice and water. Add the garlic cloves to the boiling water. After 20 seconds, add the basil and arugula and

blanch for 8 to 10 seconds. Scoop out the basil, arugula, and garlic with a large strainer and immediately plunge into the ice water.

3 Wring the herbs of the extra water and put them in a blender with the blanched garlic, olive oil, and vinegar. Purée on high until smooth and then season with salt. Set aside.

4 To make the risotto: In a medium pot, heat the chicken stock over medium-low heat.

5 In a large heavy pan or pot, heat the olive oil over medium heat. Add the onion and cook, stirring often, for 5 minutes, until soft.

6 Add the rice and cook, stirring for 2 to 3 minutes until the rice is translucent except for a white center.

7 Start adding the hot chicken stock 1 cup at a time while continuously stirring with a wooden spoon. As the stock is absorbed, add another cup. Continue until all the stock has been incorporated and the rice is cooked to al dente. This should take about 20 minutes. In the final minute, add the corn.

8 Remove from the heat and stir in the basil arugula pesto. Season with salt.

9 Seven minutes before the risotto is to be finished, put the tomatoes and corn in the oven and roast for 7 minutes, until sizzling and golden. The tomatoes will burst.

10 In a small bowl, gently toss the arugula and avocado with the olive oil and a little salt.

11 Spoon the risotto into bowls and top with some of the salad and roasted cherry tomatoes. Garnish with the roasted corn and some small fresh basil leaves, if desired.

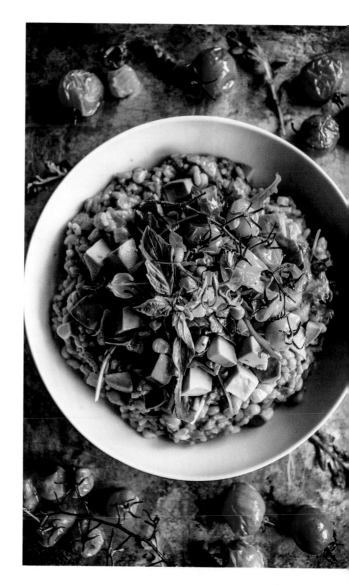

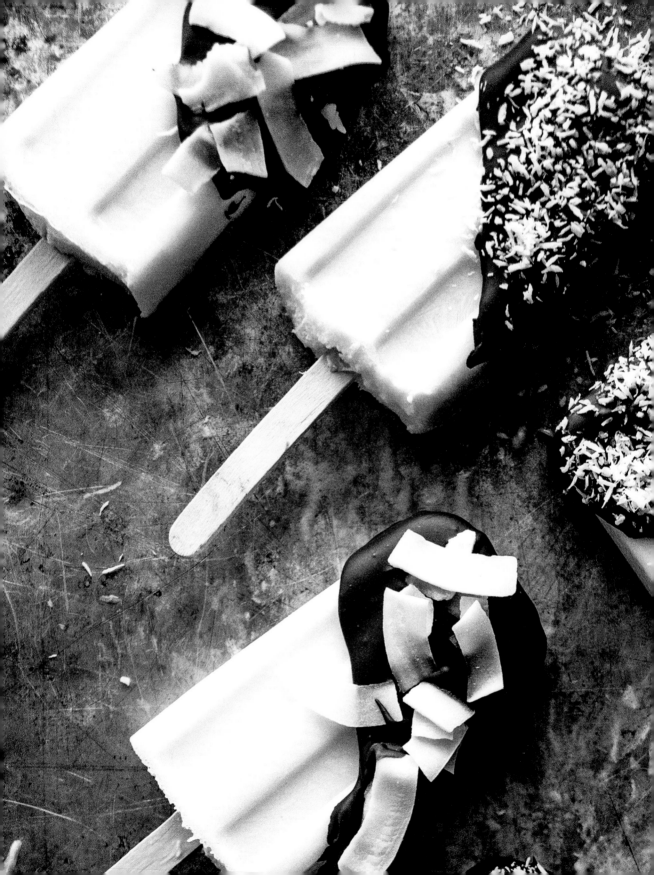

desserts

My Inner Glutton would argue that this is the most important chapter of the book, and my Inner Pastry Chef would second that argument. Treats tend to mark lots of special occasions in our lives, so having a solid collection of celebratory desserts can be the key to many happy moments. Here you'll find everything from school lunch cookies to multilayered birthday cakes and decorated cupcakes. All have been tested a few times more than necessary to make sure that each was worthy of the time, effort, and dollars required to make them.

While many of these treats are traditional, the ingredients you will use to make them will be a whole new ballgame. Gluten-free flours and oats, beet sugar, coconut oil, and chia seeds are some of the staples that have replaced my old arsenal of wheat flour, white sugar, butter, and eggs. It may take you some time to adapt, but it will be so worth it at your first bite of melt-in-your-mouth Chocolate Mousse or a warm slice of Raspberry "Buttermilk" Cake. Soon these ingredients and the way they feel and combine with one another will feel like second nature, the baking that you have always known.

◄ Chocolate-Dipped Coconut Ice Pops (page 307)

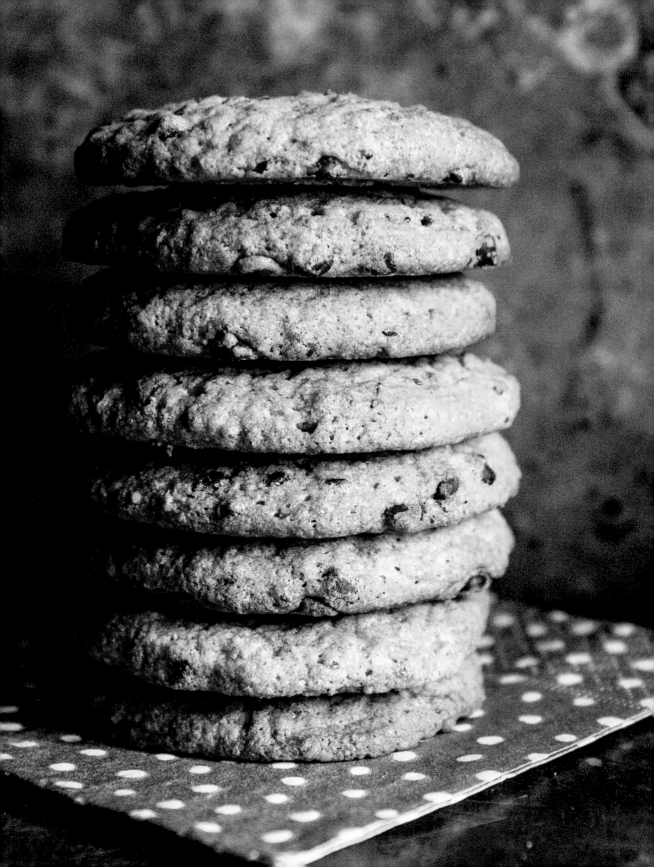

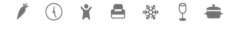

CHEWY CHOCOLATE CHIP COOKIES

PREPARATION 15 MINUTES   **COOK TIME** 12 TO 14 MINUTES   **SERVINGS** 24 COOKIES

A really good chocolate chip cookie is one of life's true simple pleasures. For me, that means it should be a bit chewy but have crisp edges—and no terrible sandy texture, please! Sweet potato purée helps me achieve all that and more, and chia seeds add a nice textural element that I enjoy. I bake double batches of these and stock the freezer with them. If you can't find the allergen-free chocolate chips, you can substitute by chopping stevia-sweetened vegan chocolate bars into small chunks.

1 tablespoon chia seeds

3 tablespoons hot water

1½ cups all-purpose gluten-free flour

½ teaspoon baking soda

½ teaspoon kosher salt

½ cup (1 stick) soy-free vegan butter

¾ cup granulated beet sugar

1 teaspoon pure vanilla extract

3 tablespoons sweet potato purée, canned or homemade (page 34)

1 cup soy-free vegan chocolate chips

1 Preheat the oven to 350°F. Line two rimmed baking sheets with silicone baking mats or parchment paper.

2 In a small bowl, combine the chia seeds and hot water. Let sit until the mixture becomes jellylike, at least 10 minutes.

3 In a separate bowl, whisk together the flour, baking soda, and salt. Set aside.

4 In the bowl of a stand mixer fitted with the paddle attachment, cream together the vegan butter and the sugar until fluffy. Add the vanilla, chia seed mixture, and the sweet potato purée and beat until well combined.

5 Add the flour mixture and beat until you have a creamy dough. Add the chocolate chips and mix them in briefly.

6 Scoop the cookie dough onto the prepared baking sheets in rounded spoonfuls (I use a 1½-inch ice cream scoop), leaving 2 inches between them (they will spread). Bake for 12 to 14 minutes, until the cookies are golden and firm. Let cool on the baking sheets for a few minutes, then transfer to wire racks to cool completely. Store the cookies in an airtight container for up to 5 days or stick them in the freezer for up to 3 months.

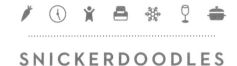

SNICKERDOODLES

PREPARATION 15 MINUTES **COOK TIME** 14 MINUTES **SERVINGS** 20 COOKIES

The perfect concoction of cinnamon and sugar takes a plain little sugar cookie from humble to great. Their crunchy sugar crust is so addictive. You'll be amazed at how quickly these disappear.

2¼ cups all-purpose gluten-free flour

1 teaspoon baking powder

1 teaspoon baking soda

½ cup coconut oil

1¼ plus ⅓ cups granulated beet sugar

1 teaspoon kosher salt

2 tablespoons sweet potato purée, canned or homemade (page 34)

3 tablespoons canned garbanzo bean liquid

2 teaspoons ground cinnamon

1 Preheat the oven to 350°F. Line two rimmed baking sheets with silicone baking mats or parchment paper.

2 In a medium bowl, whisk together the flour, baking powder, and baking soda. Set aside.

3 In the bowl of a stand mixer fitted with the paddle attachment, combine the coconut oil, 1¼ cups of the sugar, the salt, and the sweet potato purée and beat until light and fluffy. Add the garbanzo bean liquid and beat well to combine.

4 Add the flour mixture and mix well to make a sticky dough.

5 In a small bowl, stir together the remaining ⅓ cup sugar and the cinnamon.

6 Scoop the dough in rounded spoonfuls (I use a 1½-inch ice cream scoop) and drop the dough balls into the cinnamon-sugar mixture. Roll the dough ball to coat and place it on the prepared baking sheet. (These cookies will spread quite a bit, so be sure to give them room!)

7 Bake for 12 minutes, until lightly golden. Smack each cookie with the bottom of a spatula to deflate and flatten it, then let the cookies cool on the baking sheets for a few minutes. Transfer to a wire rack to cool completely. Store in an airtight container for up to 5 days or freeze for up to 3 months.

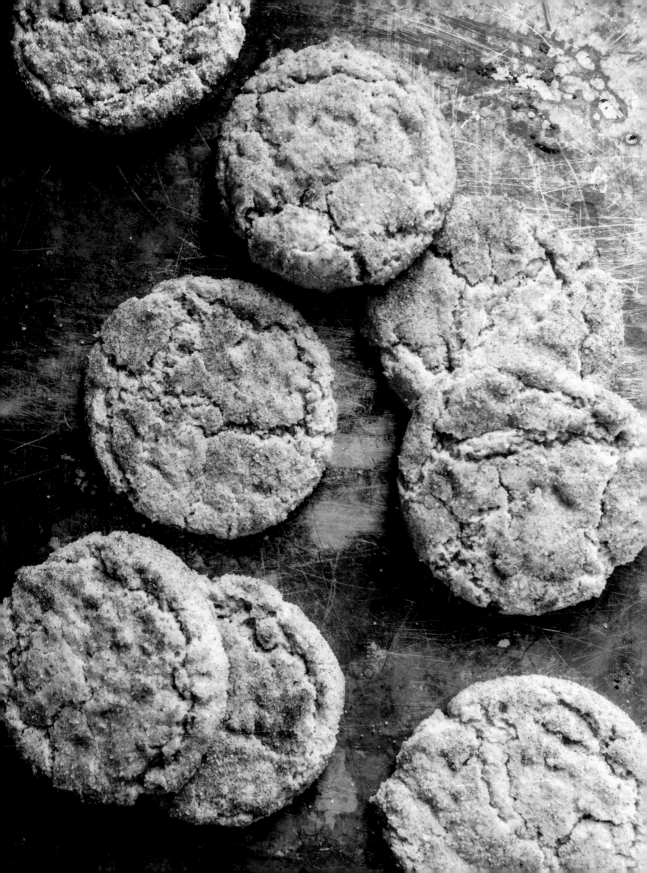

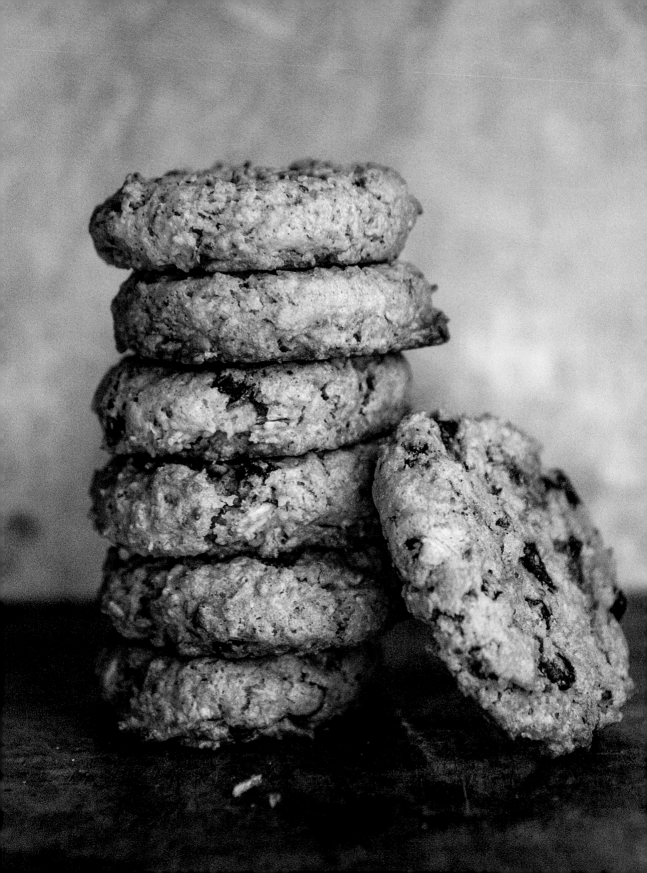

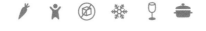

KITCHEN SINK COOKIES

PREPARATION 15 MINUTES   **COOK TIME** 18 MINUTES   **SERVINGS** 24 COOKIES

When you clean out your pantry and find the tail end of a bag of chocolate chips, half a bag of shredded coconut, and a nearly empty raisin box staring back at you, it's time to make Kitchen Sink Cookies. These are crisp, chewy, chunky cookies studded with coconut, raisins, pepitas, and melted chocolate—what's not to like?

1 tablespoon chia seeds

3 tablespoons hot water

1½ cups all-purpose gluten-free flour

1 cup gluten-free rolled oats

1 cup unsweetened shredded coconut

1 teaspoon kosher salt

½ teaspoon baking soda

½ teaspoon ground cinnamon

⅓ cup coconut oil

1 cup granulated beet sugar

1 teaspoon pure vanilla extract

¼ cup sweet potato purée, canned or homemade (page 34)

½ cup soy-free vegan chocolate chips

½ cup raisins

½ cup pepitas

1 Preheat the oven to 350°F. Line two rimmed baking sheets with silicone baking mats or parchment paper.

2 In a small bowl, combine the chia seeds and hot water. Let sit until the mixture becomes jellylike, at least 10 minutes.

3 In a large bowl bowl, whisk together the flour, oats, shredded coconut, salt, baking soda, and cinnamon. Set aside.

4 In the bowl of a stand mixer fitted with the paddle attachment, cream together the coconut oil and sugar until well combined. Add the chia

seed mixture, vanilla, and sweet potato purée and beat until incorporated.

5 Add the flour mixture and beat to make a creamy dough. Add the chocolate chips, raisins and pepitas and beat briefly to incorporate.

6 Using a 1½-inch scoop, set scoops of the cookie dough onto the prepared baking sheets, leaving 2 inches of space between them (they will spread). Bake for 16 to 18 minutes, until golden brown. Let the cookies cool on the baking sheets for a few minutes before transferring them to wire racks to cool completely. Store in an airtight container for up to 5 days or freeze for up to 3 months.

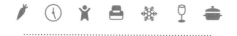

MOLASSES COOKIES

PREPARATION 10 MINUTES   **COOK TIME** 14 TO 16 MINUTES   **SERVINGS** 24 COOKIES

My family knows a thing or two about molasses cookies. We've all been making Grandma Grace's famous recipe since we were tall enough to reach the stove, and they are a fixture on our holiday tables. So when I overheard my aunt, mid-bite, confiding to a guest at one Christmas gathering that these cookies were made from her mother's recipe, I knew we had a winner.

1½ cups all-purpose gluten-free flour

½ cup gluten-free oat flour

1½ cups granulated beet sugar

1 teaspoon kosher salt

½ teaspoon baking soda

1 teaspoon baking powder

1 teaspoon ground cinnamon

1 teaspoon ground ginger

½ teaspoon ground nutmeg

½ teaspoon ground cloves

3 tablespoons canned garbanzo bean liquid

3 tablespoons sweet potato purée, canned or homemade (page 34)

2 tablespoons molasses

⅓ cup coconut oil, melted

1 Preheat the oven to 350°F. Line two rimmed baking sheets with parchment paper or silicone baking mats.

2 In the bowl of a stand mixer fitted with the paddle attachment, combine the all-purpose flour, oat flour, 1 cup of the sugar, salt, baking soda, baking powder, cinnamon, ginger, nutmeg, and cloves. Add the garbanzo bean liquid, sweet potato purée, molasses, and coconut oil and beat vigorously until the batter is thick and smooth.

3 Place the remaining ½ cup sugar in a shallow bowl.

4 Scoop the batter into rounded spoonfuls (I use a 1½-inch ice cream scoop) and drop them into the bowl of sugar. Gently roll the dough balls in the sugar and then place the cookies on the prepared baking sheets. They will spread, so leave 2 inches room between them. Bake 14 to 16 minutes, rotating the baking sheets halfway through.

5 Let the cookies cool on the baking sheets for a few minutes, then transfer them to wire racks or the countertop to cool completely. Store in an airtight container for up to 5 days or freeze for up to 3 months.

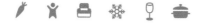

CHOCOLATE FUDGE BROWNIES

PREPARATION 15 MINUTES   **COOK TIME** 45 MINUTES   **SERVINGS** 12 BROWNIES

Few people would ever guess these super-rich and chocolaty treats were made from this ingredient list. They taste every bit the classic brownie, and if you really want to make these crazy, top them with a layer of Chocolate Ganache (page 297) or Milk Chocolate Frosting (page 292).

Nonstick cooking spray

2 cups all-purpose gluten-free flour

1½ cups granulated beet sugar

⅓ cup unsweetened cocoa powder

1½ teaspoons kosher salt

½ cup vegetable oil

2 teaspoons pure vanilla extract

⅓ cup brewed espresso or very strong coffee, at room temperature

½ cup canned garbanzo bean liquid

½ cup soy-free vegan chocolate chips

1 Preheat the oven to 325°F. Spray an 8 × 8-inch baking pan with cooking spray.

2 In the bowl of a stand mixer fitted with the paddle attachment, combine the flour, sugar, cocoa powder, and salt. With the mixer running on low, add the oil, vanilla, and espresso. Add the garbanzo bean liquid and mix until you have a uniform, thick batter. Add the chocolate chips to the mixer and briefly mix them in.

3 Pour the batter into the prepared pan and spread it evenly with a spatula. Bake for 45 minutes, until the top is firm and a toothpick inserted into the center comes out clean. Let the brownies cool completely in the pan before slicing for a clean cut.

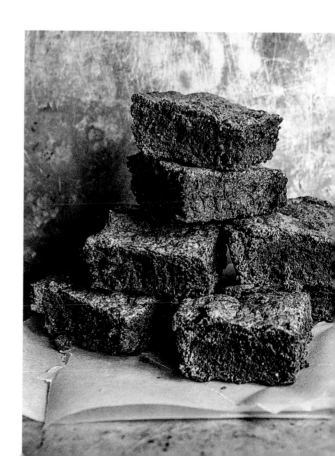

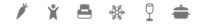

CHOCOLATE COCONUT CARAMEL BARS

PREPARATION 15 MINUTES   **COOK TIME** 35 MINUTES   **SERVINGS** 16 TO 24 BARS

A retro, indulgent cookie bar stuffed with coconut, chocolate, and caramel with a crispy cookie crust, these are my take on a magic bar. Bring these to school or the office to share and you will be very popular indeed. They also freeze well.

CRUST

Nonstick cooking spray

2¼ cups all-purpose gluten-free flour

1¼ cups beet confectioners' sugar

1 cup unsweetened shredded coconut

2 tablespoons baking powder

½ teaspoon kosher salt

½ teaspoon xanthan gum (see page 34)

1 teaspoon pure vanilla extract

11 tablespoons (½ cup plus 3 tablespoons) coconut oil

CARAMEL

½ cup coconut oil

1¼ cups granulated beet sugar

½ cup unsweetened coconut cream

2 teaspoons pure vanilla extract

1 teaspoon kosher salt

TOPPINGS

1 cup soy-free vegan chocolate chips

1 cup unsweetened shredded coconut

1 Preheat the oven to 350°F. Line a 9 ×13-inch baking pan with parchment, then coat with cooking spray.

2 To make the crust: In a food processor, combine the flour, confectioners' sugar, coconut, baking powder, salt, and xanthan gum and pulse a few times to combine. Add the vanilla and the coconut oil and pulse to create a crumbly dough.

3 Transfer the dough to the prepared pan and use your hands then a sturdy spatula to press it completely flat. Bake for 10 minutes, until lightly golden.

4 Meanwhile, make the caramel: In a small saucepan, combine the coconut oil, sugar, coconut cream, vanilla, and salt. Simmer over medium-low heat until slightly thickened, 5 minutes.

5 Remove the crust from the oven (don't turn off the oven) and use the spatula to press down on the crust firmly, releasing the steam. Pour the caramel over the crust and bake for 15 minutes more.

6 Sprinkle the caramel evenly with the chocolate chips and coconut. Bake for 5 minutes more.

7 Let the bars cool completely in the pan before cutting into bars. Store in an airtight container for up to 5 days or freeze for up to 3 months.

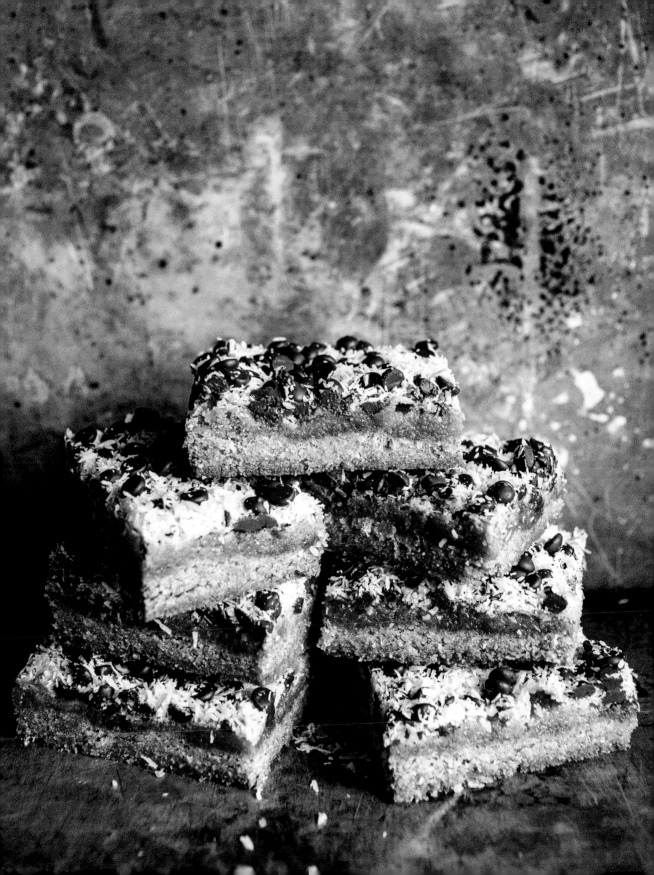

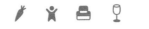

CHOCOLATE MOUSSE

PREPARATION 1 HOUR 15 MINUTES   **COOK TIME** 5 MINUTES   **SERVINGS** 2 TO 4

Old-school though this may be, I still consider it elegant and decadent, the ultimate romantic dessert for two! I was thrilled when I found a way to create a dairy-free chocolate mousse without sacrificing any flavor. Note that the cream whips up faster and more easily if you freeze the bowl that you whip it in first. Even thirty minutes in the freezer will make a big difference.

1 cup soy-free vegan dark chocolate chips (about 5 ounces)

Pinch of kosher salt

1 teaspoon pure vanilla extract

3 cups unsweetened coconut cream

Fresh raspberries, for garnish (optional)

1 In a small saucepan, combine the chocolate chips, salt, vanilla, and 1½ cups of the coconut cream. Bring just to a simmer over medium heat, then remove from the heat.

2 Whisk until the chocolate has completely melted and the mixture is very smooth. Transfer to a bowl and refrigerate for at least 1 hour, or until the mixture is very cold and has firmed up. Refrigerate the remaining 1½ cups coconut cream at the same time.

3 When the chocolate mixture is cold, place the chilled coconut cream in the bowl of a stand mixer fitted with the whisk attachment. Whip the cream until soft peaks form. Add the chilled chocolate mixture and whip until the mousse is soft, fluffy, and uniform in color.

4 Spoon the mousse into individual serving bowls, or scoop the mousse into a pastry bag fitted with a star tip and pipe the mousse into bowls or glasses. Refrigerate until ready to serve. Garnish with raspberries, if desired.

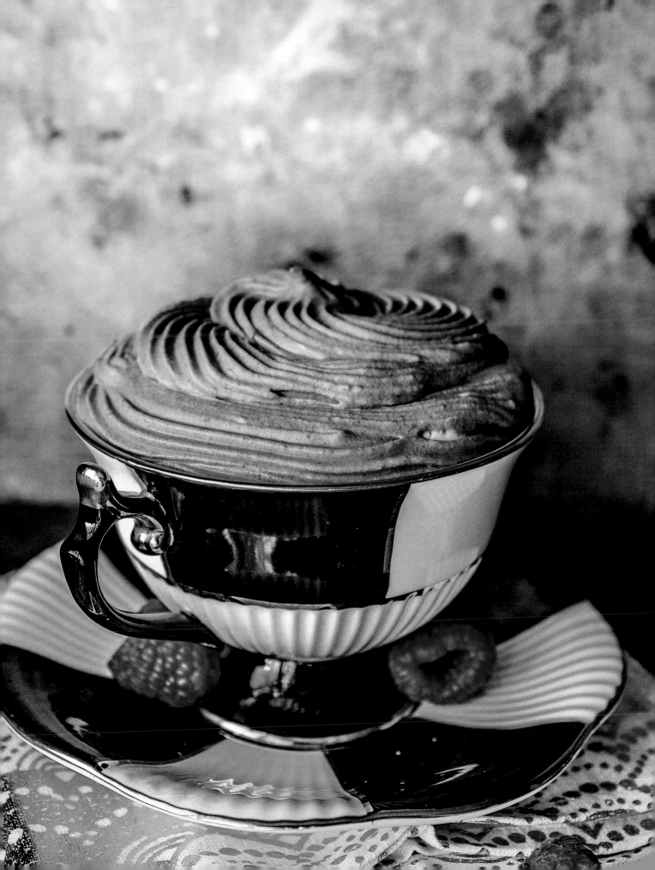

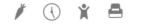

PIA'S FAMOUS CHOCOLATE BROWNIE MUG CAKE

PREPARATION 5 MINUTES **COOK TIME** 2 MINUTES **SERVINGS** 2

These jaunty mug cakes are the first dessert I came up with post–allergy diagnosis to satisfy Pia's chocolate cravings, and they are so easy that my little girls can make and microwave them all on their own. The result is a fudgy mix between a cake and a pudding, a perfect hot chocolaty dessert that takes seven minutes, max, from start to finish. Add a generous dollop of coconut whipped cream to really put this over the top. If you like, make a double batch of the batter and fill mini mason jars so you can pull one out of the fridge and microwave to order throughout the week.

½ cup all-purpose gluten-free flour

½ cup granulated beet sugar

¼ cup unsweetened cocoa powder

Pinch of kosher salt

½ cup unsweetened coconut milk

¼ cup vegetable oil

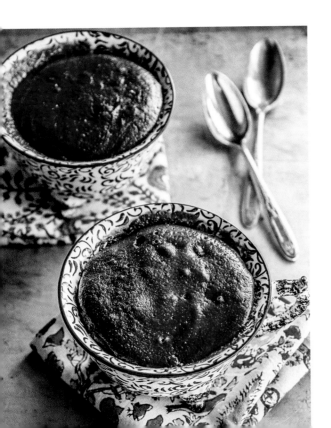

1 In a blender or food processor, combine the flour, sugar, cocoa powder, salt, coconut milk, and oil and purée until the mixture is smooth and free of lumps. Divide the batter between two microwave-safe mugs.

2 Microwave on high until the mixture is cooked through, 1 minute 40 seconds to 2 minutes. It should still be moist in the center, not dry.

3 Let cool for a minute and serve hot.

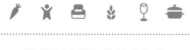

FRUIT CRISP

PREPARATION 10 MINUTES   **COOK TIME** 90 MINUTES   **SERVINGS** 12

Sorry, Grandma Grace—your fruit crisp was a beloved family recipe, but I have to admit I like this updated version even better. The coconut oil makes the topping especially crisp, and because I bake the whole thing for a long time, the fruit filling is lusciously tender. You can make this with fresh or frozen fruit, so it's practical, too. When blackberries are in season, they're my go-to fruit, but readily available Granny Smith apples are a great option any time of year. If you use apples or pears, peel them and very thinly slice them for best results.

TOPPING

1 cup all-purpose gluten-free flour

1 teaspoon baking soda

1 teaspoon kosher salt

1 teaspoon ground cinnamon

1 cup granulated beet sugar

3 cups gluten-free rolled oats

1 cup coconut oil

CRISP

8 cups fresh or frozen fruit

2 tablespoons granulated beet sugar

½ teaspoon ground cinnamon

1 Preheat the oven to 350°F. Grease a 9 × 13-inch baking dish.

2 To make the crisp topping: In a large bowl, combine the flour, baking soda, salt, cinnamon, sugar, and oats. Using a pastry cutter or two forks, cut the coconut oil into the dry ingredients until the mixture forms coarse crumbs. Set aside.

3 In a large bowl, sprinkle the fruit with the sugar and cinnamon and mix well. Spread the fruit in the prepared baking dish and sprinkle evenly with the crisp topping.

4 Bake for about 90 minutes, until the fruit is bubbling and the topping is golden brown. Let cool slightly before serving.

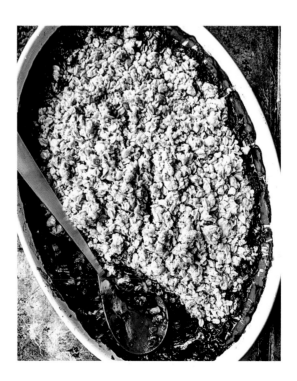

CHOCOLATE CUPCAKES WITH
FLUFFY MILK CHOCOLATE FROSTING

PREPARATION 20 MINUTES   **COOK TIME** 16 TO 18 MINUTES   **SERVINGS** 12 CUPCAKES

Every child should get to have a cupcake at least once in a while. I believe that is a fundamental right. These chocolate cupcakes are easy and foolproof and totally delicious. I customize them with sprinkles or edible flowers, depending on the occasion. They are also really easy for me to send with my children to their friends' birthday parties so that they get to have a treat, too. This batter can easily be made into a layer cake by dividing the batter between two 9-inch round cake pans and baking in a preheated 350°F oven at for 25 minutes.

CUPCAKES

1 cup unsweetened coconut milk

1 tablespoon cider vinegar

1¼ cups all-purpose gluten-free flour

1½ teaspoons xanthan gum (see page 34)

½ cup unsweetened cocoa powder

1½ teaspoons baking powder

1 teaspoon baking soda

½ teaspoon kosher salt

1 cup granulated beet sugar

⅓ cup vegetable oil

2 teaspoons pure vanilla extract

MILK CHOCOLATE FROSTING

½ cup soy-free vegan chocolate chips

1 cup (2 sticks) soy-free vegan butter, at room temperature

½ cup unsweetened cocoa powder

2½ cups confectioners' beet sugar

¼ cup unsweetened coconut milk

2 teaspoons pure vanilla extract

1 To make the cupcakes: Preheat the oven to 350°F. Line a 12-cup muffin tin with paper liners.

2 In a small bowl, combine the coconut milk and vinegar and set aside.

3 In the bowl of a stand mixer fitted with the whisk attachment, combine the flour, xanthan gum, cocoa powder, baking powder, baking soda, salt, and sugar. Add the coconut milk mixture, the oil, and the vanilla and whisk until fluffy, about 1 minute.

4 Scoop the batter into the prepared muffin tin. Bake for 16 to 18 minutes, until the cupcakes are baked through. Let the cupcakes cool completely in the tin on a wire rack before frosting.

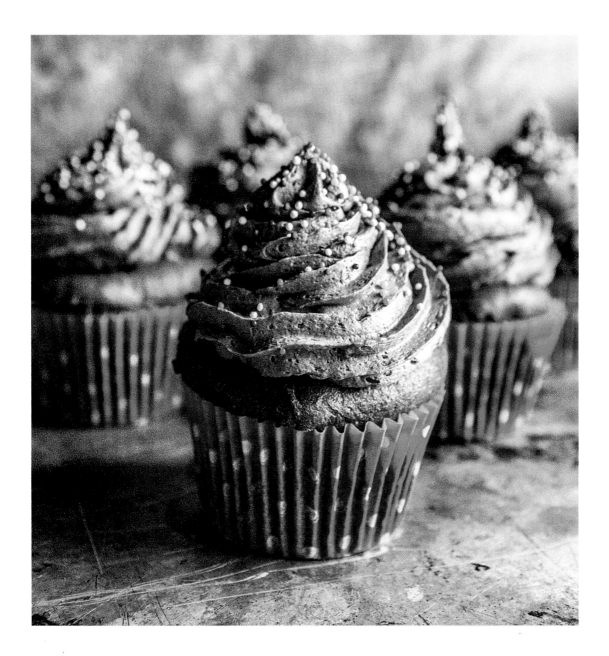

5 To make the frosting: Put the chocolate chips in a microwave-safe bowl and microwave for 60 seconds on high heat. Whisk until smooth.

6 In the bowl of a stand mixer fitted with the whisk attachment, beat together the vegan butter and cocoa powder until well combined. Add the melted chocolate and beat until smooth. Add the confectioners' sugar a little at a time to combine, and then add the coconut milk and vanilla. Beat the frosting until fluffy. Pipe or spread the frosting generously over the cooled cupcakes.

CARROT CAKE WITH
VANILLA "CREAM CHEESE" FROSTING

PREPARATION 20 MINUTES   **COOK TIME** 25 MINUTES   **SERVINGS** 12

When it comes to carrot cake, my mom and I argue over the addition of little bits of nuts and fruits and other squirrel food that she would like to see included, but my answer is NO WAY. My recipe shall include only carrots. Whatever you do from there, just don't tell me. This cake screams spring, or really just "dessert!!" You can also use this recipe to make cupcakes. Pour the batter into a 12-cup muffin tin lined with paper liners and bake in a preheated 350°F oven for 16 to 18 minutes.

CARROT CAKE

Nonstick cooking spray

1 cup unsweetened coconut milk

1 tablespoon apple cider vinegar

4½ cups all-purpose gluten-free flour

2 cups granulated beet sugar

4 teaspoons baking powder

2 teaspoons baking soda

1 tablespoon xanthan gum (see page 34)

1 tablespoon ground cinnamon

1 teaspoon ground nutmeg

2 teaspoons kosher salt

2½ cups packed grated carrots (about 3 to 4 carrots)

2 teaspoons pure vanilla extract

1 cup vegetable oil

VANILLA "CREAM CHEESE" FROSTING

1 cup (2 sticks) soy-free vegan butter

5 cups beet confectioners' sugar

1 tablespoon pure vanilla extract

1 teaspoon apple cider vinegar

3 tablespoons unsweetened coconut milk

Pinch of kosher salt

1 To make the carrot cake: Preheat the oven to 350°F. Spray two 9-inch round cake pans with cooking spray and line them with parchment paper rounds cut to fit.

2 In a small bowl, combine the coconut milk and vinegar and set aside.

3 In the bowl of a stand mixer fitted with the whisk attachment, combine the flour, sugar, baking powder, baking soda, xanthan gum, cinnamon, nutmeg, and salt. Add the carrots, and with the mixer running on low, add the vanilla, vegetable oil, and coconut milk mixture. Mix well until you have a smooth batter.

4 Divide the batter evenly between the prepared pans. Bake for 25 minutes, until a toothpick inserted into the center comes out clean. Let the cakes cool completely in the pans.

5 To make the vanilla "cream cheese" frosting: In the bowl of a stand mixer fitted with the paddle attachment, whip the vegan butter until fluffy, then slowly add the confectioners' sugar and continue beating until fluffy. Add the vanilla, vinegar, coconut milk, and a pinch of salt. Whip until fluffy.

6 Place one cake round on a cake plate and top with one-third of the frosting. Place the other round on top and frost the sides and top of the cake with the remaining frosting.

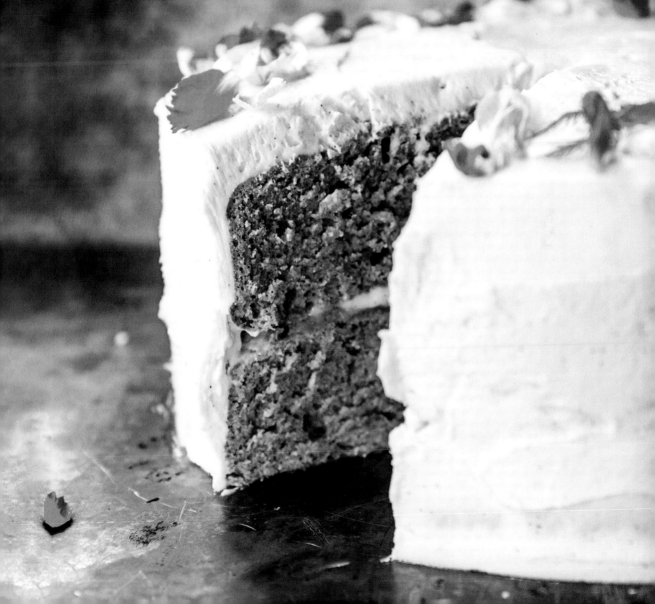

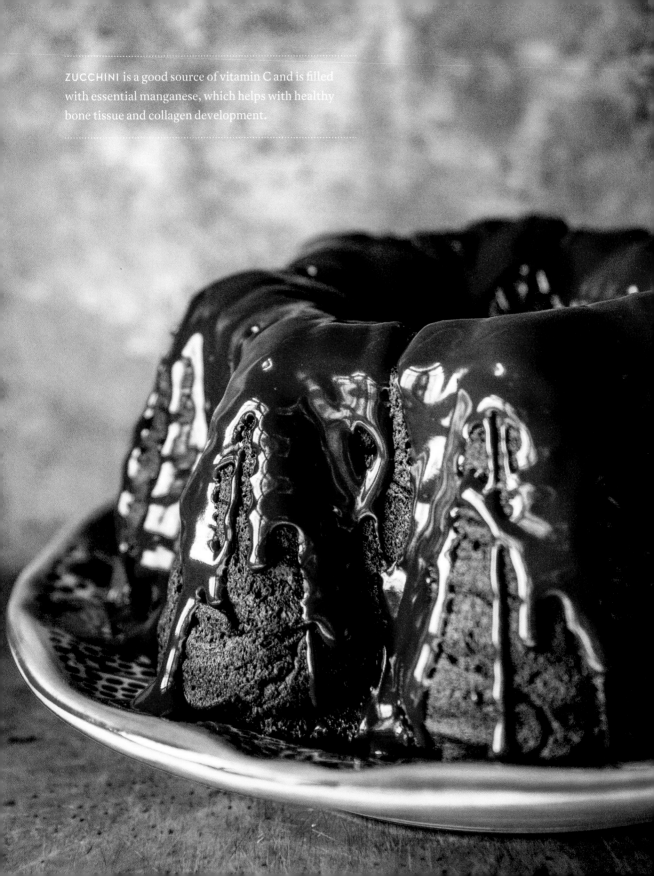

ZUCCHINI is a good source of vitamin C and is filled with essential manganese, which helps with healthy bone tissue and collagen development.

CHOCOLATE ZUCCHINI BUNDT CAKE

PREPARATION 20 MINUTES   COOK TIME 25 MINUTES   SERVINGS 12

I have always had a soft spot for baking with veggies, and zucchini is probably my favorite. When I was growing up, my mother's vegetable garden produced zucchini the size of rolling pins, and she would crank out loaf after loaf of zucchini bread and tons of cakes all summer long. I add dark chocolate and strong coffee plus a silky chocolate ganache and it makes for a perfect, moist chocolate cake that delivers great texture, flavor, and looks.

CAKE

Nonstick cooking spray

3 cups all-purpose gluten-free flour

¾ cup unsweetened cocoa powder

1½ cups granulated beet sugar

1 tablespoon baking powder

1½ teaspoons baking soda

2½ teaspoons xanthan gum (see page 34)

1 teaspoon ground cinnamon

2 teaspoons kosher salt

2 cups packed grated zucchini (about 1½ to 2 large zucchini)

1 teaspoon pure vanilla extract

¾ cup vegetable oil

¾ cup strong hot coffee

½ cup soy-free vegan chocolate chips

CHOCOLATE GANACHE

½ cup unsweetened coconut cream

1 cup soy-free vegan chocolate chips

1 To make the cake: Preheat the oven to 350°F. Spray a 10-cup Bundt pan with cooking spray.

2 In the bowl of a stand mixer fitted with the whisk attachment, combine the flour, cocoa powder, sugar, baking powder, baking soda, xanthan gum, cinnamon, and salt. Add the zucchini, and with the mixer running on low, add the vanilla, vegetable oil, and hot coffee. Mix to make a smooth batter and then mix in the chocolate chips.

3 Transfer the batter to the prepared pan. Bake until puffed and domed on top, about 50 minutes.

4 Let the cake cool completely in the pan on a wire rack before turning it out onto the rack.

5 To make the chocolate ganache: In a small saucepan, bring the coconut cream to a simmer over low heat. Remove from the heat and add the chocolate chips. Whisk until the chocolate has melted and the mixture is smooth. Set aside. The ganache will thicken as it cools.

6 Place a baking sheet under the wire rack holding the cake. Drizzle the ganache over the cake, letting the extra chocolate drip onto the baking sheet.

7 Transfer the cake to a serving plate and serve.

VANILLA-VANILLA LAYER CAKE

PREPARATION 40 MINUTES   **COOK TIME** 25 MINUTES   **SERVINGS** 12

Vanilla-vanilla is a delicious classic that will always, always make everyone happy, happy. This has graced many birthday celebrations and even a baby shower, and few guests ever suspected that it contained not a speck of butter, eggs, or wheat flour. It's a tender vanilla cake, and the absolutely delicious frosting looks lovely tinted with a few drops of color to suit your occasion.

CAKE

Nonstick cooking spray

2 cups unsweetened coconut milk

2 tablespoons apple cider vinegar

4 cups all-purpose gluten-free flour

2 cups granulated beet sugar

2 tablespoons baking powder

2 teaspoons xanthan gum (see page 34)

1 teaspoon baking soda

1 teaspoon kosher salt

½ cup vegetable oil

1 tablespoon pure vanilla extract

VANILLA FROSTING

1 cup (2 sticks) soy-free vegan butter

5 cups confectioners' beet sugar

1 tablespoon pure vanilla extract

3 tablespoons unsweetened coconut milk

Pinch of kosher salt

1 To make the cake: Preheat the oven to 350°F. Spray two 9-inch round cake pans with cooking spray and line them with parchment paper rounds cut to fit.

2 In a small bowl, combine the coconut milk and vinegar and set aside.

3 In the bowl of a stand mixer fitted with the paddle attachment, combine the flour, sugar, baking powder, xanthan gum, baking soda, and salt. Add the vegetable oil, vanilla, and coconut milk mixture and mix until the batter is fluffy.

4 Divide the batter between the prepared pans and gently smooth it to the edges with a spatula.

Bake for 25 minutes, or until the cakes are golden. Let the cakes cool completely in the pans.

5 To make the vanilla frosting: In the bowl of a stand mixer fitted with the whisk attachment, whip the vegan butter until fluffy. Slowly add the confectioners' sugar and continue beating until well combined. Add the vanilla, coconut milk, and a pinch of salt. Whip until fluffy.

6 Place one cooled cake layer on a serving plate and spread with one-third of the frosting. Place the second layer on top and frost the sides and top of the cake with the remaining frosting.

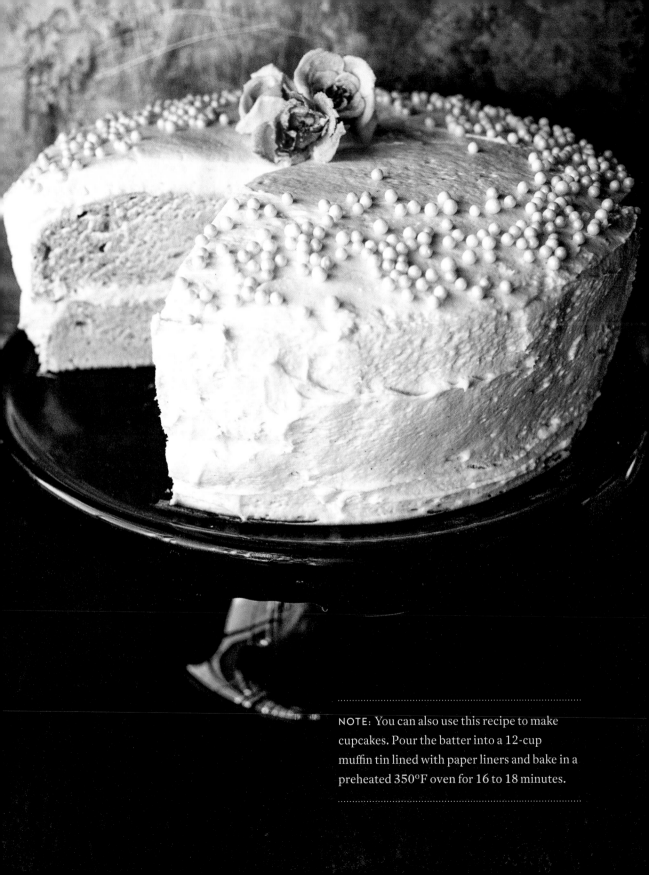

NOTE: You can also use this recipe to make cupcakes. Pour the batter into a 12-cup muffin tin lined with paper liners and bake in a preheated 350°F oven for 16 to 18 minutes.

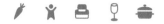

PUMPKIN LAYER CAKE WITH MAPLE FROSTING AND SALTED CARAMEL DRIZZLE

PREPARATION 20 MINUTES   **COOK TIME** 40 MINUTES   **SERVINGS** 12

The flavors of this showstopping cake are reminiscent of a maple bar doughnut and are made even more indulgent with a drizzle of salted caramel. The pumpkin purée in the cake makes for a really moist and tender crumb while keeping it from being too sweet. The fall flavors and special occasion looks of this cake make it a perfect holiday dessert, but I enjoy it any time of year.

CAKE

Nonstick cooking spray

1 cup unsweetened coconut milk

1 tablespoon apple cider vinegar

4½ cups all-purpose gluten-free flour

2 cups granulated beet sugar

4 teaspoons baking powder

2 teaspoons baking soda

1 tablespoon xanthan gum (see page 34)

1 tablespoon ground cinnamon

2 teaspoons ground nutmeg

2 teaspoons kosher salt

2 cups pumpkin purée, canned or homemade (page 34)

1 cup vegetable oil

¼ cup hot water

MAPLE FROSTING

1 cup (2 sticks) soy-free vegan butter

5 cups confectioners' beet sugar

2 tablespoons unsweetened coconut milk

2 tablespoons pure maple extract

Pinch of kosher salt

SALTED CARAMEL SAUCE

1 cup granulated beet sugar

½ teaspoon kosher salt

⅓ cup unsweetened coconut cream

1 To make the cake: Preheat the oven to 350°F. Spray two 9-inch round cake pans with cooking spray and line them with parchment paper rounds cut to fit.

2 In a small bowl, combine the coconut milk and the vinegar and set aside.

3 In the bowl of a stand mixer fitted with the whisk attachment, combine the flour, sugar, baking powder, baking soda, xanthan gum, cinnamon, nutmeg, and salt. Add the pumpkin purée and mix on medium until combined. Reduce the speed to low and add the vegetable oil, hot water, and coconut milk mixture. Mix until incorporated, then raise the speed to medium-high and whip until the batter is fluffy and uniform.

4 Divide the batter between the prepared pans and spread the batter to the edges.

5 Bake for 30 minutes, or until golden and a toothpick inserted into the centers comes out clean. Let the cakes cool completely in the pans on a wire rack.

6 To make the maple frosting: In the bowl of a stand mixer fitted with the whisk attachment, combine the vegan butter and 3 cups of the confectioners' sugar and beat on low speed until well combined. Add the remaining 2 cups confectioners' sugar, the coconut milk, maple extract, and salt. Gradually increase the speed to high and beat the frosting until it is nice and fluffy.

7 To make the salted caramel sauce: In a small saucepan, combine the sugar, salt, and ¼ cup water. Cook over medium heat, without stirring, swirling the pan gently to mix the water and sugar together, until the caramel has turned a deep golden color, about 8 minutes. Try not to get sugar granules on the side of the pan. Keep a close eye on the sugar, because it can become too dark really quickly! Pull the caramel off the heat and add the coconut cream by the spoonful, swirling to

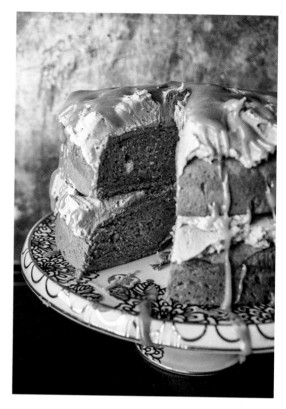

combine (don't stir!). The caramel will be a deep, smooth, amber color. Transfer the caramel to a heatproof container (mason jars work well) and let cool to room temperature. It is important that the caramel is cool, or the entire cake will melt when you pour it on.

8 Place one cooled cake layer on a serving plate and spread with one-third of the frosting. Place the second layer on top. You can use the remaining frosting to frost the sides and top of the cake or just pile it all on the top, leaving the sides of the cake unfrosted.

9 Drizzle the cake with the cooled caramel sauce and serve. (You can refrigerate the caramel in a covered container for up to 1 week. To bring it back to room temperature, microwave it for 20 seconds or heat it up in a water bath.)

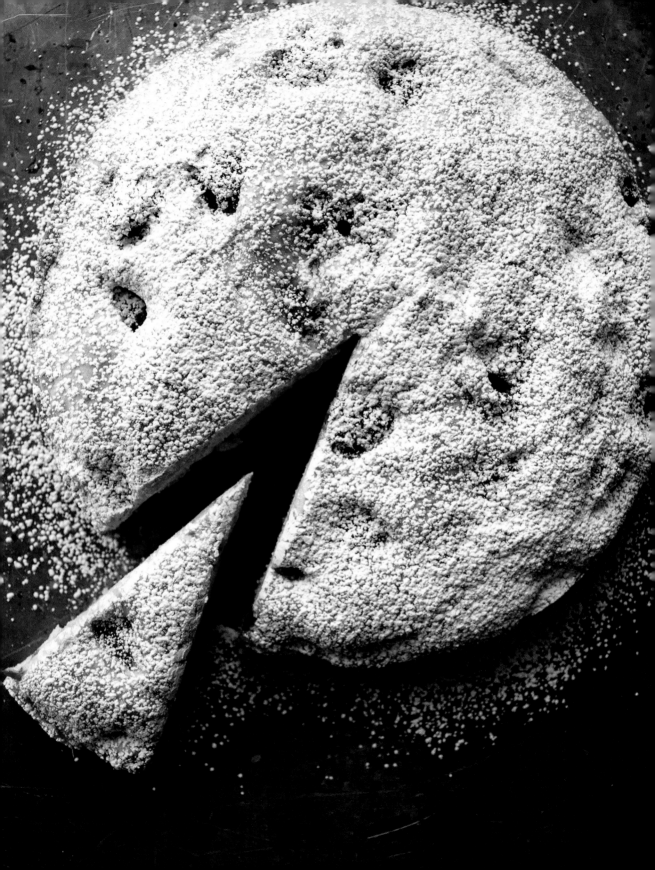

RASPBERRY "BUTTERMILK" CAKE

PREPARATION 10 MINUTES   COOK TIME 25 MINUTES   SERVINGS 8

Several years ago, I featured a recipe on my blog based on a very old recipe card for Raspberry Buttermilk Cake from my great-aunt Mary, and it has become a family staple. It has the same wonderful texture, flavor, and appealing "tang" as the original, achieved here by the addition of faux buttermilk. Because it is simple in both presentation—just a dusting of confectioners' sugar—and preparation, I affectionately refer to it as a "weeknight" cake, but the truth is, I serve this often as a breakfast cake, and would never turn down a slice with a cup of hot tea in the afternoon, either!

Nonstick cooking spray

1 cup unsweetened coconut milk

1 tablespoon apple cider vinegar

2 cups all-purpose gluten-free flour

¾ cup granulated beet sugar

1 tablespoon baking powder

1 teaspoon xanthan gum (see page 34)

½ teaspoon kosher salt

¼ cup coconut oil, melted

2 teaspoons pure vanilla extract

½ cup raspberries or other fresh fruit

Confectioners' sugar, for serving

1 Preheat the oven to 350°F. Spray a 9-inch round cake pan with cooking spray.

2 In a small bowl, combine the coconut milk and the vinegar and set aside.

3 In a large bowl, whisk together the flour, beet sugar, baking powder, xanthan gum, and salt. Make a well in the center and add the coconut oil, vanilla, and coconut milk mixture. Stir until smooth, then very gently fold in the raspberries.

4 Transfer the batter to the prepared pan and gently smooth it to the edges of the pan.

5 Bake for 25 minutes, until the cake is golden on top and a toothpick inserted into the center comes out clean. Let the cake cool in the pan on a wire rack for at least 20 minutes, then invert it onto a serving plate. Sprinkle with confectioners' sugar, slice, and serve.

STRAWBERRY-COCONUT SHORTCAKES

PREPARATION 15 MINUTES   **COOK TIME** 15 MINUTES   **SERVINGS** 6

Strawberry shortcake is *the* quintessential summer dessert, appropriate for both big crowds and small dinner parties. With a tender, flaky coconut shortcake; creamy, rich coconut whipped cream; and juicy macerated strawberries, you get a little bit of heaven in every bite. Make sure that you serve these the same day you make them, for freshness.

COCONUT WHIPPED CREAM

2 (15-ounce) cans unsweetened coconut cream, chilled

2 tablespoons beet confectioners' sugar (optional)

MACERATED STRAWBERRIES

4 cups thinly sliced fresh strawberries

1 tablespoon granulated beet sugar

1 teaspoon fresh lemon juice

COCONUT SHORTCAKES

6 tablespoons unsweetened coconut milk, plus more for brushing the shortcakes

2 teaspoons apple cider vinegar

2 cups all-purpose gluten-free flour, plus more for forming the shortcakes

½ cup plus 1 tablespoon unsweetened shredded coconut

½ cup plus 1 tablespoon granulated beet sugar

2 teaspoons baking powder

½ teaspoon baking soda

½ teaspoon xanthan gum (see page 34)

½ teaspoon kosher salt

6 tablespoons (¾ stick) soy-free vegan butter, cut into chunks

1 To make the coconut whipped cream: In the bowl of a stand mixer fitted with a whisk attachment, combine the chilled coconut cream and the confectioners' sugar (if using). Whip until the coconut cream forms soft peaks. Immediately place the whipped cream in the refrigerator; it will thicken further as it chills.

2 To make the macerated strawberries: In a medium bowl, combine the strawberries, sugar, and lemon juice. Set aside at room temperature.

3 To make the coconut shortcakes: Preheat the oven to 400°F. Line a rimmed baking sheet with a silicone baking mat or parchment paper.

4 In a small bowl, combine the coconut milk and the vinegar and set aside.

5 In a food processor, combine the flour, ½ cup of the shredded coconut, ½ cup of the sugar, the baking powder, baking soda, xanthan gum, and salt. Pulse to mix thoroughly. Add the vegan butter and pulse until it is completely

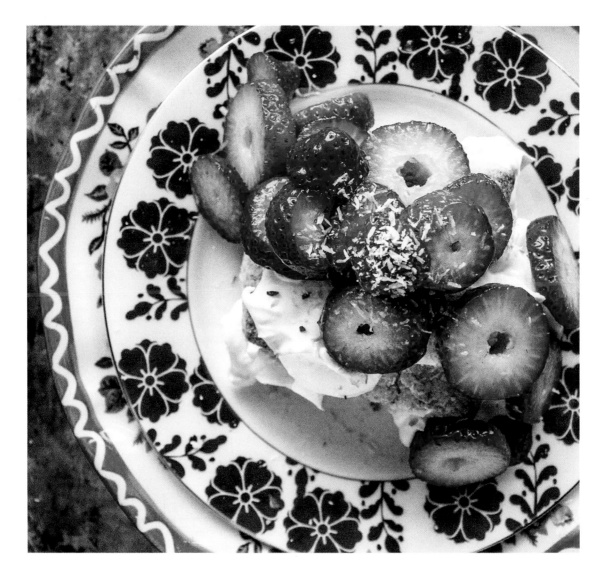

incorporated into the dry ingredients. Add the coconut milk mixture and pulse to make a wet and slightly sticky dough.

6 Dump the dough onto a very lightly floured countertop. Shape the dough into a disc 1½ to 2 inches thick. Dip a sharp knife into the flour on the counter and slice the disc into 6 equal wedges.

7 Transfer the shortcakes to the prepared baking sheet and brush the tops lightly with coconut

milk. Sprinkle with the remaining 1 tablespoon sugar and remaining 1 tablespooon shredded coconut.

8 Bake the shortcakes for 14 to 15 minutes, until lightly golden on the edges. Let them cool before splitting them open horizontally and filling with generous amounts of macerated strawberries and chilled coconut whipped cream.

BERRY SORBET

PREPARATION 15 MINUTES, PLUS 6 TO 8 HOURS FREEZING TIME
COOK TIME 5 MINUTES SERVINGS 6

Sorbet is one of the simplest things to make—no ice cream maker required—and the end result is as beautiful as it is delicious. This is a wonderful recipe to experiment with; you can swap out the berries for anything from pears to passion fruit.

2 cups plus 1 tablespoon granuated beet sugar

4 cups fresh or frozen berries

1 teaspoon fresh lemon juice

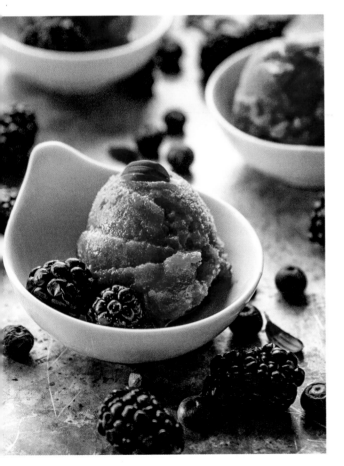

1 In a medium saucepan, combine 2 cups of the sugar and 2 cups water and bring to a simmer over medium heat. Simmer for about 5 minutes, stirring to make sure that the sugar has dissolved. Set the simple syrup aside to cool.

2 In a food processor, combine the berries with the remaining 1 tablespoon sugar and the lemon juice. Purée until smooth. Pass the purée through a fine-mesh sieve into a bowl, using a rubber spatula to press on the solids. Stir the purée into the simple syrup.

3 Transfer the sorbet base to a freezer-safe container and freeze for at least 6 to 8 hours. Let the sorbet soften on the counter briefly before scooping and serving.

CHOCOLATE-DIPPED COCONUT ICE POPS

PREPARATION 8 HOURS FREEZING TIME   **COOK TIME** 5 MINUTES   **SERVINGS** 10

These fancy grown-up pops are like a frozen coconut candy bar. They are so pretty and elegant that I have even served them to dinner party guests—much to their delight! (Photograph on page 276.)

2 cups unsweetened coconut milk

1 cup unsweetened coconut cream

½ cup unsweetened shredded coconut

½ cup granulated beet sugar

10 ounces soy-free vegan dark chocolate

1 teaspoon coconut oil

Toasted unsweetened shredded coconut, for garnish

1 In a small saucepan, combine the coconut milk, coconut cream, shredded coconut, and sugar and bring to a boil over medium heat. Reduce the heat to low and simmer until the sugar has dissolved, 2 to 3 minutes. Set aside to cool slightly.

2 Transfer the coconut mixture to a blender and purée on high until smooth. Pour the purée into 10 ice pop molds and add wooden sticks. Freeze overnight.

3 Place a baking sheet in the freezer for at least 30 minutes.

4 In a microwave-safe bowl, combine the chocolate and coconut oil. Microwave on high until the chocolate is mostly melted, about 75 seconds, then whisk until smooth. Let the chocolate cool a little.

5 Put a sheet of wax paper or parchment paper on the chilled baking sheet. Remove the pops from the molds and place them on the baking sheet. Pour the melted chocolate over half of each pop while holding them over the bowl of melted chocolate (to catch the extra chocolate). Sprinkle them with toasted shredded coconut and place them back on the on the baking sheet. When you are all done, store the pops on the baking sheet in the freezer.

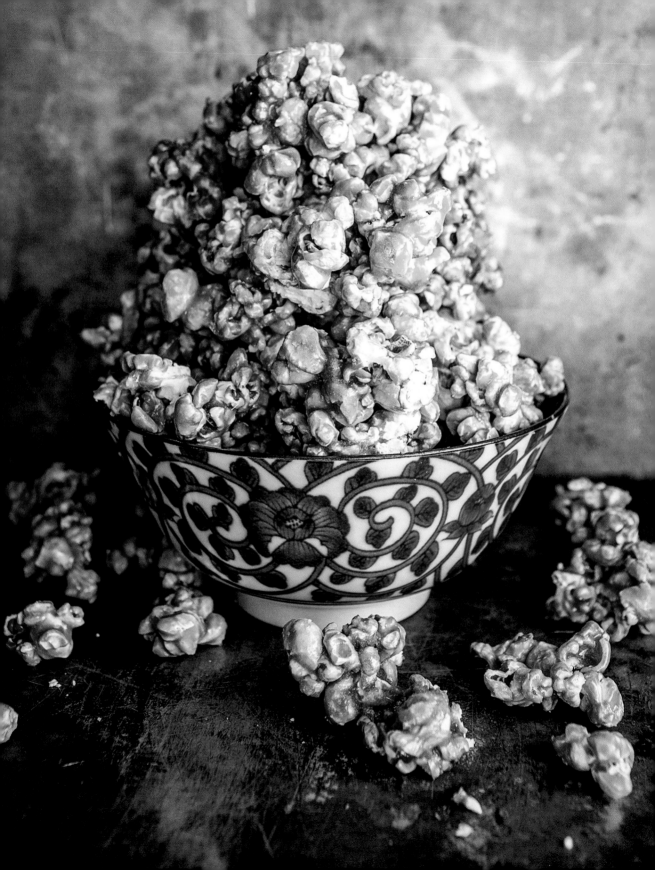

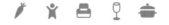

SALTED CARAMEL CORN

PREPARATION 5 MINUTES · **COOK TIME** 30 MINUTES · **SERVINGS** 12

Crispy, crunchy, salty, sugary-sweet caramel corn is my Kryptonite—it deprives me of all my powers to resist its charms. I make this for tailgating parties as well as for Halloween and other fun occasions when we need a sweet snack. It's surprisingly easy and stores really well. While it is not difficult to make, it is critically important that you make the caramel in a dry pot (NO water!) and that you don't rinse the wooden spoon and then put a damp spoon into the caramel. Any extra moisture will cause the caramel coating to be crisp rather than glossy (although it is still delicious that way!).

¼ cup plus ⅓ cup coconut oil

½ cup unpopped popcorn kernels

1 teaspoon pure vanilla extract

½ teaspoon baking soda

1 cup granulated beet sugar

½ cup pure maple syrup

1 teaspoon kosher salt, plus more for serving

1 Preheat the oven to 250°F. Line a rimmed baking sheet with parchment paper.

2 In a large pot, melt ¼ cup of the coconut oil over medium heat. Add the popcorn kernels, cover the pot, and cook, moving the pan often, until the time between pops is about 10 seconds. Immediately remove from the heat and transfer the popcorn to a large bowl. Rinse out and dry the pot well and return it to the stovetop.

3 In a small bowl, combine the vanilla and the baking soda and set aside. Add the sugar, maple syrup, remaining ⅓ cup coconut oil, and salt to the pot. Whisk the ingredients together and simmer over medium heat, stirring continuously, until lightly golden, 4 to 5 minutes. Be very careful not to let it burn or smoke around the edges.

4 Turn off the heat under the caramel and add the vanilla–baking soda mixture to the pot (the baking soda will make it froth). Whisk until the caramel is smooth. Immediately pour the popcorn into the caramel and use a dry wooden spoon or spatula to stir and coat the popcorn with the caramel as thoroughly as you can.

5 Transfer the caramel corn to the prepared baking sheet and bake for 10 minutes. Stir the popcorn, then return to the oven and bake for 10 minutes more. Remove from the oven, sprinkle with a little salt, and let cool.

6 Store the caramel corn in an airtight container for up to 2 weeks.

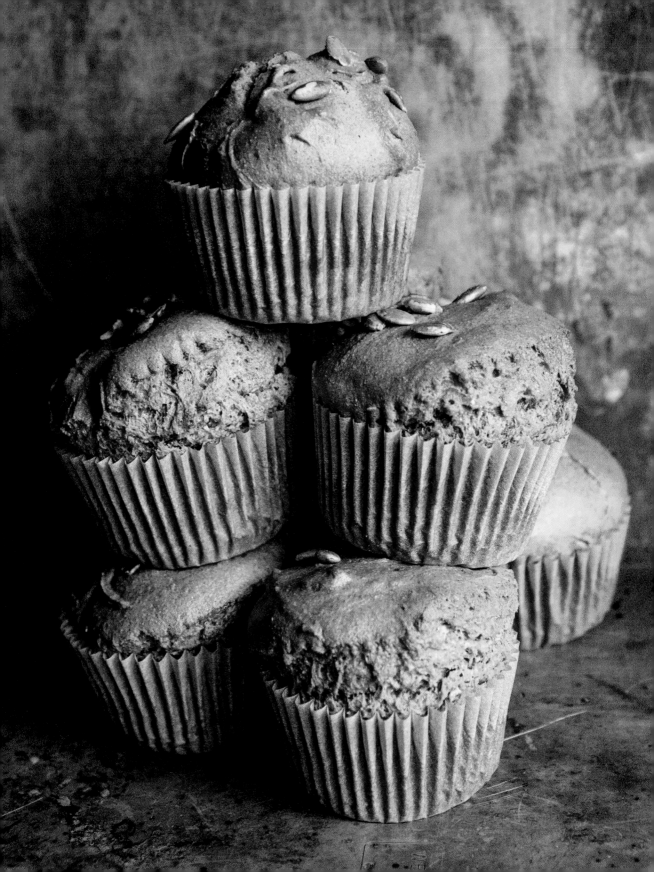

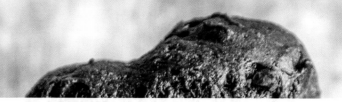

breakfast

Allergies put a major crimp in my morning-meal love. If I couldn't have eggs, cereal, toast, pancakes, or waffles, and coffee with cream, then what on earth was the point of getting out of bed?

When I finally stopped feeling sorry for myself and started getting creative, I discovered a whole world of breakfast possibilities: our mornings are full of quinoa breakfast bowls, baked oatmeal, and, of course, a rainbow of delicious smoothies. It is hard to beat the ease and convenience of a good smoothie—the kids and I can drink them in the car on the way to school when we're running late—not to mention the nutrition factor (you can sneak really good things into a smoothie, like aloe or spinach, without anyone knowing). But when I have a little more time on the weekends, or have made the effort to prep ahead of time, we can have fresh home-baked treats made with allergen-free ingredients that rival anything we were accustomed to eating first thing in the a.m.

Pumpkin Muffins (page 327) and Double Chocolate Sweet Potato Muffins (page 329)

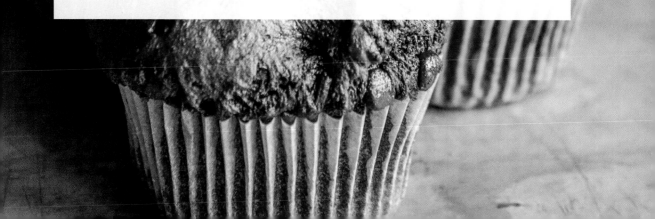

SMOOTHIES

PREPARATION 5 MINUTES   COOK TIME N/A   SERVINGS 2

GREEN SMOOTHIE

Even my children love these! The frozen peaches and coconut milk bring out the natural sweetness in the vegetables, and balances their grassy freshness.

1 cup frozen peaches

½ cup packed spinach leaves

½ cup cucumber chunks

¼ cup packed fresh parsley

2 tablespoons fresh lemon juice

1 cup unsweetened coconut milk

Combine all of the ingredients in a blender and purée on high until smooth. Divide the smoothie between two glasses and serve immediately. For a less pulpy smoothie, strain the smoothie through a fine-mesh strainer.

BERRY POMEGRANATE SMOOTHIE

This smoothie has an especially vibrant color and doesn't contain any kind of milk—it's just fruit and juice. The slushy consistency is especially welcome on a hot afternoon.

1 cup frozen raspberries

1½ cups frozen strawberries

1 banana

1½ cups pure pomegranate juice

Pomegranate seeds, for garnish (optional)

Combine the raspberries, strawberries, banana, and pomegranate juice in a blender and purée on high until smooth. Serve immediately, garnished with pomegranate seeds, if desired.

TROPICAL SMOOTHIE

All of the sweet flavors of the tropics come together in this easy breakfast or snack. I like to garnish it with a little extra pineapple or chopped strawberries.

1½ cups unsweetened coconut milk

1 banana

½ cup frozen pineapple

½ cup frozen mango

¼ cup frozen strawberries

Combine all of the ingredients in a blender and purée on high until smooth. Divide the smoothie between two glasses and serve immediately.

BLUEBERRY COCONUT SMOOTHIE

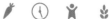

This beautiful smoothie happens to be especially thick and sweet and sometimes I even add a dollop of vanilla whipped coconut cream to make it feel like a decadent dessert.

1½ cups unsweetened coconut milk

1 banana

1 cup fresh or frozen blueberries

2 teaspoons agave

Coconut Whipped Cream (page 304),

toasted coconut flakes and blueberries for garnish (optional)

Combine all of the ingredients in a blender and purée on high until smooth. Divide the smoothie between two glasses and top with Coconut Whipped Cream, toasted coconut flakes, and blueberries, if desired.

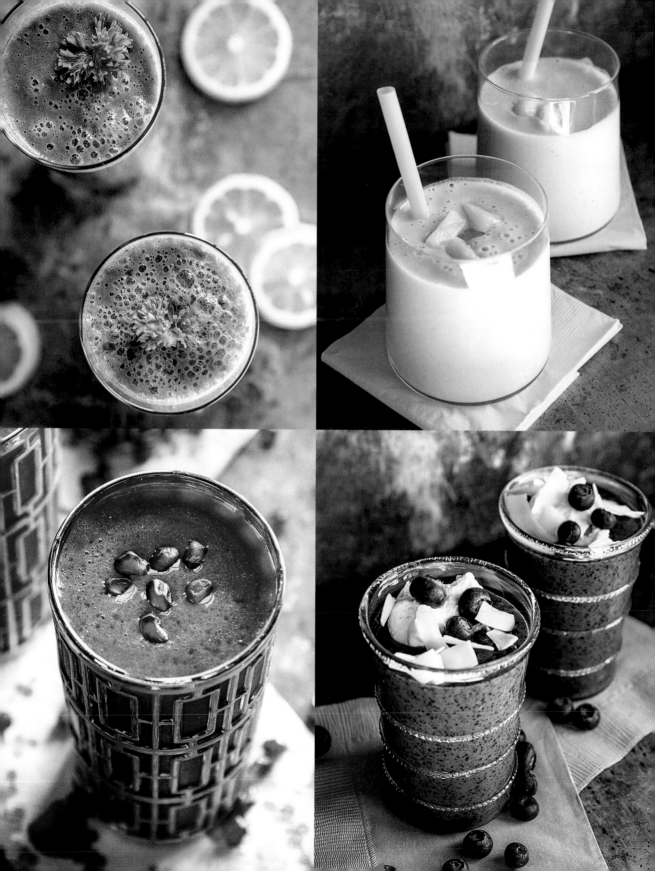

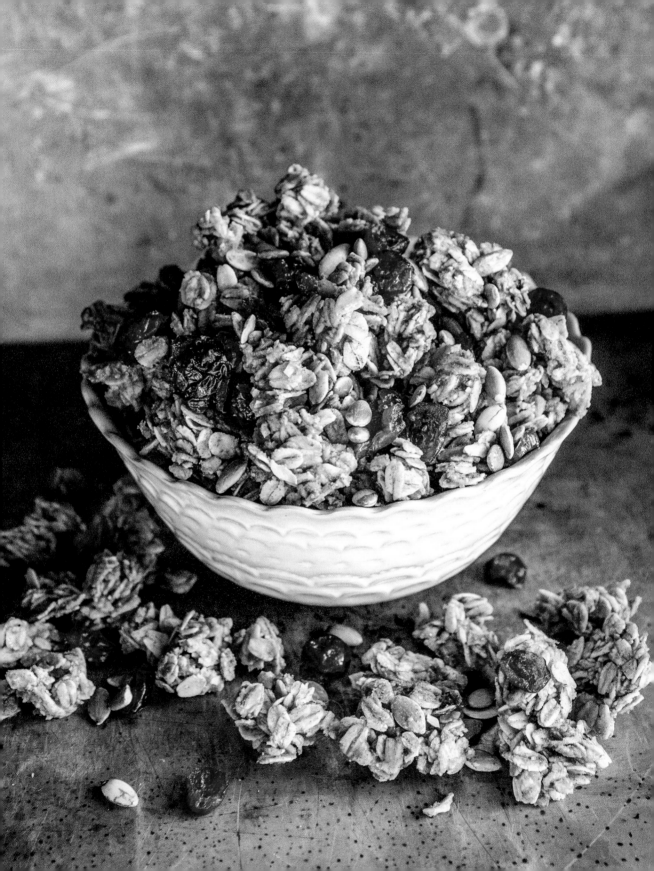

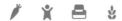

SWEET POTATO GRANOLA

PREPARATION 10 MINUTES   **COOK TIME** 40 MINUTES   **SERVINGS** 6

This is a lightly sweet and spiced granola that can not only be served for breakfast with coconut milk or yogurt, but also works well in snack-size portions for school. I will often grab a handful on the way to the gym for fast and healthy fuel.

5 cups gluten-free rolled oats

1 tablespoon ground cinnamon

½ teaspoon ground nutmeg

½ teaspoon ground ginger

1 cup granulated beet sugar

1½ teaspoons kosher salt

1 cup sweet potato purée, canned or homemade (page 34)

½ cup vegetable oil

¼ cup pure maple syrup

½ cup dried cranberries

½ cup roasted and salted pepitas

1 Preheat the oven to 325°F.

2 In a large bowl, combine the oats, cinnamon, nutmeg, ginger, sugar, and salt.

3 In a medium bowl, whisk together the sweet potato purée, oil, and maple syrup. Add the sweet potato mixture to the oat mixture and mix well with a spatula.

4 Transfer the mixture to a rimmed baking sheet and spread it out in an even layer. Bake the granola for 20 minutes. Remove from the oven and stir very thoroughly. Return the granola to the oven for 20 minutes more, until it is golden brown.

5 Sprinkle with the cranberries and pepitas and let cool completely on the baking sheet. If you let it cool without stirring it, you will get a chunkier granola.

6 Store in an airtight container for up to 3 weeks.

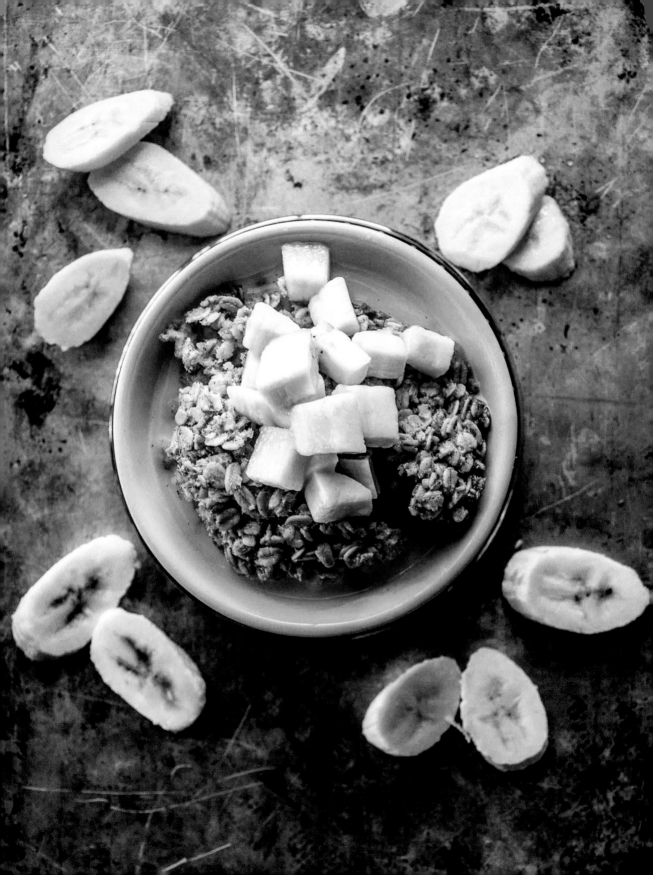

BAKED BANANA OATMEAL

PREPARATION 10 MINUTES   COOK TIME 30 MINUTES   SERVINGS 6

This is so simple. I love it because you can make it the night before and just heat it up in the oven or the microwave in the morning. The first time I made it, I didn't expect too much because it was so easy, but then my little girls went nuts for it and have requested it many times since. I like to dress it up by serving it hot with some chilled coconut milk, dried or fresh fruit, and toasted coconut.

Nonstick cooking spray

1 cup mashed ripe banana (about 1 large banana)

½ cup granulated beet sugar

2 tablespoons coconut oil, melted

2 teaspoons ground cinnamon

½ teaspoon ground nutmeg

1 teaspoon kosher salt

2 teaspoons baking powder

3 cups gluten-free rolled oats

1 cup unsweetened coconut milk, plus more for serving

1 teaspoon pure vanilla extract

Fresh fruit or agave, for serving (optional)

1 Preheat the oven to 350°F. Spray an 8 × 8-inch baking dish with cooking spray.

2 In a large bowl, combine the mashed banana, sugar, and coconut oil and beat with a wooden spoon until smooth. Add the cinnamon, nutmeg, salt, baking powder, and oats and stir until incorporated. Add the coconut milk and vanilla and mix well.

3 Transfer to the prepared pan and bake for 30 minutes.

4 Serve hot, topped with fresh fruit and agave, if desired.

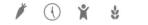

CREAMY COCONUT OATMEAL

PREPARATION 2 MINUTES   **COOK TIME** 15 MINUTES   **SERVINGS** 2

On cold mornings, you want "something to stick to your bones," as my mom always said. A bowl of these creamy coconut oats is even more tasty or "special," as Coco would say, with a topping of fresh fruit, toasted coconut, and agave.

2 cups unsweetened coconut milk

1 cup gluten-free rolled oats

¼ cup granulated beet sugar

¼ cup unsweetened shredded coconut

½ teaspoon ground cinnamon

Pinch of kosher salt

Fresh blueberries, agave, coconut milk, and toasted coconut, for garnish

1 In a small saucepan, bring the coconut milk to a simmer over medium heat. Add the oats, sugar, coconut, cinnamon, and salt and stir. Reduce the heat to medium-low and cook until the coconut milk has been absorbed and the oatmeal is creamy, about 15 minutes.

2 Serve immediately, topped with fresh blueberries, agave, coconut milk, and toasted coconut.

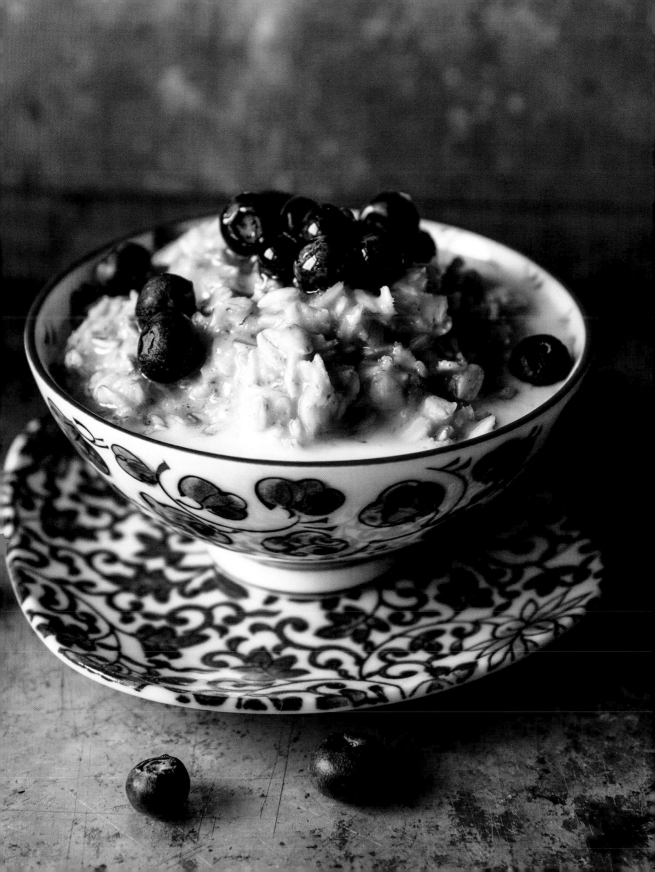

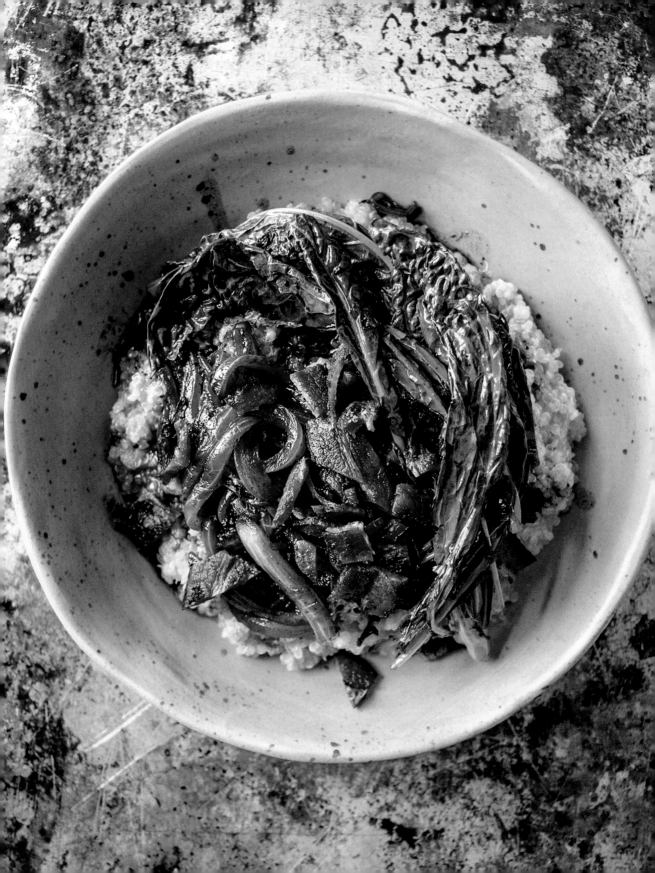

SAVORY QUINOA BREAKFAST BOWL WITH BACON, ONIONS, AND GREENS

PREPARATION 10   COOK TIME 45 MINUTES   SERVINGS 4 TO 6

Quinoa cooked into a savory steamed porridge topped with crispy bacon, soft red onions, and hearty Tuscan kale is a rich and hearty breakfast that will keep you full for hours. It's also a great candidate for brunch or even dinner!

3½ cups chicken broth

2 cups unsweetened coconut milk (from a carton)

1 teaspoon kosher salt, plus more as needed

2 cups quinoa, uncooked

6 thick-cut strips of bacon

1 red onion, julienned

1 tablespoon olive oil

4 cups trimmed and chopped Tuscan kale

1 In a medium pot bring 3 cups of the chicken broth, 1 cup of the coconut milk, and the salt to a boil. Stir in the quinoa and bring back to a boil, then cover the pot and turn the heat to low.

2 Simmer the covered quinoa for 20 minutes, and then let sit for another 10 minutes on the stove without the heat on. Remove the lid and stir in the remaining cup of coconut milk, which should absorb right into the quinoa and give it more of a creamy consistency. Season to taste with kosher salt.

3 While the quinoa is simmering, cook the bacon in a large pan over medium heat, flipping often until the bacon is crispy and the fat has rendered, about 7 minutes. Set the bacon aside and add the red onions to the bacon fat. Cook on medium-low heat, stirring often for 10 minutes. Add the remaining ½ cup of chicken broth and deglaze the pan, scraping up all of the little browned bits. Continue to cook another 10 minutes until the liquid has cooked down to a sauce-like consistency and the onions are very soft and brown. Season to taste with salt.

4 Scoop the quinoa into bowls and top with a generous spoonful of the onions.

5 In the same pan, quickly heat the oil over high heat. Add the kale and sauté for 1 minute, until just wilted. Sprinkle with kosher salt. Divide the kale among the serving bowls, crumble some bacon over each portion, and serve hot.

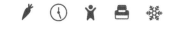

WAFFLES

PREPARATION 10 MINUTES   **COOK TIME** 3 MINUTES   **SERVINGS** 4 TO 6 WAFFLES

Waffles forever remind me of my dad. They were his best claim to "cooking" when I was growing up, and I can't make a single batch of these without thinking of him. These waffles now star as breakfast many mornings of the week, thanks to the freeze-and-toast method we often use. They also tend to make at least a monthly appearance at "Breakfast for Dinner" nights, with some fresh fruit and an ample portion of bacon. I went through several recipes to get here, the final and best addition being the beer. It gives them a yeasty flavor that is just right, as well as enough lift to keep the waffles light and fluffy.

These waffles can be frozen and reheated in the toaster, or you can refrigerate the batter overnight. If you are going to freeze and retoast them, cook them only until pale golden, not golden brown.

1 cup unsweetened coconut milk

1 tablespoon apple cider vinegar

¼ cup granulated beet sugar

½ cup gluten-free rolled oats

2 cups all-purpose gluten-free flour

2 teaspoons baking powder

1 teaspoon kosher salt

¼ cup coconut oil, melted

½ cup gluten-free beer

Nonstick cooking spray

Pure maple syrup, warmed, for serving

Fresh or cooked fruit, for serving (optional)

1 Preheat a waffle iron.

2 In a small bowl, combine the coconut milk and vinegar and set aside.

3 In a large mixing bowl combine the sugar, oats, flour, baking powder, and salt. Add the coconut milk mixture, the coconut oil, and beer and beat with a whisk until you have a smooth batter (studded with the oats).

4 Spray the waffle iron with cooking spray and spoon the batter into the hot waffle iron. Cook until golden brown, about 3 minutes. Transfer to a plate and serve hot with warm maple syrup and fruit, if desired. You can keep the finished waffles warm in a 300°F oven until ready to serve.

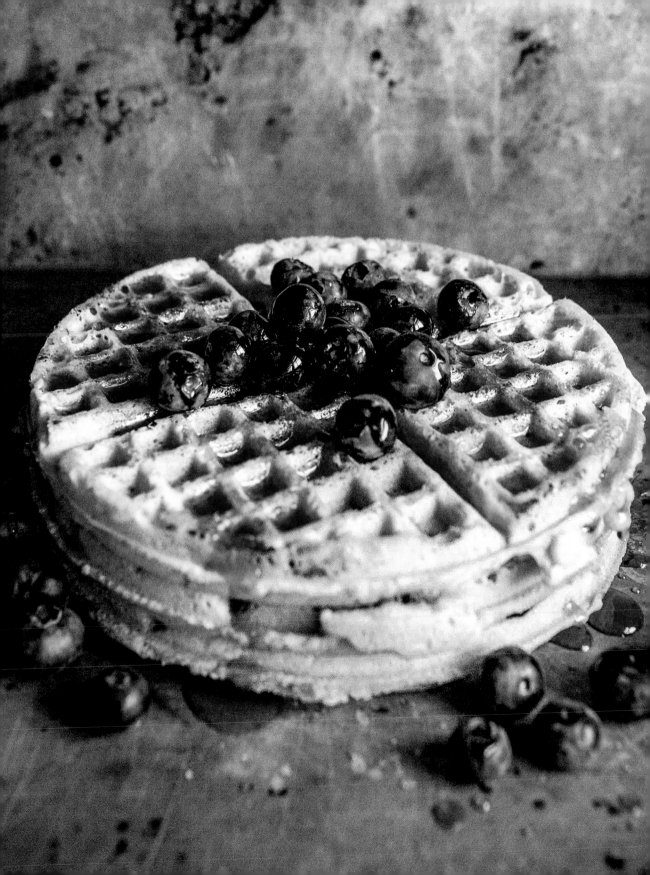

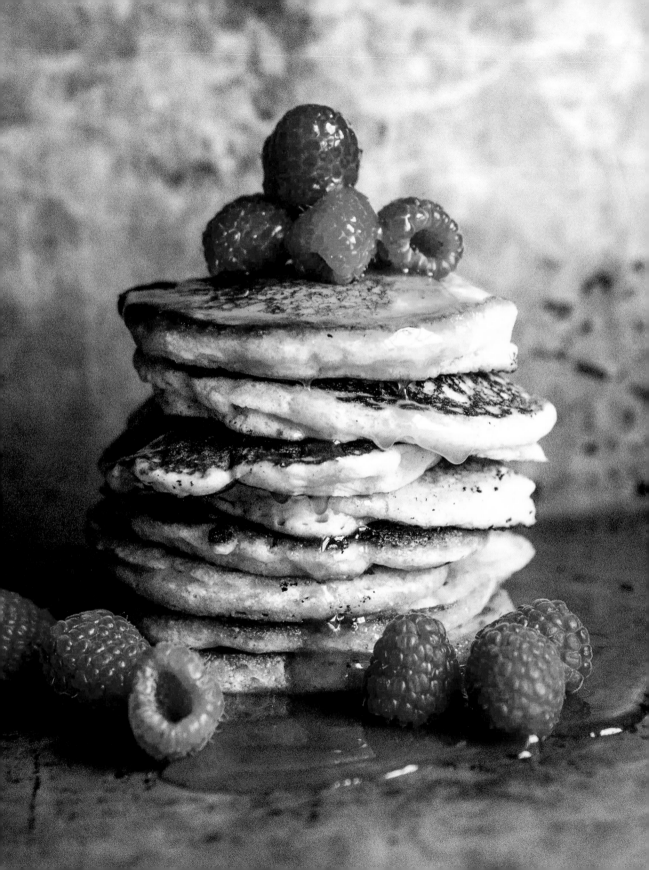

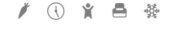

"BUTTERMILK" PANCAKES

PREPARATION 15 MINUTES   COOK TIME 10 MINUTES   SERVINGS 4

Buttermilk pancakes = comfort food. And this is the best "faux" buttermilk pancake recipe you are going to find. They are nice and thin and not too sweet, with just enough tang from the faux buttermilk. Drizzle these with maple syrup to get the full, dazzling effect of perfect pancakes.

1 cup unsweetened coconut milk

1 tablespoon apple cider vinegar

1 cup all-purpose gluten-free flour

2 tablespoons granulated beet sugar

2 teaspoons baking powder

1 teaspoon kosher salt

1 tablespoon coconut or vegetable oil, melted, plus more for the pan

Pure maple syrup, for serving

1 pint fresh raspberries, for serving

1 In a small bowl, combine the coconut milk and vinegar and set aside.

2 In a large bowl, whisk together the flour, sugar, baking powder, and salt until well combined. Add the coconut milk mixture and the melted coconut oil and whisk until smooth.

3 Heat a griddle or nonstick pan over medium-high heat and grease the griddle with the coconut oil.

4 Pour 3 to 4 tablespoons of the batter into the pan to form pancakes and cook for about 2 minutes, or until you see little bubbles forming on the edges of the pancakes. Flip them and cook for a minute more.

5 Serve the pancakes hot, with maple syrup and a sprinkling of raspberries.

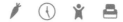

PUMPKIN PANCAKES
WITH COCONUT MAPLE SYRUP

PREPARATION 15 MINUTES   **COOK TIME** 10 MINUTES   **SERVINGS** 4

When I posted the recipe for The Best Pumpkin Pancakes on my blog, it received hundreds of thousands of views and people loved them. This is my new (and very close to the original) version of those pancakes. They have a nice tang from the faux buttermilk and are more pumpkiny in flavor than sweet, making them a perfect foil for the creamy coconut maple syrup. (Photograph on page 14.)

PANCAKES

¾ cup unsweetened coconut milk

1 teaspoon apple cider vinegar

1 cup all-purpose gluten-free flour

2 tablespoons granulated beet sugar

2 teaspoons baking powder

1 teaspoon kosher salt

½ cup canned pumpkin purée

COCONUT MAPLE SYRUP

½ cup pure maple syrup

¼ cup unsweetened coconut cream

• • •

Coconut or vegetable oil

1 In a small bowl, combine the coconut milk and vinegar and set aside.

2 In a medium bowl, whisk together the flour, sugar, baking powder, and salt. Add the pumpkin purée and the coconut milk mixture and whisk until smooth.

3 To make the coconut maple syrup: In a small saucepan, heat the syrup until bubbles form around the edges of the pan. Remove from the heat and whisk in the coconut cream. Transfer to a pitcher.

4 Heat a griddle or nonstick pan over medium-high heat. Grease the griddle with coconut oil.

5 Pour 3 to 4 tablespoons of the batter into the pan to form pancakes and cook for about 2 minutes, or until you see little bubbles forming on the edges of the pancakes. Flip them and cook another minute. Serve immediately, or keep hot in a 200°F oven until ready to serve. Serve hot, with the coconut maple syrup.

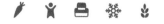

PUMPKIN MUFFINS

PREPARATION 15 MINUTES   **COOK TIME** 17 MINUTES   **SERVINGS** 12 MUFFINS

Pumpkin muffins were the very first gluten-, dairy-, and egg-free baked good I ever attempted, and I'm happy to say we've come a long way, baby, since those dense and heavy hockey pucks (if hockey pucks could crumble)! These are fluffy, moist, and tender, with a nice chew to them. Basically, they are amazing (photograph on page 310).

½ cup unsweetened coconut milk

2 teaspoons apple cider vinegar

2 cups all-purpose gluten-free flour

1 cup granulated beet sugar

1½ teaspoons baking powder

1 teaspoon baking soda

1 teaspoon kosher salt

1½ teaspoons xanthan gum (see page 34)

1 tablespoon ground cinnamon

½ teaspoon ground cloves

½ teaspoon ground nutmeg

1 cup canned pumpkin purée

¼ cup coconut oil, melted

¼ cup pepitas

1 Preheat the oven to 350°F. Line a 12-cup muffin tin with paper liners.

2 In a small bowl, combine the coconut milk and vinegar and set aside.

3 In the bowl of a stand mixer fitted with the whisk attachment, combine the flour, sugar, baking powder, baking soda, salt, xanthan gum, cinnamon, cloves, and nutmeg and mix on low speed. Add the pumpkin purée, coconut oil, and coconut milk mixture and mix until well combined and fluffy.

4 Spoon the batter into the prepared muffin tin, filling each liner three-quarters full, and sprinkle with the pepitas. Bake for 15 to 17 minutes, until fluffy and golden. Let the muffins cool in the pan for a few minutes before transferring to a wire rack to cool completely.

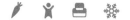

RASPBERRY OATMEAL STREUSEL MUFFINS

PREPARATION 15 MINUTES   **COOK TIME** 25 MINUTES   **SERVINGS** 12 MUFFINS

The first time I was pregnant, a whole-milk latte and a raspberry oatmeal streusel muffin were my midmorning treat, a habit that stuck with me long after the pregnancy! That seems like a different life, but I still really love myself a raspberry oatmeal streusel muffin, especially now that I can enjoy it with no guilt or ill effects. These are way better than the originals ever were.

STREUSEL TOPPING

⅔ cup gluten-free rolled oats

¼ cup granulated beet sugar

¼ teaspoon baking soda

½ teaspoon ground cinnamon

¼ teaspoon kosher salt

¼ cup coconut oil

MUFFINS

½ cup unsweetened coconut milk

2 teaspoons apple cider vinegar

2 cups all-purpose gluten-free flour

2 tablespoons gluten-free rolled oats

½ cup granulated beet sugar

2 teaspoons baking powder

1 teaspoon baking soda

1½ teaspoons xanthan gum (see page 34)

1 teaspoon kosher salt

1 cup unsweetened applesauce

¼ cup coconut oil, melted

1 cup fresh raspberries

1 Preheat the oven to 350°F. Line a 12-cup muffin tin with paper liners.

2 To make the streusel topping: In a medium bowl, combine the oats, sugar, baking soda, cinnamon, and salt. Add the solid coconut oil and cut or pinch it into the dry ingredients until you have pea-size chunks. Set aside.

3 To make the muffins: In a small bowl, combine the coconut milk and vinegar and set aside.

4 In a large bowl, combine the flour, oats, sugar, baking powder, baking soda, xanthan gum, and salt. Add the applesauce, coconut oil, and coconut milk mixture and stir until well combined. It will be a very fluffy batter. Very gently fold in the raspberries.

5 Scoop the batter into the prepared muffin tin and spoon the streusel evenly over the batter. Bake for about 25 minutes, until golden and puffed up. Let cool in the tin for a few minutes before serving warm or at room temperature.

DOUBLE CHOCOLATE
SWEET POTATO MUFFINS

PREPARATION 15 MINUTES   **COOK TIME** 17 MINUTES   **SERVINGS** 12 MUFFINS

These muffins are so deeply chocolaty and moist with sweet potato that they could easily be dessert-worthy. Even your pickiest eaters will not be able to stop at just one. (Photograph on page 311.)

½ cup unsweetened coconut milk

2 teaspoons apple cider vinegar

1½ cups all-purpose gluten-free flour

½ cup unsweetened cocoa powder

1 cup granulated beet sugar

1½ teaspoons baking powder

1 teaspoon baking soda

1 teaspoon kosher salt

1½ teaspoons xanthan gum (see page 34)

½ teaspoon ground cinnamon

1 cup sweet potato purée, canned or homemade (page 34)

¼ cup coconut oil, melted

¼ cup soy-free vegan chocolate chips

1 Preheat the oven to 350°F. Line a 12-cup muffin tin with paper liners.

2 In a small bowl, combine the coconut milk and vinegar and set aside.

3 In the bowl of a stand mixer fitted with the whisk attachment, combine the flour, cocoa powder, sugar, baking powder, baking soda, salt, xanthan gum, and cinnamon and mix on low speed. Add the sweet potato purée, coconut oil, and coconut milk mixture. Mix until the batter is fluffy and well combined. Add the chocolate chips to the mixer and briefly mix them in.

4 S.coop the batter into the prepared muffin tin. Bake for 15 to 17 minutes, until a toothpick inserted into the center of a muffin comes out clean.

5 Let the muffins cool in the tin on a wire rack.

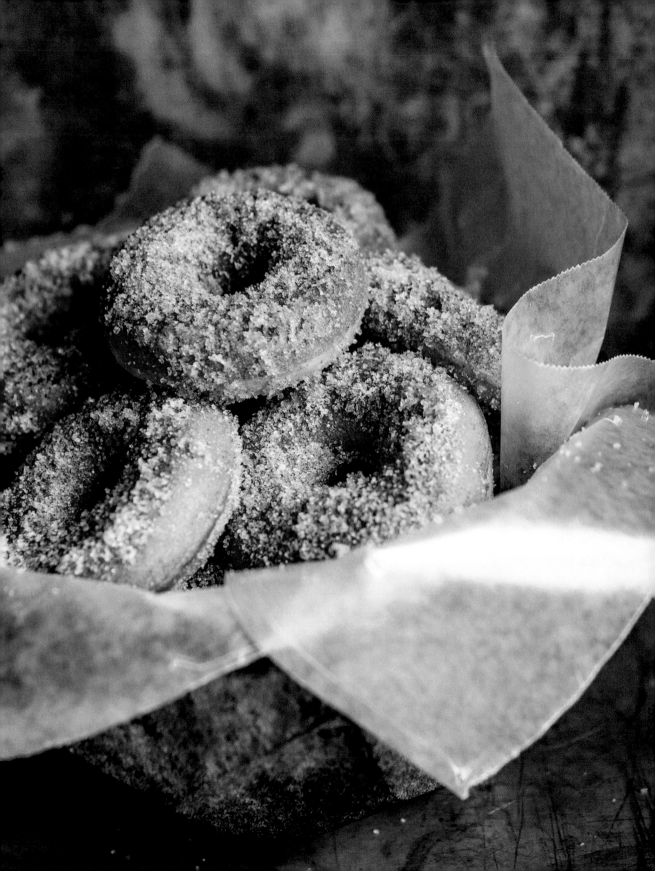

APPLESAUCE CINNAMON-SUGAR DOUGHNUTS

PREPARATION 10 MINUTES **COOK TIME** 10 MINUTES
SERVINGS 10 LARGE OR 16 TO 18 MINI DOUGHNUTS

These hot, sugary, little melt-in-your-mouth doughnuts are completely addictive and blow people's minds. I have made these for everything from breakfast to snacks and even brought out a hot batch for dessert at a dinner party. (And, yes, they were a major hit!)

Nonstick cooking spray

¾ cup unsweetened coconut milk

1 teaspoon apple cider vinegar

1½ cups all-purpose gluten-free flour

1 cup granulated beet sugar

1 teaspoon baking powder

½ teaspoon baking soda

¼ teaspoon xanthan gum (see page 34)

½ teaspoon kosher salt

½ teaspoon ground nutmeg

⅓ cup unsweetened applesauce

2 tablespoons coconut oil, melted

1 teaspoon ground cinnamon

1 Preheat the oven to 350°F. Spray a doughnut pan or mini doughnut pan with cooking spray.

2 In a small bowl, combine the coconut milk and vinegar and set aside.

3 In a medium bowl, combine the flour, ½ cup of the sugar, the baking powder, baking soda, xanthan gum, salt, and nutmeg. Add the applesauce and the melted coconut oil to the coconut milk mixture, then add them to the flour mixture. Mix well until you have a thick batter. Scoop the batter into a large resealable plastic bag with one corner snipped off or a pastry bag fitted with a plain round tip. Pipe the batter into the prepared pan.

4 Bake for 10 minutes for full-size doughnuts or 5 minutes for minis, until the doughnuts are golden. Turn the doughnuts out onto a wire rack to cool.

5 In a small bowl, combine the remaining ½ cup sugar and the cinnamon. Spray or brush the still-hot doughnuts with coconut oil and then roll them in the cinnamon sugar.

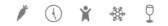

BLACKBERRY SCONES
WITH VANILLA GLAZE

PREPARATION 20 MINUTES · COOK TIME 12 MINUTES · SERVINGS 6 SCONES

I really enjoy how these scones have a nice rise and traditional crumbly texture while retaining a tender center. You can substitute any kind of fruit.

SCONES

6 tablespoons unsweetened coconut milk

2 teaspoons apple cider vinegar

2 cups all-purpose gluten-free flour, plus more as needed

½ cup plus 1 tablespoon granulated beet sugar

2 teaspoons baking powder

½ teaspoon baking soda

½ teaspoon xanthan gum (see page 34)

½ teaspoon kosher salt

6 tablespoons (¾ stick) cold soy-free vegan butter, cut into chunks

½ cup fresh blackberries

VANILLA GLAZE

¾ cup beet confectioners' sugar

1 tablespoon unsweetened coconut milk

½ teaspoon pure vanilla extract

1 Preheat the oven to 400°F. Line a rimmed baking sheet with parchment paper.

2 In a small bowl, combine the coconut milk and vinegar and set aside.

3 In a food processor, combine the flour, ½ cup of the sugar, the baking powder, baking soda, xanthan gum, and salt. Pulse to combine. Add the vegan butter and pulse until it is completely incorporated. Add the coconut milk mixture and pulse until you have a wet and slightly sticky dough.

4 Transfer the dough to a lightly floured countertop. Shape the dough into a disc.

5 Dip a sharp knife into flour and slice through the disc horizontally. Flip the top over and set the blackberries in the middle of the bottom disc. Replace the top disc and pinch the edges together to encase the berries.

6 Slice the disc into 6 wedges. Transfer them to the prepared baking sheet and sprinkle the tops with the remaining 1 tablespoon sugar.

7 Bake the scones for 12 minutes, until they are pale golden brown on the edges. Let cool for a few minutes, then transfer to a wire rack set over a rimmed baking sheet.

8 To make the vanilla glaze: In a small bowl, whisk together the glaze ingredients until smooth.

9 Drizzle the glaze over the scones and serve immediately.

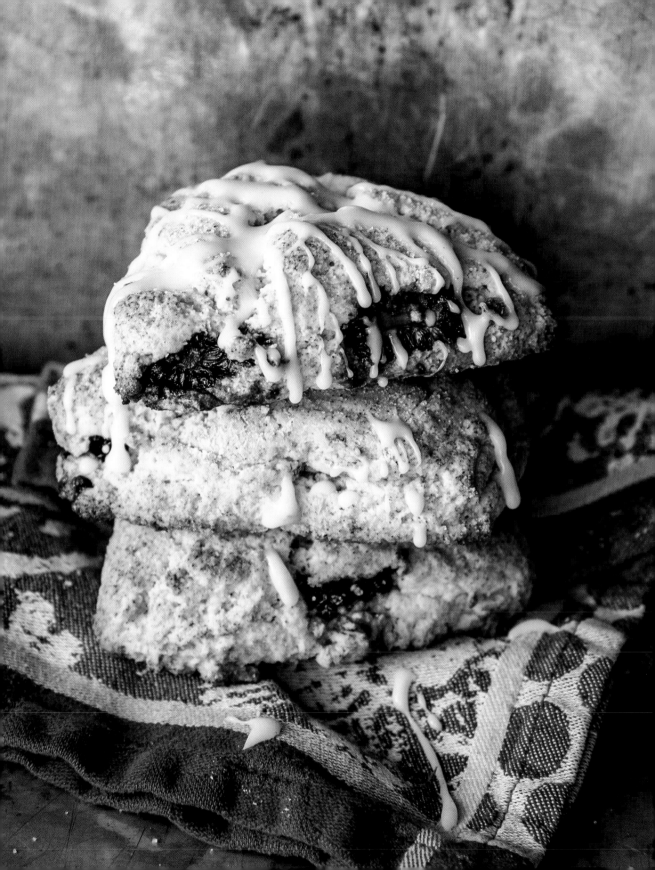

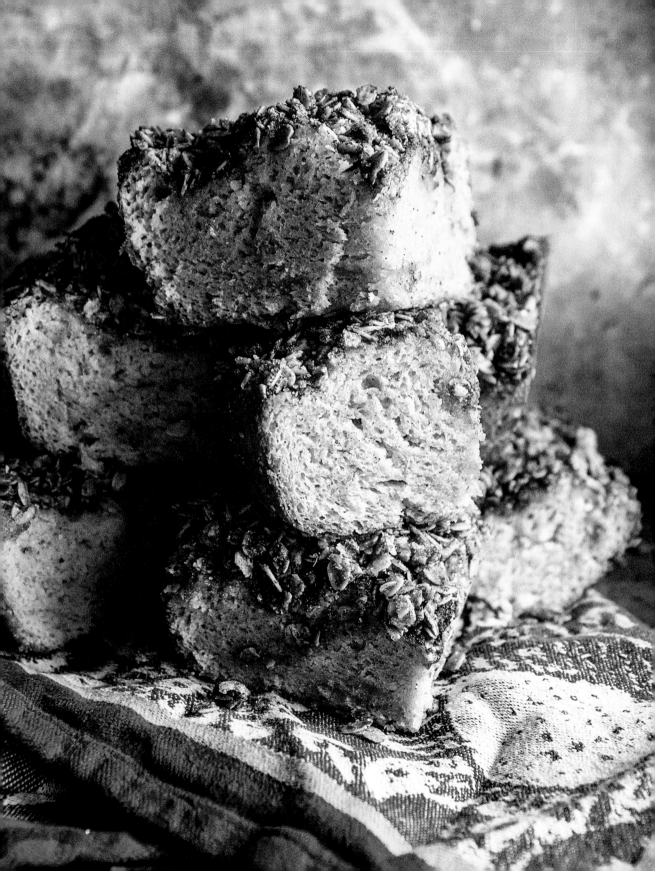

CINNAMON STREUSEL COFFEE CAKE

PREPARATION 15 MINUTES   **COOK TIME** 50 MINUTES   **SERVINGS** 6 TO 8

You can't go wrong with this nostalgic classic coffee cake recipe. The tender crumb and wonderfully crisp and sweet spiced topping will make this a weekend breakfast staple.

COFFEE CAKE

Nonstick cooking spray

1 cup unsweetened coconut milk

1 tablespoon apple cider vinegar

2 cups all-purpose gluten-free flour

1 cup granulated beet sugar

1 tablespoon baking powder

1 teaspoon xanthan gum (see page 34)

½ teaspoon kosher salt

1 teaspoon ground nutmeg

¼ cup coconut oil, melted

1 tablespoon pure vanilla extract

STREUSEL TOPPING

1 cup gluten-free rolled oats

¼ cup granulated beet sugar

¼ teaspoon baking soda

1 teaspoon ground cinnamon

¼ teaspoon kosher salt

¼ cup coconut oil

• • •

Beet confectioners' sugar, for dusting

1 Preheat the oven to 350°F. Spray an 8 × 8-inch cake pan with cooking spray.

2 In a small bowl, combine the coconut milk and vinegar and set aside.

3 In the bowl of a stand mixer fitted with the whisk attachment, combine the flour, sugar, baking powder, xanthan gum, salt, and nutmeg and mix well. Add the coconut oil, vanilla, and coconut milk mixture and beat until smooth.

4 Transfer the batter to the prepared pan and gently smooth to the edges of the pan using a spatula.

5 To make the streusel topping: In a medium bowl, mix together the oats, sugar, baking soda, cinnamon, and salt. Using your hands or a fork, cut in the coconut oil until the topping holds together in small chunks.

6 Sprinkle the streusel topping evenly over the batter. Bake for 45 to 50 minutes, until golden or until a toothpick inserted into the center comes out clean.

7 Let the cake cool in the pan for at least 20 minutes, then dust with confectioners' sugar, cut into squares in the pan, and serve.

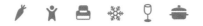

LEMON-BLUEBERRY COFFEE CAKE

PREPARATION 20 MINUTES   **COOK TIME** 60 MINUTES   **SERVINGS** 10 TO 12

If you're looking for something tasty for Easter or Mother's Day or a baby or wedding shower, look no further. This lovely tender, sweet, and tart lemon cake with juicy little bursts of blueberry and a pretty lemon glaze is perfect for celebrating something great!

COFFEE CAKE

Nonstick cooking spray

1½ cups unsweetened coconut milk

1½ tablespoons apple cider vinegar

2 tablespoons fresh lemon juice

3 cups all-purpose gluten-free flour

1¼ cups granulated beet sugar

1 tablespoon plus 2 teaspoons baking powder

1½ teaspoons xanthan gum (see page 34)

1 teaspoon kosher salt

Zest of 2 lemons

⅔ cup coconut oil, melted

1 teaspoon pure vanilla extract

1 cup fresh blueberries

LEMON GLAZE

Zest of 2 lemons

2 teaspoons fresh lemon juice

2 teaspoons unsweetened coconut milk

1 cup beet confectioners' sugar

1 Preheat the oven to 350°F. Spray a 10-cup Bundt pan with cooking spray.

2 In a small bowl, combine the coconut milk, vinegar, and lemon juice and set aside.

3 In a large bowl, combine the flour, sugar, baking powder, xanthan gum, salt, and lemon zest and whisk well. Make a well in the center and add the coconut oil, vanilla, and coconut milk mixture. Stir until you have a smooth batter. Very gently fold in the blueberries.

4 Transfer the batter to the prepared pan and gently smooth the batter to the edges of the pan with a spatula. Bake for 60 minutes, until a skewer inserted into the cake comes out clean. Let the cake cool in the pan for at least 20 minutes, then turn it out onto a wire rack set over a rimmed baking sheet.

5 To make the lemon glaze: In a small mixing bowl, whisk together the zest of one lemon, lemon juice, coconut milk, and confectioners' sugar until smooth.

6 Drizzle with the glaze, sprinkle with the remaining lemon zest, then slice and serve.

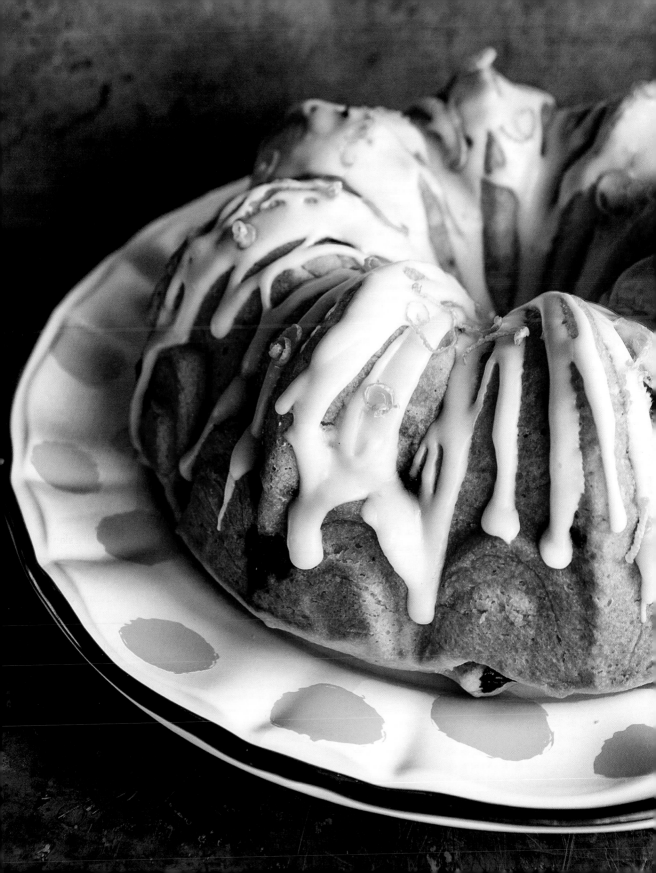

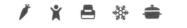

BANANA BREAD

PREPARATION 10 MINUTES   **COOK TIME** 60 MINUTES   **SERVINGS** 8

During the colder months when there isn't a ton of fresh fruit, you'll find this becomes a go-to recipe. It works as an after-school snack, breakfast on the go, and "dessert" in a school lunch.

Nonstick cooking spray

2½ cups all-purpose gluten-free flour

1 cup granulated beet sugar

2 teaspoons baking powder

1 teaspoon baking soda

1½ teaspoons xanthan gum (see page 34)

¾ teaspoon ground cinnamon

1 teaspoon kosher salt

1½ cups mashed ripe banana (about 2 bananas)

2 teaspoons pure vanilla extract

½ cup vegetable oil

½ cup unsweetened coconut milk

1 Preheat the oven to 350°F. Spray a 9 × 5-inch loaf pan with coconut oil spray.

2 In the bowl of a stand mixer fitted with the whisk attachment, combine the flour, sugar, baking powder, baking soda, xanthan gum, cinnamon, and salt. Add the mashed banana, vanilla, vegetable oil, and coconut milk and mix until well combined.

3 Transfer the batter to the prepared pan. Bake for 60 minutes, until a toothpick inserted into the center comes out clean.

4 Let the bread cool in the pan until warm or room temperature before turning it out and slicing. Store in an airtight container at room temperature for up to 1 week (though it will never last that long!).

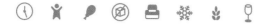

CHICKEN MANGO BREAKFAST SAUSAGE

PREPARATION 15 MINUTES   **COOK TIME** 10 MINUTES   **SERVINGS** 4 TO 6

Some people like sweet in the morning, others like savory. Others still like to start the day with protein. This dish will satisfy one and all, and is also extremely versatile. You could swap apples or red bell pepper for the mango, or swap turkey or pork for the ground chicken, or play around with other herbs such as sage or thyme. Serve these sausages with breakfast potatoes or any baked good.

2 teaspoons plus
2 tablespoons vegetable oil

½ cup very finely diced
yellow onion

13 ounces ground chicken

½ cup finely diced fresh
mango

1 tablespoon minced seeded
red Fresno chile

1 tablespoon minced fresh
chives

2 tablespoons dehydrated
potato flakes

1 teaspoon kosher salt

1 In a heavy skillet, heat the 2 teaspoons of the oil over medium heat. Add the onion and sauté for 5 minutes, until soft and tender.

2 Scrape the onion into a medium bowl. Add the chicken, mango, chile, chives, potato flakes, and salt. Using clean hands, mix everything together really well.

3 Form the mixture into 6 equal-size patties. Set them on a plate or a sheet of wax paper.

4 Heat the same skillet or griddle over high heat. When the pan is really hot, reduce the heat to medium and add the remaining 2 tablespoons oil. Gently place the patties in the pan and cook until golden brown, about 3 minutes. Flip the patties and cook on the other side for 2 to 3 minutes, or until they are just cooked through. Serve hot.

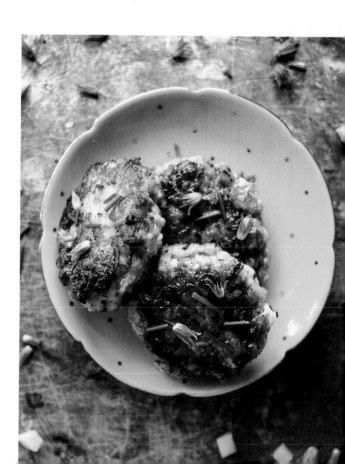

acknowledgments

I owe many thanks to the people who helped and inspired me during the creation of this book:

To the people who come to my blog each day, it seems like *everything* has changed over in my little neck of the woods, and I love how many of you stayed and learned with me and have hopefully added more healthy dishes to your repertoires. I get more excited about this way of cooking by the day, continuing to grow and improve in ways that I can share with you, which is a great source of joy in my life.

Pia and Coco, you were the inspiration for this book and the reasons I knew I couldn't rest until I had tried to help other children like you. Thank you for your patience while I worked long hours and for being my cheerleaders and my "kiss and a hug" every day. Thank you for letting me share your personal stories so that we could help others. XOXO

To Pete, my love, thank you so much for supporting me every step of the way through this book and through this transition. Thank you for living in a house without baguettes, eggs, and cheese so that you don't upset your children! Thank you for greeting with nothing but kind words a kitchen and a wife that often look like we got stuck in a blender. Mostly, just thank you for being you.

My mother, Susan, is a tireless supporter, a shoulder to cry on, and my therapist. Mom and Dad, I love you for always helping me to believe in what I am doing and for instilling so much strength and perseverance.

Mom, my sister Julie, Sue, Susie, Katie, and Jessica were all my recipe testers. Thank you all so much. I couldn't have done this without your time and feedback.

My enthusiastic and unflagging taste-testers Lilly and Judy also happen to be pillars of help and support. Thank you both for always having such a great attitude.

Janis Donnaud, you are the very best and I am extremely grateful to have you in my corner. Thank you so much for your guidance and intuition, which are always spot on.

A tremendous thank-you to my editor, Pam Krauss, who has pushed me creatively and technically further than I ever imagined I could go. I am so happy that you could see the vision for this book and for this movement. I hope that we are able to reach and help many people with this book. And to the whole Penguin Random House publishing team that helped put this book together—Erica Gelbard, La Tricia Watford, Terry Deal, Anne Kosmoski, Farin Schlussel, Claire Vaccaro, Justin Thrift, Erica Rose—I send my thanks.

Kelly Baker, thank you for helping to get my children healthy and for being a tremendous resource in the writing of this book.

Joe, thank you for helping me find a happy place of self-care when the stress was at its worst!

Leslie Eliel, thank you for helping me form these life-transitioning ideas into a game plan long before I realized what I was doing!

To my friends and family who make me laugh when I've had a long week, support me by helping me with my kids (thank you, Tula!), and cook and test and have us to dinner, I love you—thank you so much.

index

Page numbers in **bold** indicate tables; those in *italics* indicate photographs.

A

ADD/ADHD, **13,** 17, 19
advocating health, 38, 40, 42, *42*
agave, 35
alcoholic drinks, gluten-free, **54**
"allergies," 10, 16
    See also food allergies
aloe vera, 36
Alzheimer's disease, 34, 264
Amazon, 34, 35, 46
American restaurants, 44
anaphylaxis, 16, 17, **24, 25,** 43
antibiotics, 11, 12, 35
appetizers, 121–43
apple cider vinegar, 35
apples, 27, 28
Applesauce Cinnamon-Sugar
    Doughnuts, *330, 331*
appliances and tools, 31, 37, 47
Apricot Chicken Wings, 134, *135*
aquafaba (garbanzo liquid), 35
arthritis, **13,** 17, 19, 142, 159, 209, 264
artichokes
    Frisée & Artichoke Salad,
        240–41, *241*
    Lemon-Artichoke Hummus, *124,*
        125
    Roasted Red Pepper Pizza,
        Artichoke Hearts, *7,* 197
"artificial flavorings," 29
artificial sweeteners, 23
arugula
    Arugula Basil Pesto, 274–75, *275*
    Beet Pizza with Baby Arugula,
        194, *195*

Roasted Squash and Arugula
    Salad, 106, *107*
Asian Chicken Salad, Ginger
    Vinaigrette, 89, 90, *91*
Asian condiments, 28
Asian Pulled Pork, 231, 245
Asian Salmon Burgers, 189, 202–3,
    203
Asian Vegetable Noodle Soup,
    58, 80
Asparagus & Pea Salad, *88,* 115
asthma, 14, 20, **24, 25,** 142, 159
avocados, 27
    Brussels Sprouts, Bacon, Red
        Onion, & Avocado, 148, *149*
    Endive Avocado Salad, *116,* 117
    Red Cabbage, Bacon, and
        Avocado Slaw, *98,* 99
    Rosemary Chicken Salad with
        Avocado and Bacon, 92, *93*
    Tomatillo-Avocado Sauce, 264
avoid-and-reintroduce, 15, 21

B

bacon, **51**
    Brussels Sprouts, Bacon, Red
        Onion, & Avocado, 148, *149*
    Hot Spinach, Strawberry, and
        Bacon Salad, 102, *103*
    Pasta with Bacon, Spinach, and
        Chives, *214,* 215
    Red Cabbage, Bacon, and
        Avocado Slaw, *98,* 99
    Roasted Honey, Harissa, and
        Bacon Carrots, 146, *147*
    Rosemary Chicken Salad with
        Avocado and Bacon, 92, *93*
    Savory Quinoa Breakfast Bowl,
        Bacon, *320,* 321

Sweet Potato Salad with Bacon,
    145, 160, *161*
Baked Banana Oatmeal, *316,* 317
baked goods, 31–32, 34, **34,** 35, **35,
    51,** 175–87
Baker, Kelly, 13
Balsamic Vinaigrette, *98,* 99
Banana Bread, 338
Banana Oatmeal, Baked, *316,* 317
bananas, 22, 27
bananas, rice, applesauce, toast
    (B.R.A.T.) diet, 12
Bánh Mì Salad, 94, *95*
Bars, Chocolate Coconut Caramel,
    286, *287*
basil
    Arugula Basil Pesto, 274–75, *275*
    Basil-Mint Vinaigrette, 114, *114*
    Basil–Pumpkin Seed Pesto, 150,
        151
    Hot Basil Vinaigrette, *216,* 217
    Red Pepper Basil Sauce, 208–9,
        209
    Strawberry-Basil Salsa, 231, 262,
        263
beans, 27
    See also black beans; chickpeas;
        white beans
beef, 27, **51**
    Beef Stew, 258, *259*
    Beer-Braised Brisket, 231, 252,
        253
    Classic Beef Chili, 82, *83*
    Grilled Skirt Steak, 250, *251*
    Meat Loaf, 231, 257
    Old-Fashioned Spaghetti and
        Meatballs, *210,* 212–13
    Shredded Beef Tostadas, 231,
        254, 255–56
    Steak Lettuce Tacos, 52, 121,
        132–33, *133*

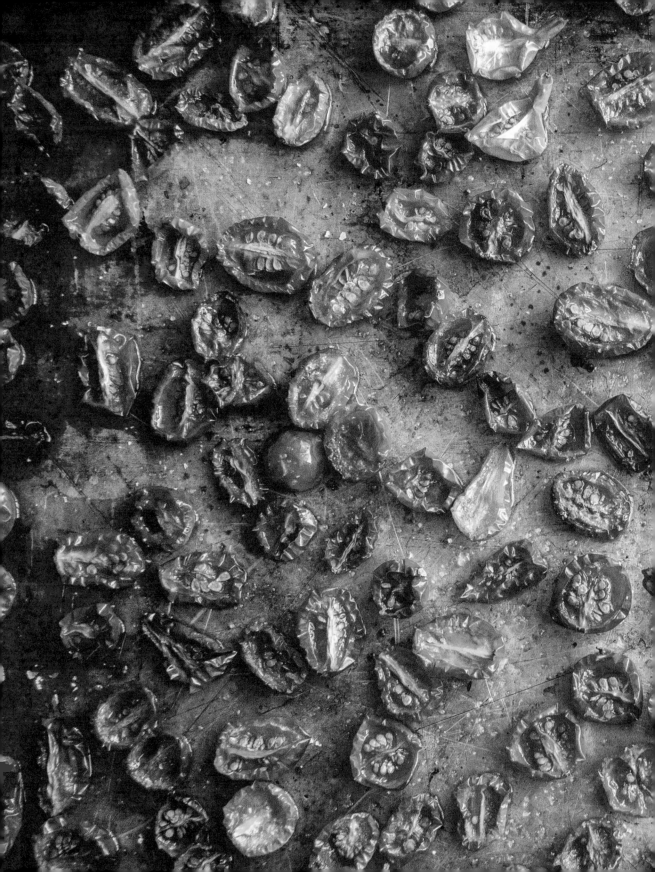